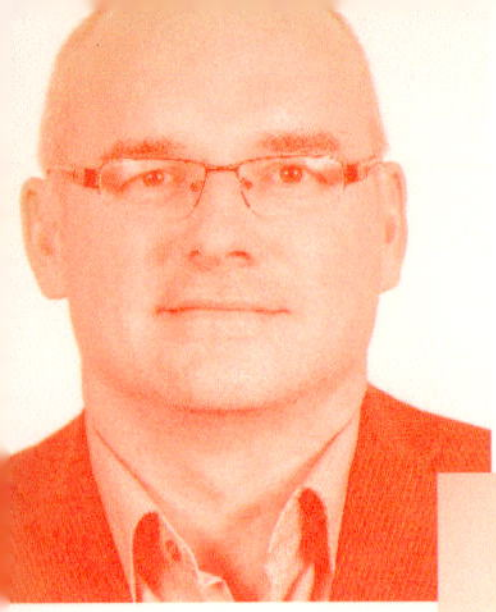
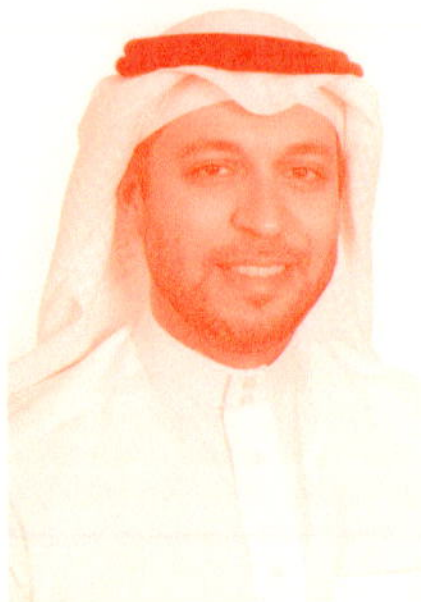
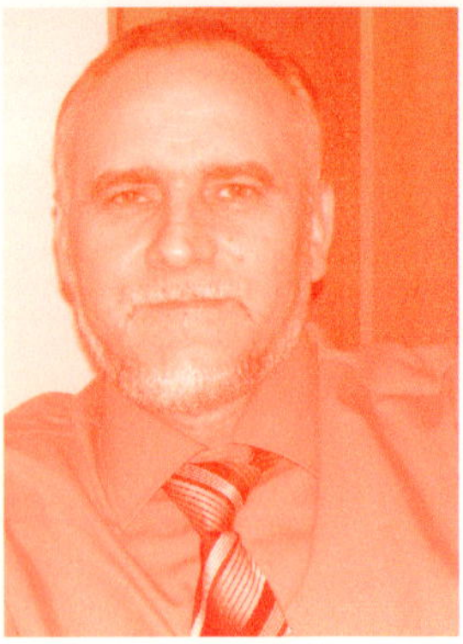
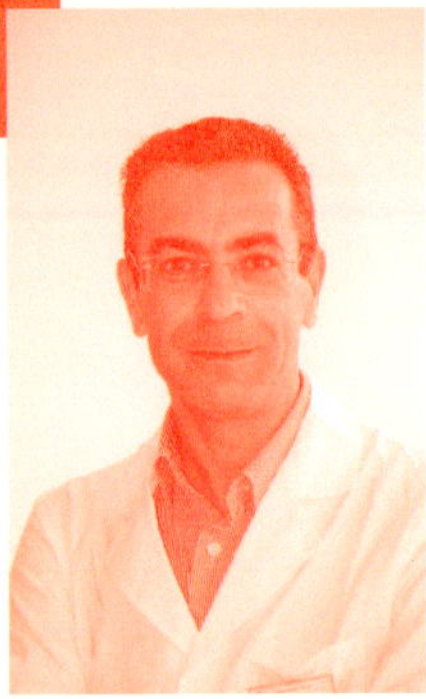
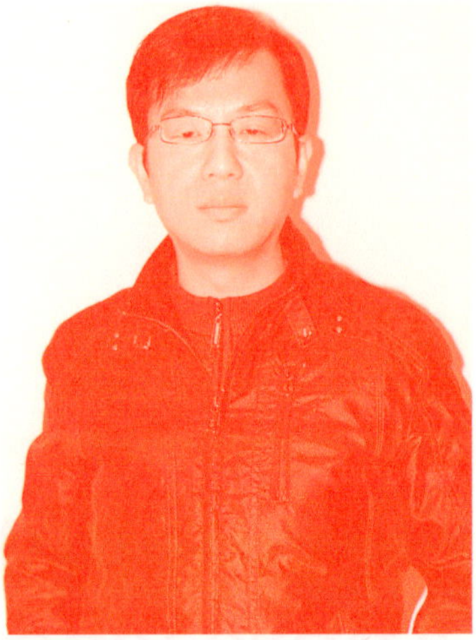
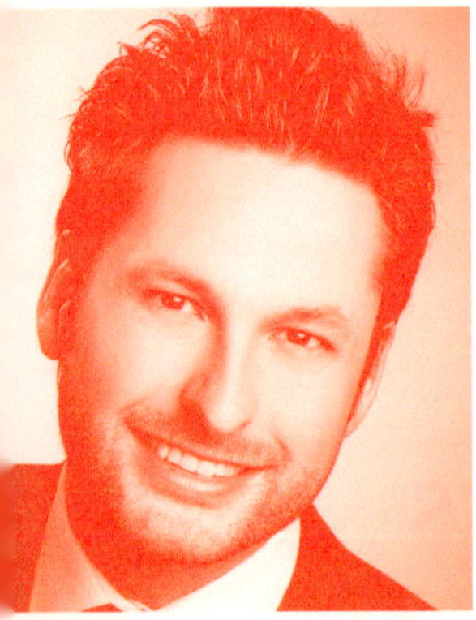
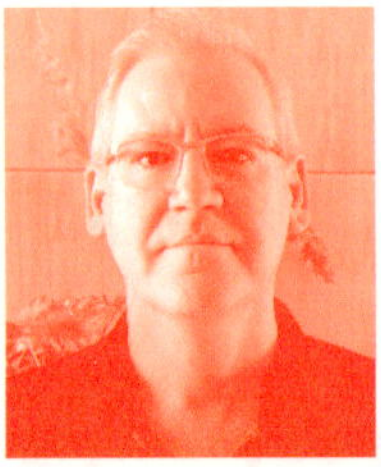

IntechOpen

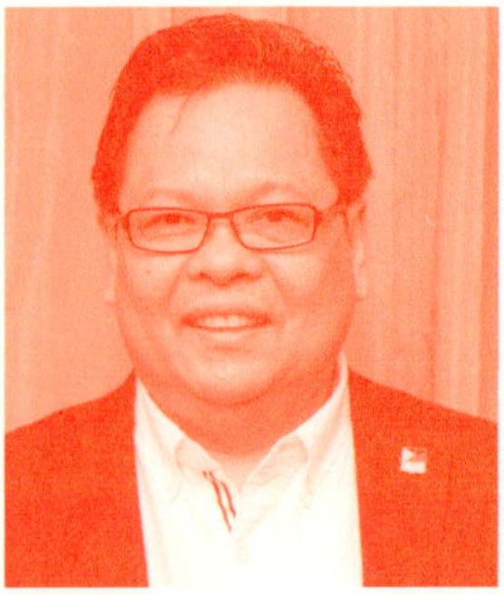
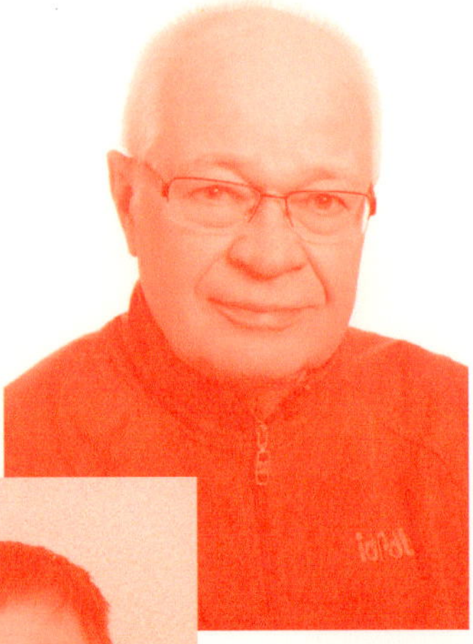
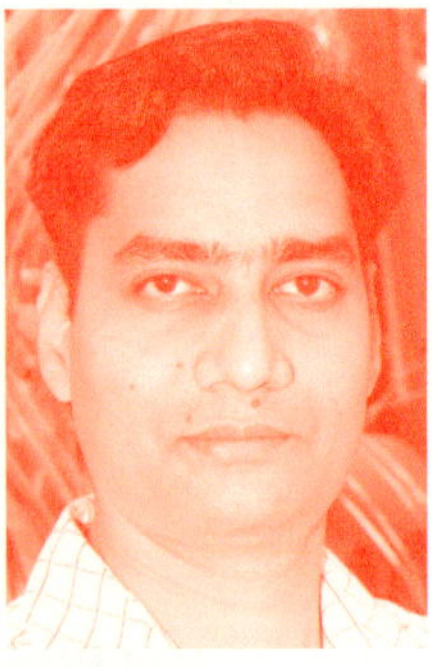
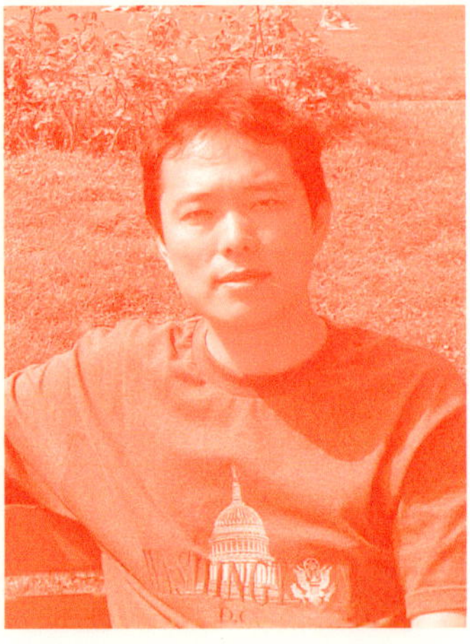
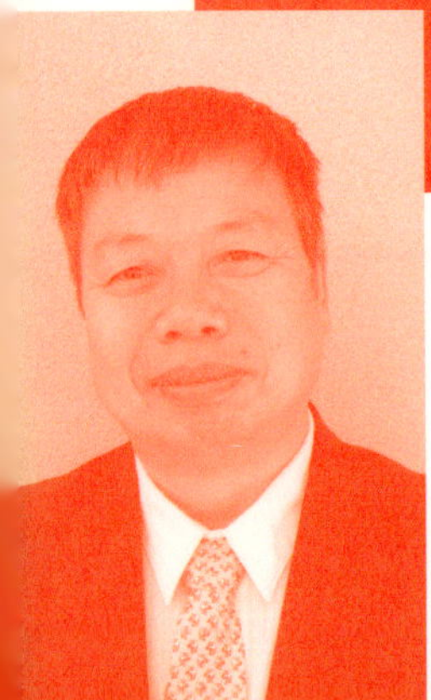
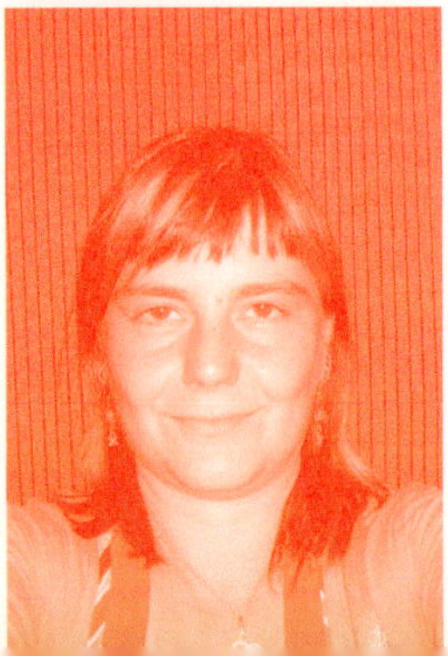

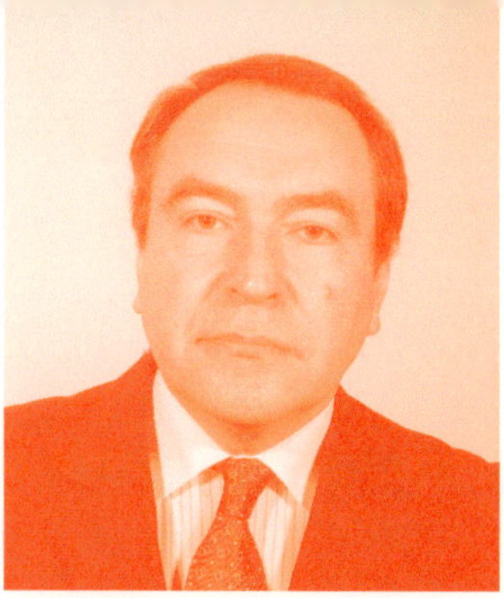
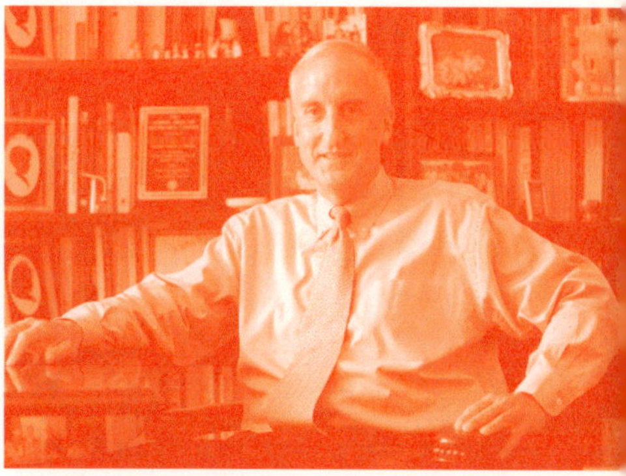
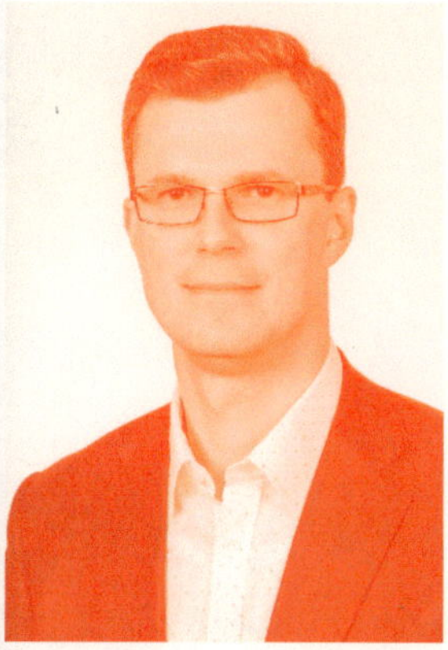
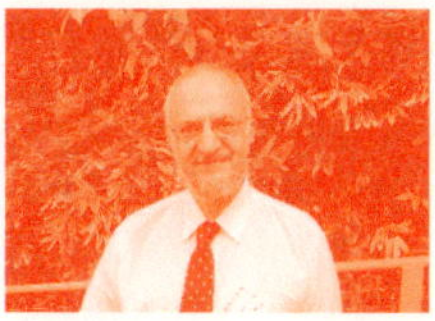
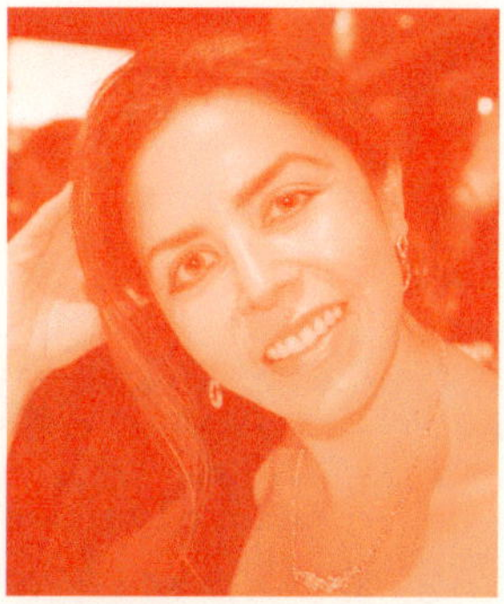

Supporting open minds since 2005

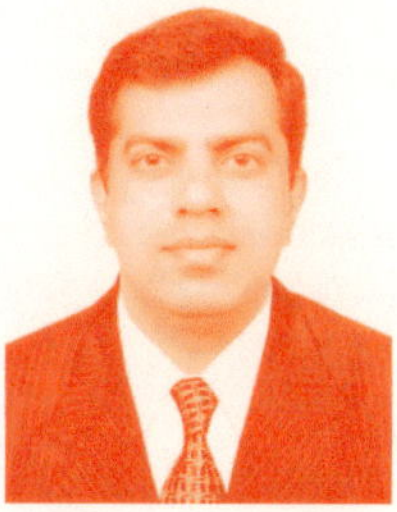
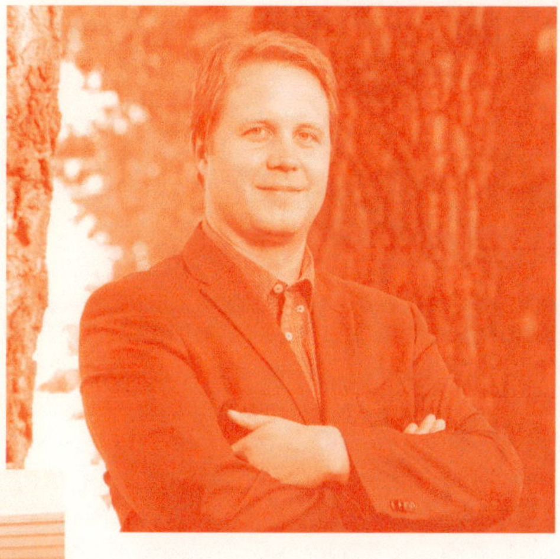
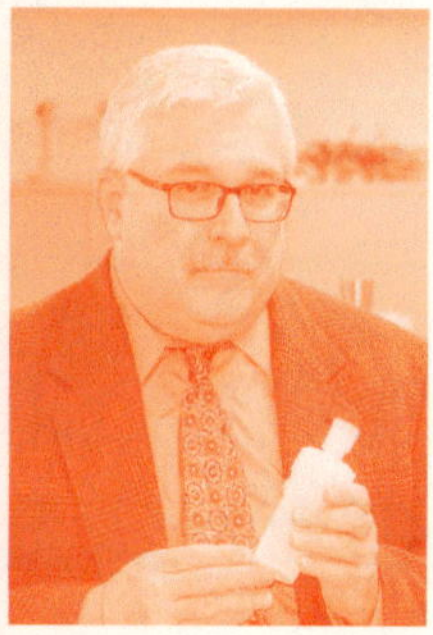
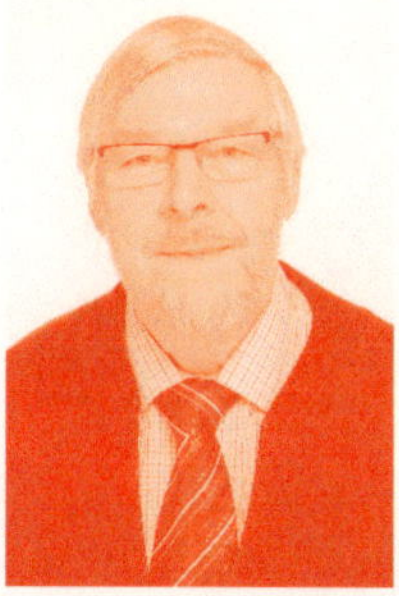
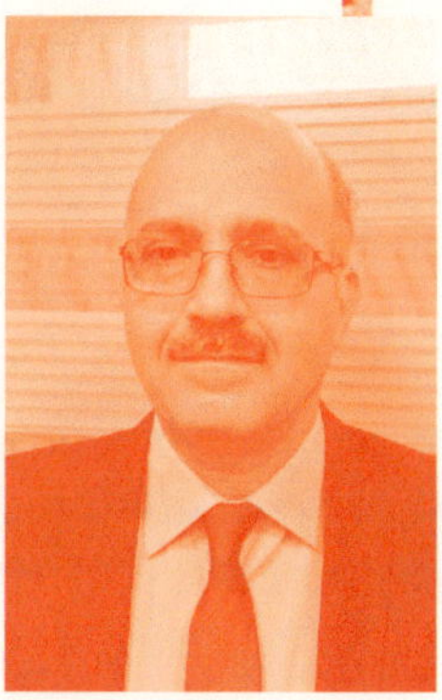
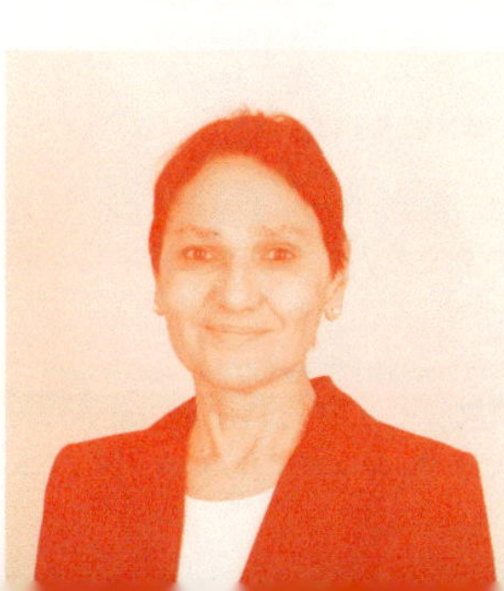
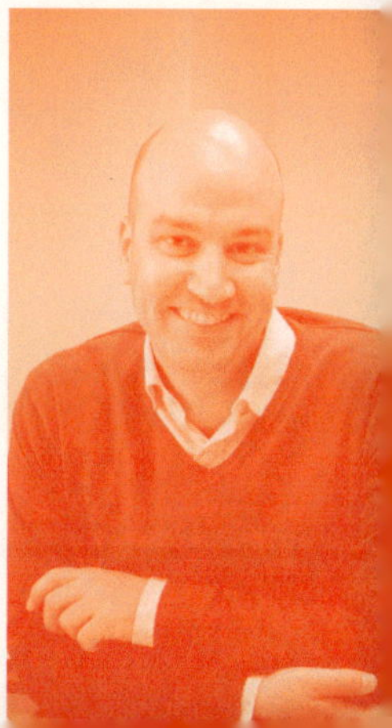

Neuroprotection - New Approaches and Prospects
http://dx.doi.org/10.5772/intechopen.77918
Edited by Matilde Otero-Losada, Francisco Capani and Santiago Perez Lloret

Contributors
Patrice Mendel Nzogang, Martial Boris Donkeng, Oxana Klementieva, Han-A Park, Katheryn Broman, Abigail Davis, Jordan May, Patrizia Polverino De Laureto, Luana Palazzi, Laura Acquasaliente, José Juan Antonio Ibarra Arias, Roxana Rodríguez-Barrera, Marcela Garibay Lopéz, Fatma Soylemez, Cagatay Han Turkseven, Cenk Suphioglu, Samuel King, Evgeniya Pushchina, Matilde Otero-Losada, María Inés Herrera, Lucas Udovin, Nicolás Toro Urrego, Juan P. Luaces, Francisco Capani, Andrea Aguilar, Tamara Kobiec, Santiago Perez Lloret, Rodolfo Alberto Kölliker Frers, Marco Fidel Avila-Rodriguez, Ianara Costa, Fausto Guzen, Elaine Pedrosa, Ana Paula Bezerra, Luciana Fernandes, José Rodolfo Cavalcanti, Marco Freire, Dayane Araújo, Amália Rego, Irami Araújo Filho, Francisco Irochima Pinheiro, Tatiana Gudasheva, Polina Povarnina, Ksenia Koliasnikova, Anna Tallerova, Larisa Kolik, Sergey Seredenin, Tatiana Antipova, Anna Nadorova, Sergey Nikolaev, Yulia Firsova, Melanie Tessa Saavedra Navarrete, Maria Yolanda Cruz Martinez, Mustapha Muzaimi, Che Mohd Nasril Che Mohd Nassir, Wai Yee Fung, Kah Hay Yuen, Hafizah Abdul Hamid, Alice Câmara, Anatoly A. Varaksin, Dmitry K. Obukhov

First published in London, United Kingdom, 2020 by IntechOpen
IntechOpen is the global imprint of INTECHOPEN LIMITED, registered in England and Wales, registration number: 11086078, 5 Princes Gate Court, London, SW7 2QJ, United Kingdom
Printed in Croatia

British Library Cataloguing-in-Publication Data
A catalogue record for this book is available from the British Library

Additional hard and PDF copies can be obtained from orders@intechopen.com

Neuroprotection - New Approaches and Prospects
Edited by Matilde Otero-Losada, Francisco Capani and Santiago Perez Lloret
p. cm.
Print ISBN 978-1-83880-439-8
Online ISBN 978-1-83880-440-4
eBook (PDF) ISBN 978-1-83969-261-1

For EU product safety concerns:
IN TECH d.o.o., Prolaz Marije Krucifikse Kozulić 3, 51000 Rijeka, Croatia, info@intechopen.com or visit our website at intechopen.com.

Meet the editors

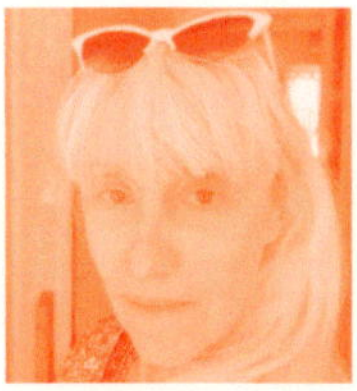

Dr. Matilde Otero-Losada graduated from the School of Pharmacy and Biochemistry, University of Buenos Aires (UBA), Argentina. She obtained a SciD in Neuropharmacology from the same univeristy and completed a PhD in Psychiatry at Wolverhampton University, England. Her following studies in psychometrics and statistical methods, radioisotopes and radiochemistry, and signal processing and microcomputers, took her to the University of California San Diego (UCSD) for training in human psychophysics. Back to Argentina, she carried on studying smell, taste, and trigeminal perception at the Hospital de Clínicas, UBA. She is devoted to the diagnosis, counseling, support, and treatment of people with olfactory and neurocognitive disorders. Focused on the study of metabolic syndrome, soft drinks, and cardiovascular-renal morbidity for the last ten years, in the last two years she is back to her roots in neuroscience. Dr. Otero-Losada has published more than ninety 90 papers in prestigious, indexed journals and authored several book chapters. She is a senior researcher at the National Research Council (Argentina) and a reviewer and praised editor of books and scientific journals, acknowledged for her stylish writing and editing skills.

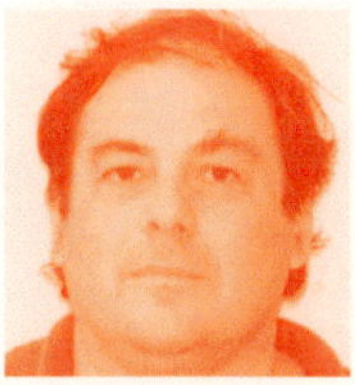

Dr. Francisco Capani graduated from the School of Medicine, University of Buenos Aires (UBA), Argentina, and completed his doctoral studies in Neuroscience at the Institute of Cell Biology and Neuroscience "Prof. E. De Robertis," School of Medicine (UBA), Argentina. He completed his postdoctoral studies abroad at the University of California San Diego (UCSD-NCMIR) and the Karolinska Institute, Department of Neuroscience. Over an eight-year period, his research focused on synaptic organization, combining electron tomography, 3D reconstruction, and correlative light and electron microscopy techniques. Upon his return to Argentina in 2006, he devoted his study to the mechanisms involved in the pathophysiology of the perinatal asphyxia supported by his broad experience in electron microscopy. Dr. Capani has published 115 papers in recognized journals and has been an invited speaker at several international conferences.

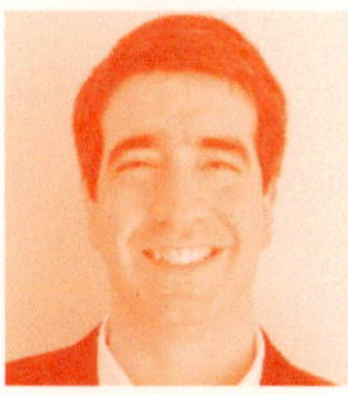

Santiago Perez-Lloret is a leading expert in neurophysiology and neuropharmacology with more 100 papers published in international medical journals (H-index = 34). He has recently edited the book *Clinical Trials in Parkinson's Disease*. After obtaining his MD and PhD, he pursued master courses in pharmacoepidemiology, clinical pharmacology, and biostatistics at the Universities of Bordeaux and Paris. Dr. Perez-Lloret is Assistant Professor of Neurophysiology at the University of Buenos Aires, and a senior researcher at the National Research Council. He is also an associate editor for *Frontiers in Pharmacology*. He is a member of the Education Committee of the International Parkinson's Disease and Movement Disorder Society (MDS).

Contents

Preface

Over the past several years, a substantial amount of information supporting new therapeutic approaches for neuroprotection has been generated. Neuroprotective strategies are developed to slow down or conceivably stop neurological disease progression and prevent the development of upsetting or painful disability. The development of new approaches and improvement of current ones are the major unmet medical needs in the treatment of neurological disorders like Parkinson's disease (PD), multiple sclerosis, hypoxic-ischemic encephalopathy following perinatal asphyxia, traumatic brain injury, chronic cerebral hypoxia in metabolic syndrome, mitochondrial dysfunction, and so.

Nearly 25%–30% of the world population is affected by neurological diseases, exerting great financial strain on the healthcare system. The costs are estimated at around $800 billion annually, which is expected to exponentially increase as the population ages and more people become at high risk of debilitating neurological diseases.

The book was conceived and developed to revisit, discuss, and compile some promising current approaches in neuroprotection, as well as to consider current goals and prospects.

A varied spectrum of neuroprotective strategies has been suggested including combined antioxidative–anti-inflammatory treatments, ozone autohemotherapy, hypothermia, cell therapy, the administration of neurotrophic factors, hemofiltration, and others. Distressingly, none of the currently available neuroprotective approaches has so far proven to prolong either life span or the cardinal symptoms of patients suffering from brain injury. Moreover, translational studies are still lacking.

The book is organized into three sections. Section I "Neuroprotection in Alzheimer's and Parkinson's Diseases" discusses the neuroprotective properties of cannabinoids, peptides, polyphenols, medicinal plants' extracts and essential oils, and others. Section II "Neuroprotection in Cerebral Ischemia and Other Neurological Diseases" deals with topics like protein misfolding as a novel neuroprotective target, the neuroprotective potential of vitamin E, neuroactive steroids, and so on. Section III "Mechanisms of Action of Other Potential Neuroprotective Treatments" approaches subjects like the neuroprotective potential of glyproline proampakine, aptamers, lifestyle factors, and mitochondrial dynamics, hydrogen sulfide, and anti-inflammatory agents.

Matilde Otero-Losada
Biomedical Research Center,
Interamerican Open University (CAECIHS-UAI),
National Research Council (CONICET),
Buenos Aires, Argentina

Santiago Pérez-Lloret
Biomedical Research Center,
Interamerican Open University (CAECIHS-UAI),
National Research Council (CONICET),
Buenos Aires, Argentina

Faculty of Medical Sciences,
Pontificia Universidad Católica Argentina,
Buenos Aires, Argentina

Francisco Capani
Biomedical Research Center,
Interamerican Open University (CAECIHS-UAI),
National Research Council (CONICET),
Buenos Aires, Argentina

Instituto Universitario de Ciencias de la Salud,
Fundación H.A Barceló,
Buenos Aires, Argentina

Department of Biology,
John F. Kennedy University,
Buenos Aires, Argentina

Facultad de Medicina,
Universidad Autónoma de Chile,
Santiago, Chile

Section 1

Neuroprotection in Alzheimer's and Parkinson's Diseases

Chapter 1

Neuroprotective Properties of Cannabinoids in Cellular and Animal Models: Hypotheses and Facts

Lucas D. Udovin, Andrea Aguilar, Tamara Kobiec, María I. Herrera, Santiago Perez Lloret, Nicolás Toro Urrego and Rodolfo A. Kölliker Frers

Abstract

Progressive neuronal loss is a typical characteristic of neurodegenerative diseases. In Parkinson's disease, the loss of dopaminergic neurons in the basal ganglia results in impaired mobility and flawed muscle control. The loss of cholinergic neurons largely in the basal forebrain contributes to memory and attention deficits and the overall cognitive impairment in Alzheimer's disease. This being said, neuroprotective drugs should be expected to preserve and/or restore the functions affected by neuronal loss, and substantially prevent cell death. The endocannabinoid system, comprising lipid mediators able to bind to and activate cannabinoid receptors, has emerged as a therapeutic target of potential interest in a variety of central nervous system diseases. Palmitoylethanolamide (PEA) is one of the most important endocannabinoids, which has a key role in modulating oxidative stress and inflammatory response with neuroprotective potential in neurological disorders. Neurodegenerative diseases undergo varied, progressive stages. The current therapeutical approaches are beginning to fall short when it comes to meet the expected results, urging to either develop or identify or develop new effective treatments. This chapter discusses the neuroprotective potential of new drugs, aiming to shed some light on their proposed mechanism of action and their effect in cellular and animal models of neurodegeneration.

Keywords: Parkinson's disease, Alzheimer's disease, endocannabinoids, palmitoylethanolamide (PEA), dopaminergic neurons

1. Introduction

The palmitoylethanolamide (PEA) is an endogenous biologically active lipids belonging to the family of the endogenous cannabinoid. PEA has many uses in a range of therapeutics areas, such as: neurological diseases, neurodegeneration, and pain.

Several studies have been carried out to define the molecular mechanism of PEA. However, at time, it was proposed that the existence of a mechanism

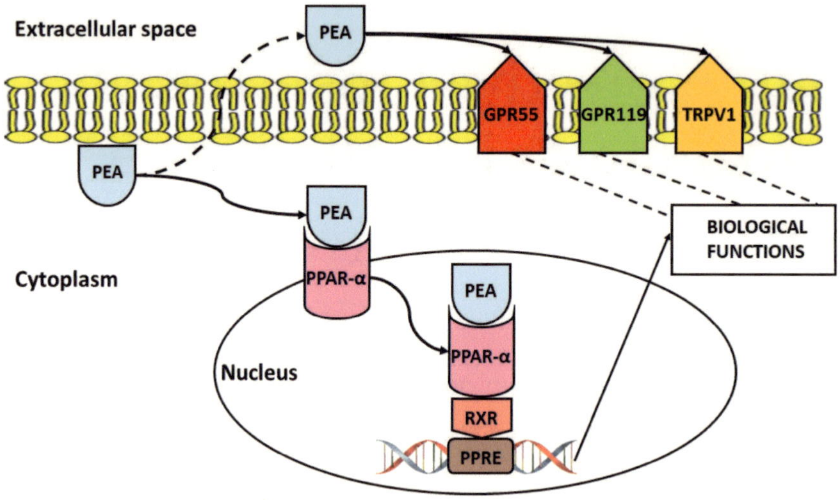

Figure 1.
Scheme of the performance of the PEA through the union to its different receptors. The PEA, through PPARα, mainly performs metabolic functions such as the regulation of lipid metabolism and exerts neuroprotective functions due to the reduction of transcription of various proinflammatory cytokines. After the binding of PEA to PPARα in the nucleus, it heterodimerizes with the RXR receptor, to then join specific DNA sequences called PPRE. These PPRE modulate transcription of target genes that control a wide variety of activities metabolic and physiological. On the other hand, it has been hypothesized that the PEA can also exercise its biological functions through different transmembrane receptors like GPR55, GPR119, and TRPV1, although this issue is still controversial.

receptor-dependent, and several studies demonstrated that PEA can act via direct activation of two different receptors: the orphan GPCR 55 (GPR55) [1] and the PPAR-α [2]. It was discovered that there is a wide variety receptors capable of interacting with PEA. All of them are belonged to these two receptors families, **Figure 1.**

Other supposition postulated that PEA could also be a cannabinoid receptor type 2 (CB2) receptor agonist; however, studies suggested that it has very weak affinity for this receptor [3]. In other hand, the transient receptor potential vanilloid receptor type 1 (TRPV1) channels can be activated for PEA in an indirectly way, **Figure 1**. These receptors are important targets of many endocannabinoids.

All data, which will be shown in this chapter, suggest that the action mechanism of PEA operates for several different ways. In the central and the peripheral nervous system, these mechanisms have collaborative interactions essential for the most important therapeutic effects of PEA.

2. Receptors of PEA

GPR55 and PPAR-α are the two most important receptors for PEA. GPR55 is a receptor belongs to the large family of GPCRs. It is expressed in brain areas, including the hippocampus, striatum, cortex, forebrain, and cerebellum. It has been reported that GPR55 utilizes the high concentration of intracellular to trigger a cascade of signalling events [4]. NF-κB, cAMP, MAPK, ERK1/2, and transcriptional regulators such as nuclear factor of activated T-cells (NFAT) are involved to GPR55 activation [5]. Other receptor belongs to the family of GPCR is GPR119, which can recognize oleoylethanolamide (OEA) and PEA. However, these two acylethanolamides do not interact with classical cannabinoid receptors such as CB1 and CB2 [6].

PPAR-α belongs to the family of PPARs and acts as a nuclear receptor protein. PPAR-α is present in many tissues and organs; liver, intestine, heart, muscle, brain, kidney, and adipose tissue. Also, this receptor is present in cells of the immune system PPAR-α. Their main functions are involved in the control of inflammatory processes and in the transcription factor regulating gene expression. In the same way, it is accepted that the binding of PEA to PPAR-α induces a heterodi-merization event with the retinoic acid receptor (RXR), forming the activated receptor complex, which decrease the transcription of pro-inflammatory genes [7].

Both receptors have recently emerged as a putative target for the treatment of pain, inflammation, and neurodegenerative diseases [8].

3. Other components involved indirectly in the mechanism of PEA

TRPV1 channel belongs to a subfamily of transient receptor potential channels (TRP channels). It is called 'the capsaicin receptor.' This is conformed by intramembrane loop linking the transmembrane domains, forming the pore channel region [9]. TRPV1 is present in sensory nerve fibres and dorsal root ganglia, keratinocytes, in brain neurons, and other cell types [10–13]. TRPV1 is activated by stimulation of the non-selective ion channel, permeable to cations. Also, it is activated by exogenous or endogenous chemical compounds [9, 14].

The changes in the phosphorylation state of TRPV1 induced by regulatory proteins (including PKA, PKC, ATP, phosphorinositide binding protein (PIRT) and phosphatidylinositol 4,5-bisphosphate (PIP2)) influent in the function of the receptor [15, 16]. The changes in the phosphorylation state produce an activation of TRPV1, then this trigger the signaling cascade to pain transmission, neurotoxicity, and inflammation [13, 17]. The high concentration of intracellular Ca^{2+} produces the stimulation of two processes very important. On the one hand, the stabilization of the channel by locked conformational. On the other hand, the inactivation of TRPV1 channel by Ca^{2+}-dependent phosphatases, such as calcineurin, which dephosphorylate it [15, 16]. This process contributes to the anti-inflammatory and analgesic actions of TRPV1 [16, 17].

There are many hypotheses about the mechanisms for the action of PEA with TRPV1 channels. One of them proposes that TRPV1 channels can be indirectly activate via PPAR-α due the action of PEA. Other mechanism proposes an indirectly activation of TRPV1 through the allosteric effects produce for PEA. It could increase AEA - or 2-AG induced activation and desensitization at TRPV1 channels [10, 18, 19].

The cannabinoid receptors types 1 and 2 (CB1 and CB2) are members of the G protein coupled receptor (GPCR) family that were identified over 20 years ago. [20, 21]. The CB1 receptor is often expressed in the brain, in the peripheral nervous system and presynaptic terminals. Also, it is expressed in almost all mammalian tissue and organs [22]. Its activation usually inhibits neurotransmitter release; the CB1 activation inhibits adenylate cyclase activity with the subsequent stimulates MAPK activity or reduction of intracellular levels of cAMP [23]. Consequently to the coupling of CB1 to PKB (Akt), phosphoinositide 3-kinase and PLC/inositol1, 4,5-trisphosphate/PKC (PLCβ/IP3/PKC) pathways [24, 25].

The CB2 receptors are involved in the activated astrocytes and microglia in the brain, where are expressed in low concentration [26]. However, this receptor is expressed in peripheral organs and cells of the immune system [16, 27–29]. One of the most important functions of the CB2 receptor is controlling the inflammatory responses [16, 30]. The CB2 receptor activation promotes MAPK activity and inhibits adenylate cyclase activity [31].

CB1 and CB2 can be indirectly activated by PEA through several of the mechanisms, although they are not direct targets [3, 12, 19, 32].

4. Brain injury and hypoxia ischemia

There are different causes of brain injury. However, none of them have a specific and efficient treatment to reverse its effects. The hypoxia-ischemia (HI) is one of the most important causes of neuronal damage and this will be the focus of this section.

HI impairs normal blood flow and reduces the oxygen and glucose supply to cells. This affects the cellular energy demand through alterations of aerobic metabolism, mitochondrial oxidative phosphorylation, and the anaerobic glycolysis [33]. Even though a HI event affects the heart, liver, kidneys, gut, and every other organ, it poses the central nervous system (CNS) to severe danger, as shown in human and animal models [33, 34]. The mechanism of brain injury involves a series of events referred to as the "excito-oxidative cascade"; it triggers the activation of excitatory glutamate receptors leading to excessive neuronal calcium influx. Calcium flooding through NMDA channels activates nitric oxide synthase raising the concentration of the free radical nitric oxide to toxic levels. The increase of both nitrogen- and oxygen-free radical species generated during the post-hypoxic re-oxygenation phase impairs the function of the enzymes associated with oxidative phosphorylation

Hypoxia-ischemia		
Model	**Global**	**Focal**
Animal (mouse/rat)	• Bilateral common carotid artery (CCA) occlusion combined with systemic hypotension, hypoxia or anoxia: this model results in variable ischemia depending on how long hypotension, hypoxia or anoxia last in neonatal rats	• Permanent middle cerebral artery (MCA) occlusion: electrocauterization of the MCA proximal to the origin of the lateral lenticulostriate arteries
	• Four vessel occlusions: A cauterizing needle causes blood electrocoagulation in the vertebral arteries, with clamps around the CCAs. The experimenter manipulates the clamps through an incision in the neck of adult rats, tightening the clamps 24 h later	• Transient middle cerebral artery (MCA) occlusion: Ligation with surgical clips or sutures
	• Uterus horns immersion: It consists of removing uterus horns containing fetuses from ready-to-deliver rats and immersing them in a water bath at 37°C for 5–20 min. The degree of HI is proportional to the immersion span	• Non-invasive model using intraluminal sutures: It consists of inserting a nylon filament through the proximal external carotid artery to occlude the MCA. Reperfusion follows later suture removal
Cell culture	• Cell culture models. There are a few cell cultures models that mimic the hypoxic–ischemic injury. Among them, oxygen and glucose deprivation (OGD) is a widely used in vitro model of ischemia that results in apoptotic and necrotic cell death	

Table 1.
Animals and cellular models to hypoxia-ischemia: in the table are showed the most used models for global and focal hypoxia ischemia.

and electron transport. Calcium toxicity is also mediated by activation of other enzymes including caspases, calpains and other proteases, and lipases, which attack mitochondria and other cellular machinery. As a result, the damaged mitochondria release signals leading to apoptosis or programmed cell death as long as the energy supplies persist, and otherwise to necrosis and destruction of cellular membranes when energy becomes exhausted. Impairment of mitochondrial oxidative phosphorylation results in lactic acid accumulation, which may be less toxic in the neonatal brain compared with the adult brain.

The extent of damage to the central nervous system determines whether global or focal HI takes place. The focal hypoxia-ischemia occurs when an end artery is exclusively occluded. However, the spread of damage depends on the duration and degree of the occlusion and on how well the collateral irrigation copes with metabolic demands. In two brain areas, the core and the penumbra are found the most evident effect of damage. In the core area, the collateral blood supply is reduced and shows the most severe and irreversible lesions. The penumbra surrounds the core area and receives collateral irrigation, reducing its vulnerability to the occlusion. Consequently, penumbra cells either recover from the transient damage or start a series of events that ultimately lead to cell death [35].

Global cerebral HI remains a superlative cause of perinatal brain injury, ultimately leading to neurologic dysfunction, which becomes manifest as cerebral palsy, mental retardation, and epilepsy [36, 37]. Encephalopathy following perinatal HI occurs in 1–3 per 1000 term births in the United Kingdom [38]. Similarly, stroke affects 15 million people worldwide each year and is the leading cause of disability in the United States of America [39].

Different models are used to investigate the pathophysiology of HI. Even though none of them strictly reproduce the clinical conditions, however, they are used to study cellular and molecular mechanisms underlying HI and test the potential therapeutic agents, **Table 1.**

5. PEA and Hypoxia—Ischemia

From the 1970s, our understanding of the pathogenesis of the hypoxia-ischemia (HI) brain injury has grown considerably [40], both in the physiological and molecular aspects. This progress has taken us closer to develop different therapies to prevent or minimize neuronal HI damage. In this regard, the hypothermia, nitric oxide synthase inhibitors, and neuronal growth factors that help neuronal survival and may play a role in rescuing brain tissue and promoting brain growth following injury and blocking HI apoptosis by caspase inhibition [36]. Hypothermia is one of the few strategies applied in the clinical treatment of perinatal brain injury due to both HI and stroke [41]. With the advance in molecular science, pharmacology, and genomics, new therapeutic approaches are arising. Accordingly, pharmacogenomics has gathered the interest of many groups allowing individualized treatment and maximizing therapeutic effects while minimizing side effects [42].

The treatment with PEA has been used in cellular and animal models. Rats were exposed to neonatal anoxia-ischemia (AI) and then treated with vehicle or PEA showed that neonatal AI was associated with decreased locomotion, as well as recognition and spatial memory impairments. Furthermore, these deficits were accompanied with enhanced neuroinflammation and astrogliosis, as well as a decreased PPARα expression. PEA treatment was able to prevent neuroinflammation, reduce astrogliosis, and preserve cognitive functions [43]. In addition, it has also been shown that in a mice model of perinatal hypoxic-ischemic (HI) encephalopathy, PEA exert neuroprotective effects on cultured cortical neurons being mediated by TRPV4 receptor, and cotreatment with OEA and PEA is able to enhance neuroprotective effects of the acylethanolamides [18]. A neuroprotective function of injected PEA and OEA has been substantiated in mice with transient middle cerebral artery occlusion [44, 45], but both in the OEA and in the PEA, the mechanism by which they would be exercising their neuroprotective actions would be through PPARα activation [44]. Besides, PEA may potentiate microglial cell motility after focal cerebral ischemia by an apparent non-cannabinoid receptor-mediated mechanism [46]. PEA exerts neuroprotection and reduces inflammatory secondary events associated with brain ischemia reperfusion injury (middle cerebral artery occlusion (MCAo)), in rats subjected to MCAo and treated with PEA in conjunction with Luteolin post-ischemia showed reduced edema and brain infract volume, improved neurobehavioral functions, and reduced expression of pro-inflammatory markers and astrocyte markers. In the same sense, a cohort of 250 stroke patients undergoing neurorehabilitation on either an inpatient or an outpatient basis that were treated for 60 days with a pharmaceutical preparation of PEA and luteolin improved the neurological status, impairment of cognitive abilities, the degree of spasticity, pain, and independence in daily living activities [47]. PEA-mediated improvements in tissues histology shown by reduction of lesion size and improvement in apoptosis level (assayed by Bax and Bcl-2) further support the efficacy of PEA therapy in MCAo mice. PEA treatment blocked infiltration of astrocytes and restored MCAo-mediated reduced expression of PAR, nitrotyrosine, iNOS, chymase, tryptase, growth factors (BDNF and GDNF), and GFAP and also inhibited the MCAo-mediated increased expression of pJNK, NF-kB, and degradation of IkB-a, as well as improved neurobehavioral functions as evaluated by motor deficits [48]. In perinatal asphyxia (PA) murine model, PEA attenuated PA-induced cellular and molecular hippocampal damage and its corresponding behavioral alterations. PEA treatment improved dendritic cytoskeleton alteration in CA1 hippocampal area evidenced by the increase of MAP-2 and the reduction of pNF-H/M immunostaining and protein expression levels, as well as, vertical exploration impairments and anxiety-related behaviors [49]. On the other hand, in a cellular oxygen and glucose deprivation (OGD) model that mimics brain-ischemia, PEA and luteolin pre-treatment synergistically prevented the OGD-induced degranulation of mast cells and reduced the neurotoxic potential of MC/9 cells conditioned medium as well as pure neurons susceptibility to OGD [50].

6. PEA and neurodegenerative diseases

Many neurodegenerative diseases are characterized by loss of the functions of the nervous system causes for neuronal disorders or damage. The most frequently diseases are Alzheimer's disease (AD) and Parkinson's disease (PD). The effect of the damage can lead to loss of the mobility, behavioral disorders, and dementia.

The effects of PEA were demonstrated in several assays. To AD, for example, it was registered in a mouse model, that administration of the PEA produces a reduction in the behavioral impairments [51].

In assays in vivo using adults' male rats, which consisted in the intrahippocampal injection of amyloid-β1–42 (Aβ1–42) peptide, the administration of PEA affected in: the high transcription and expression of GFAP and S100β (activators of astrocytes), the increased expression of BACE1 and APP (amyloidogenic), and phosphorylated τ proteins. Also, PEA changed the altered expression of microtubule-associated protein (MAP-2) and cognitive functions induced [52].

An animal PD model that use the injection of the neurotoxin 1-methyl-4-phenyl-1,2,3,6-tetrahydropyridine (MPTP) has been showed the neuroprotective actions of PEA [53]. A treatment with PEA neutralizes the activation of astrocytes and expression of iNOS protein, the loss of nigrostriatal neurons, and the expression of microtubule-associated, produced by MPTP in the model. In other hand, PEA decreased the motor dysfunctions associated to the MPTP effects. The activation of PPAR-α was a key piece in the PEA effects [53]. On the other hand, in cellular models, PEA has been shown to have protective effect on SH-SY5Y neuroblastoma against 6-OHDA damage, partly by inhibiting endoplasmic reticulum stress detrimental response [54].

Therapeutic effects of PEA have also been reported in several chronic models of MS, such as chronic relapsing experimental autoimmune encephalomyelitis (CREAE), Theiler's murine encephalomyelitis virus-induced demyelinating disease (TMEV-IDD), and myelin oligodendrocyte glycoprotein-induced experimental autoimmune encephalomyelitis (MOG-EAE). In an animal model of chronic relapsing experimental allergic encephalomyelitis induced by repeated administration to mice of syngenic spinal cord homogenate emulsified in Freund's complete adjuvant, it was demonstrated that PEA alleviated the spasticity found in the hind limbs [55] and also in TMEV-IDD, respectively [56]. These effects of PEA are due in large part to their anti-inflammatory effects. In both CREAE and TMEV-IDD, a reduction in proinflammatory cytokines was observed, accompanied by a decrease in damage and axonal demyelination [56, 57]. On the other hand, in a mouse, significantly reduces the development of clinical signs in the MOG model of EAE accompanied

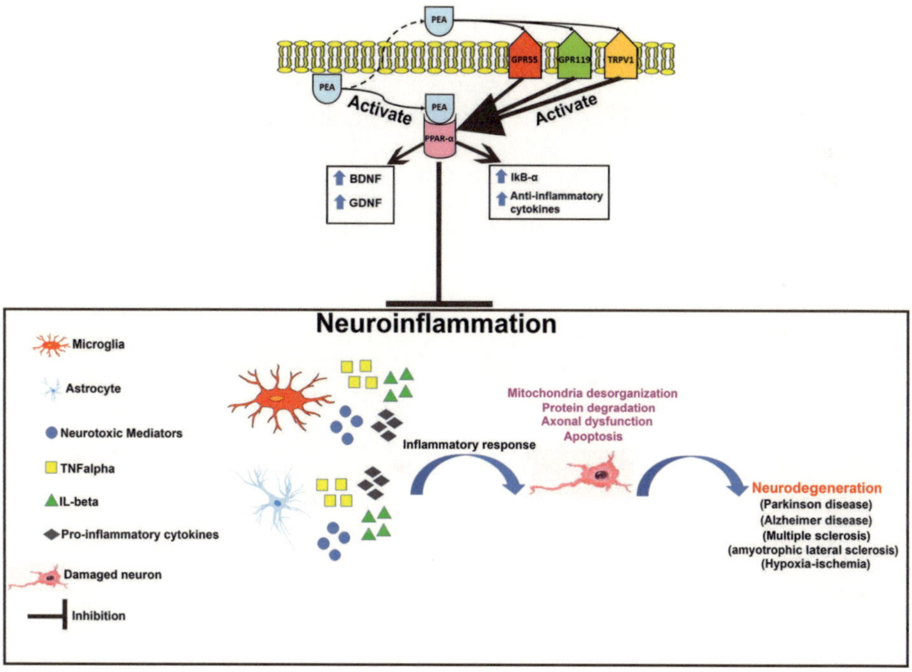

Figure 2.
Schematic representation of inhibitory effect of palmitoylethanolamide (PEA) on neuroinflammation in neurodegenerative disorders such us hypoxia-ischemia. Neuroinflammation is a common process both for neurodegenerative diseases and for hypoxia-ischemia. This process consists of an inflammatory response carried out by both astrocytes and microglia cells through the release of proinflammatory cytokines, neurotoxic mediators, TNFalpha, and IL-beta. These latter throughout the activation of their own receptors trigger intracellular mechanisms conveying in protein degradation, mitochondria desorganization, axonal dysfunction, and apoptosis, with consequent neurodegeneration at the basis of diseases like Parkinson, Alzheimer, multiple and amyotrophic lateral sclerosis and hypoxia-ischemia. The PEA through the PPARα activation inhibits the neuroinflammatory process through the increase in the production of anti-inflammatory cytokines, the synthesis of IkB-α, as well as, favoring the increase of the synthesis of neurotrophic mediators such as: GDNF and BDNF.

by a reduction in transcript expression of the acute-phase protein SAA1, TNF-α, IL-1β, IFN-γ, and NLRP3 proinflammatory proteins and TLR2, Fpr2, CD137, CD3-γ, TCR-ζ chain, and CB2 receptors [58]. In addition, PEA and PPAR-α (peroxisome proliferator-activated receptor-α agonist) have been effective in reducing symptoms of central neuropathic pain in patients with multiple sclerosis [59].

All these evidences suggest that PEA is a central and promising target in the development of new neuroprotective agents, being PPAR-α the main mechanism by which this neuroprotection would be being exercised. The block or mimic PEA effects were evidenced for the use of PPAR-α agonists and antagonists, supporting this idea [7, 60, 61]. **Figure 2** schematizes how the mechanism of action of PEA is in neurodegenerative diseases such as hypoxia-ischemia.

7. Conclusion

PEA is involved in several processes: lipidic metabolism, proinflammatory cytokine genes transcription, signaling cascade, and proliferation. PEA is expressed in brain, skin, liver, intestine, heart, muscle, kidney, and adipose tissue.

It plays a protective role in several neurological disorders and ischemic brain injury. In vivo assays with PEA treatment showed an improve of the neuroinflammation, reduce astrogliosis, and preserve cognitive functions by PPAR-α activation. In vitro assays, pretreatment with PEA and a flavonoid prevent the degranulation of mast cells and reduce the neurotoxic potential of MC/9 cells in OGD model.

PEA treatment could be a potential alternative therapy than hypothermia. This is because the hypothermia is an unspecific treatment and PEA acts under specific mechanism. However, this sort of therapy is still incipient, to say the least, and further investigations should pursue on focusing in the main downstream effectors involved in HI.

Author details

Lucas D. Udovin[1*], Andrea Aguilar[1], Tamara Kobiec[2], María I. Herrera[2], Santiago Perez Lloret[1], Nicolás Toro Urrego[1] and Rodolfo A. Kölliker Frers[1,3]

1 Institute of Cardiological Research, University of Buenos Aires, National Research Council (ININCA-UBA-CONICET), Buenos Aires, Argentina

2 Centro de Investigaciones en Psicología y Psicopedagogía (CIPP), Pontificia Universidad Católica Argentina, Buenos Aires, Argentina

3 Hospital Ramos Mejía, Buenos Aires, Argentina

*Address all correspondence to: lucas2304@hotmail.com

References

[1] Ryberg E, Larsson N, Sjögren S, Hjorth S, Hermansson N-O, Leonova J, et al. The orphan receptor GPR55 is a novel cannabinoid receptor. British Journal of Pharmacology. 2007;**152**(7):1092-1101

[2] Lo Verme J, Fu J, Astarita G, La Rana G, Russo R, Calignano A, et al. The nuclear receptor peroxisome proliferator-activated receptor-α mediates the anti-inflammatory actions of palmitoylethanolamide. Molecular Pharmacology. 2005;**67**(1):15 LP-19 LP

[3] Sugiura T, Kondo S, Kishimoto S, Miyashita T, Nakane S, Kodaka T, et al. Evidence that 2-arachidonoylglycerol but not N-palmitoylethanolamine or anandamide is the physiological ligand for the cannabinoid CB2 receptor. Comparison of the agonistic activities of various cannabinoid receptor ligands in HL-60 cells. The Journal of Biological Chemistry. 2000;**275**(1):605-612

[4] Lauckner JE, Jensen JB, Chen H-Y, Lu H-C, Hille B, Mackie K. GPR55 is a cannabinoid receptor that increases intracellular calcium and inhibits M current. Proceedings of the National Academy of Sciences of the United States of America. 2008;**105**(7):2699-2704

[5] Henstridge DC, Febbraio MA. Adiponectin sparks an interest in calcium. Cell Metabolism. 2010;**11**:447-449

[6] Godlewski G, Offertáler L, Wagner JA, Kunos G. Receptors for acylethanolamides—GPR55 and GPR119. Prostaglandins & Other Lipid Mediators. 2010;**89**:105-111

[7] LoVerme J, La Rana G, Russo R, Calignano A, Piomelli D. The search for the palmitoylethanolamide receptor. Life Sciences. 2005;**77**(14):1685-1698

[8] Yang H, Zhou J, Lehmann C. GPR55—a putative "type 3" cannabinoid receptor in inflammation. Journal of Basic and Clinical Physiology and Pharmacology. 2016;**27**(3):297-302

[9] Caterina MJ, Schumacher MA, Tominaga M, Rosen TA, Levine JD, Julius D. The capsaicin receptor: A heat-activated ion channel in the pain pathway. Nature. 1997;**389**(6653): 816-824. DOI: 10.1038/39807

[10] Cristino L, de Petrocellis L, Pryce G, Baker D, Guglielmotti V, Di Marzo V. Immunohistochemical localization of cannabinoid type 1 and vanilloid transient receptor potential vanilloid type 1 receptors in the mouse brain. Neuroscience. 2006;**139**(4):1405-1415

[11] Marzo V, Starowicz K, Cristino L. TRPV1 receptors in the central nervous system: Potential for previously unforeseen therapeutic applications. Current Pharmaceutical Design. 2008;**14**(1):42-54

[12] Petrosino S, Iuvone T, Di Marzo V. N-palmitoyl-ethanolamine: Biochemistry and new therapeutic opportunities. Biochimie. 2010;**92**(6):724-727

[13] Edwards J. TRPV1 in the central nervous system: Synaptic plasticity, function, and pharmacological implications. Progress in Drug Research. 2014;**68**:77-104

[14] Iannotti FA, Hill CL, Leo A, Alhusaini A, Soubrane C, Mazzarella E, et al. Nonpsychotropic plant cannabinoids, cannabidivarin (CBDV) and cannabidiol (CBD), activate and desensitize transient receptor potential vanilloid 1 (TRPV1) channels in vitro: Potential for the

treatment of neuronal hyperexcitability. ACS Chemical Neuroscience. 2014;**5**(11):1131-1141. DOI: 10.1021/cn5000524

[15] Cortright DW, Szallasi A. Biochemical pharmacology of the vanilloid receptor TRPV1: An update. European Journal of Biochemistry. 2004;**271**:1814-1819

[16] Iannotti FA, Di Marzo V, Petrosino S. Endocannabinoids and endocannabinoid-related mediators: Targets, metabolism and role in neurological disorders. Progress in Lipid Research. 2016;**62**:107-128

[17] Nagy I, Friston D, Valente JS, Torres Perez JV, Andreou AP. Pharmacology of the capsaicin receptor, transient receptor potential vanilloid type-1 ion channel. Progress in Drug Research. 2014;**68**:39-76

[18] Portavella M, Rodriguez-Espinosa N, Galeano P, Blanco E, Romero JI, Holubiec MI, et al. Oleoylethanolamide and palmitoylethanolamide protect cultured cortical neurons against hypoxia. Cannabis Cannabinoid Research. 2018;**3**(1):171-178

[19] Petrosino S, Puigdemont A, Della Valle MF, Fusco M, Verde R, Allara M, et al. Adelmidrol increases the endogenous concentrations of palmitoylethanolamide in canine keratinocytes and down-regulates an inflammatory reaction in an in vitro model of contact allergic dermatitis. Veterinary Journal. 2016;**207**:85-91

[20] Matsuda LA, Lolait SJ, Brownstein MJ, Young AC, Bonner TI. Structure of a cannabinoid receptor and functional expression of the cloned cDNA. Nature. 1990;**346**(6284):561-564

[21] Munro S, Thomas KL, Abu-Shaar M. Molecular characterization of a peripheral receptor for cannabinoids. Nature. 1993;**365**(6441):61-65

[22] Pertwee RG. Pharmacology of cannabinoid CB1 and CB2 receptors. Pharmacology & Therapeutics. 1997;**74**(2):129-180

[23] Turu G, Hunyady L. Signal transduction of the CB1 cannabinoid receptor. Journal of Molecular Endocrinology. 2010;**44**(2):75-85

[24] Gomez del Pulgar T, Velasco G, Guzman M. The CB1 cannabinoid receptor is coupled to the activation of protein kinase B/Akt. The Biochemical Journal. 2000;**347**(Pt 2):369-373

[25] Sanchez MG, Ruiz-Llorente L, Sanchez AM, Diaz-Laviada I. Activation of phosphoinositide 3-kinase/PKB pathway by CB(1) and CB(2) cannabinoid receptors expressed in prostate PC-3 cells. Involvement in Raf-1 stimulation and NGF induction. Cellular Signalling. 2003;**15**(9):851-859

[26] Stella N. Cannabinoid and cannabinoid-like receptors in microglia, astrocytes, and astrocytomas. Glia. 2010;**58**(9):1017-1030

[27] Izzo AA. Cannabinoids and intestinal motility: Welcome to CB2 receptors. British Journal of Pharmacology. 2004;**142**(8):1201-1202

[28] Pertwee RG. GPR55: A new member of the cannabinoid receptor clan? British Journal of Pharmacology. 2007;**152**(7):984-986

[29] Campora L, Miragliotta V, Ricci E, Cristino L, Di Marzo V, Albanese F, et al. Cannabinoid receptor type 1 and 2 expression in the skin of healthy dogs and dogs with atopic dermatitis. American Journal of Veterinary Research. 2012;**73**(7):988-995

[30] Basu S, Dittel BN. Unraveling the complexities of cannabinoid receptor 2

(CB2) immune regulation in health and disease. Immunologic Research. 2011;**51**(1):26-38

[31] Demuth DG, Molleman A. Cannabinoid signalling. Life Sciences. 2006;**78**(6):549-563

[32] Di Marzo V, Melck D, Orlando P, Bisogno T, Zagoory O, Bifulco M, et al. Palmitoylethanolamide inhibits the expression of fatty acid amide hydrolase and enhances the anti-proliferative effect of anandamide in human breast cancer cells. The Biochemical Journal. 2001;**358**(Pt 1):249-255

[33] de Groot H, Rauen U. Ischemia-reperfusion injury: Processes in pathogenetic networks: A review. Transplantation Proceedings. 2007;**39**(2):481-484

[34] Kalogeris T, Baines CP, Krenz M, Korthuis RJ. Cell biology of ischemia/reperfusion injury. International Review of Cell and Molecular Biology. 2012;**298**:229-317

[35] Dugan LL, Choi DW. Hypoxia-ischemia and brain infarction. In: Siegel GJ, Agranoff BW, Albers RW, et al., editors. Basic Neurochemistry: Molecular, Cellular and Medical Aspects. 6th ed. Lippincott-Raven; 1999

[36] Johnston MV, Trescher WH, Ishida A, Nakajima W. Neurobiology of hypoxic-ischemic injury in the developing brain. Pediatric Research. 2001;**49**(6):735-741

[37] Vannucci SJ, Willing LB, Goto S, Alkayed NJ, Brucklacher RM, Wood TL, et al. Experimental stroke in the female diabetic, db/db, mouse. Journal of Cerebral Blood Flow and Metabolism. 2001;**21**(1):52-60

[38] Uria-Avellanal C, Robertson NJ. Na(+)/H(+) exchangers and intracellular pH in perinatal brain injury. Translational Stroke Research. 2014;**5**(1):79-98

[39] Wang C, Jie C, Dai X. Possible roles of astrocytes in estrogen neuroprotection during cerebral ischemia. Reviews in the Neurosciences. 2014;**25**(2):255-268

[40] Dietrich WD. Neurobiology of stroke. International Review of Neurobiology. 1998;**42**:55-101

[41] Liu L, Yenari MA. Clinical application of therapeutic hypothermia in stroke. Neurological Research. 2009;**31**(4):331-335

[42] Ross OA, Worrall BB, Meschia JF. Advancing stroke therapeutics through genetic understanding. Current Drug Targets. 2007;**8**(7):850-859

[43] Holubiec MI, Romero JI, Suarez J, Portavella M, Fernandez-Espejo E, Blanco E, et al. Palmitoylethanolamide prevents neuroinflammation, reduces astrogliosis and preserves recognition and spatial memory following induction of neonatal anoxia-ischemia. Psychopharmacology. 2018;**235**(10):2929-2945

[44] Sun Y, Alexander SPH, Garle MJ, Gibson CL, Hewitt K, Murphy SP, et al. Cannabinoid activation of PPAR alpha; a novel neuroprotective mechanism. British Journal of Pharmacology. 2007;**152**(5):734-743

[45] Schomacher M, Muller HD, S ommer C, Schwab S, Schabitz W-R. Endocannabinoids mediate neuroprotection after transient focal cerebral ischemia. Brain Research. 2008;**1240**:213-220

[46] Franklin A, Parmentier-Batteur S, Walter L, Greenberg DA, Stella N. Palmitoylethanolamide increases after focal cerebral ischemia and potentiates microglial cell motility. The Journal of Neuroscience. 2003;**23**(21):7767-7775

[47] Caltagirone C, Cisari C, Schievano C, Di Paola R, Cordaro M, Bruschetta G, et al. Co-ultramicronized palmitoylethanolamide/luteolin in the treatment of cerebral ischemia: From rodent to man. Translational Stroke Research. 2016;7(1):54-69

[48] Ahmad A, Genovese T, Impellizzeri D, Crupi R, Velardi E, Marino A, et al. Reduction of ischemic brain injury by administration of palmitoylethanolamide after transient middle cerebral artery occlusion in rats. Brain Research. 2012;**1477**:45-58

[49] Herrera MI, Udovin LD, Toro-Urrego N, Kusnier CF, Luaces JP, Capani F. Palmitoylethanolamide ameliorates hippocampal damage and behavioral dysfunction after perinatal asphyxia in the immature rat brain. Frontiers in Neuroscience. 2018;**12**:145

[50] Parrella E, Porrini V, Iorio R, Benarese M, Lanzillotta A, Mota M, et al. PEA and luteolin synergistically reduce mast cell-mediated toxicity and elicit neuroprotection in cell-based models of brain ischemia. Brain Research. 2016;**1648**(Pt A):409-417

[51] D'Agostino G, Russo R, Avagliano C, Cristiano C, Meli R, Calignano A. Palmitoylethanolamide protects against the amyloid-beta25-35-induced learning and memory impairment in mice, an experimental model of Alzheimer disease. Neuropsychopharmacology. 2012;**37**(7):1784-1792

[52] Scuderi C, Stecca C, Valenza M, Ratano P, Bronzuoli MR, Bartoli S, et al. Palmitoylethanolamide controls reactive gliosis and exerts neuroprotective functions in a rat model of Alzheimer's disease. Cell Death & Disease. 2014;**5**:e1419

[53] Esposito E, Impellizzeri D, Mazzon E, Paterniti I, Cuzzocrea S. Neuroprotective activities of palmitoylethanolamide in an animal model of Parkinson's disease. PLoS One. 2012;**7**(8):e41880

[54] Avagliano C, Russo R, De Caro C, Cristiano C, La Rana G, Piegari G, et al. Palmitoylethanolamide protects mice against 6-OHDA-induced neurotoxicity and endoplasmic reticulum stress: In vivo and in vitro evidence. Pharmacological Research. 2016;**113** (Pt A):276-289

[55] Baker D, Pryce G, Croxford JL, Brown P, Pertwee RG, Makriyannis A, et al. Endocannabinoids control spasticity in a multiple sclerosis model. The FASEB Journal: Official Publication of the Federation of American Societies for Experimental Biology. 2001;**15**(2):300-302

[56] Loria F, Petrosino S, Mestre L, Spagnolo A, Correa F, Hernangomez M, et al. Study of the regulation of the endocannabinoid system in a virus model of multiple sclerosis reveals a therapeutic effect of palmitoylethanolamide. The European Journal of Neuroscience. 2008;**28**(4):633-641

[57] Rahimi A, Faizi M, Talebi F, Noorbakhsh F, Kahrizi F, Naderi N. Interaction between the protective effects of cannabidiol and palmitoylethanolamide in experimental model of multiple sclerosis in C57BL/6 mice. Neuroscience. 2015;**290**:279-287

[58] Contarini G, Franceschini D, Facci L, Barbierato M, Giusti P, Zusso M. A co-ultramicronized palmitoylethanolamide/luteolin composite mitigates clinical score and disease-relevant molecular markers in a mouse model of experimental autoimmune encephalomyelitis. Journal of Neuroinflammation. 2019;**16**(1):126

[59] Kopsky DJ, Hesselink JMK. Multimodal stepped care approach with acupuncture and PPAR-alpha agonist

palmitoylethanolamide in the treatment of a patient with multiple sclerosis and central neuropathic pain. Acupuncture in Medicine. 2012;**30**(1):53-55

[60] Sheu MY, Fowler AJ, Kao J, Schmuth M, Schoonjans K, Auwerx J, et al. Topical peroxisome proliferator activated receptor-alpha activators reduce inflammation in irritant and allergic contact dermatitis models. The Journal of Investigative Dermatology. 2002;**118**(1):94-101

[61] Lo Verme J, Fu J, Astarita G, La Rana G, Russo R, Calignano A, et al. The nuclear receptor peroxisome proliferator-activated receptor-alpha mediates the anti-inflammatory actions of palmitoylethanolamide. Molecular Pharmacology. 2005;**67**(1):15-19

Chapter 2

An Alternate View of Neuroprotection with Peptides in Alzheimer's Disease

Samuel King and Cenk Suphioglu

Abstract

Neuroprotection plays a crucial role in everyday life, maintaining a clean environment in the central nervous system to allow for normal functioning. In Alzheimer's disease and other neurodegenerative disorders, neuroprotection may have two roles. Under standard circumstances, the immune system protects the CNS, but sometimes it can exacerbate the pathophysiology of some diseases through neuroinflammation leading to further degeneration. Alzheimer's disease is fast getting out of control, with no new approvals in therapeutics since 2003, and of those approved, all target symptomatic treatment. Initiated by a microglial response to Aβ plaques, therapeutic development should focus on the amyloid cascade as a neuroprotective measure for Alzheimer's disease. This chapter will examine the status of the types of therapeutics in clinical trials for Alzheimer's disease, offering insights into peptides as an area of opportunity for neuroprotection and detailing considerations for the use of peptides in Alzheimer's disease.

Keywords: Alzheimer's disease, peptides, neuroinflammation, therapeutic development, CNS indications

1. Introduction

The central nervous system (CNS) consists of the brain and spinal cord, playing the role of control centre in the body. It is responsible for sending and integrating signals from around the body and coordinating activity. Protecting the CNS is crucial to sustaining life. Without this system, normal day-to-day functions such as breathing and eating would be compromised. Arguably, the most important organ in the CNS is the brain. This is protected from external physical injury by the skull and meninges, which provide a buffer against forceful trauma to the head. How does the brain protect itself from internal injury, such as a microbiological threat or other small molecules that invade the sterile environment? Bacteria, viruses and misfolded proteins are as much of a threat as physical impacts. However, there is no durable exterior to protect from these internal attacks. The next line of defence is the immune system, a complex network of specialised cells that aim to protect the body against these biological threats.

The immune response is key to maintaining the delicate environment of the CNS. However, the neuroprotective properties of the immune system may also be detrimental to the surrounding neurons. Immune cells release chemical mediators such as cytokines and histamine to damage foreign cells, but these mediators also damage sensitive structures that make up the brain. This process occurs in disorders where degeneration of cellular tissue in the brain is present. Disorders such as Alzheimer's disease (AD), Parkinson's disease (PD), Huntington's disease (HD) and Amyotrophic Lateral Sclerosis (ALS) all exhibit progressive degeneration of specific neuronal cell populations [1, 2]. All four diseases are commonly found to exhibit misfolding, aggregation and accumulation of specific proteins. This hallmark feature is now widely accepted as a possible cause for these diseases and other neurodegenerative disorders [3–5]. Deposition of amyloid-forming proteins functions as the initiating step for neuroinflammation [6] activating pattern recognition receptors (PRRs) on microglia, the resident macrophages in the brain [6, 7]. To protect the brain, microglia recognise fragments of these misfolded proteins and secrete cytokines and chemokines. The release of these pro-inflammatory immunomodulators mediates neuroinflammation, attracting other immune cells such as astrocytes and perivascular macrophages to aid in innate immunity [8]. In most cases, activated microglia will clear the build-up of the pathogenic proteins resolving the immune response and subsequent inflammation.

In a typical immune response where resolution is achieved, clearance of the localised inflammation allows the surrounding tissue to return to normal conditions. When the immune response is not resolved, inflammation persists in the local area, potentially becoming toxic to neighbouring cells. Prolonged inflammation in a sensitive environment such as the CNS is highly likely to cause damage to neurons and other nearby cells, leading to local degeneration of tissue. Damage-associated molecular patterns (DAMPs) released from neurons in the inflamed area are recognised by PRRs on primed microglia. This further stimulates the release of pro-inflammatory molecules [9]. This persistent self-propagating cycle of inflammation and necrosis causes the chronic inflammation that exacerbates the pathology of the disease. The notion that neuroprotection does more damage than it prevents has been explored recently, with some proposing that inflammation is the causative agent of neurodegeneration [10, 11]. To prevent neurodegeneration found in diseases like AD, neuroprotective therapeutics must be developed in order to prevent further inflammation and damage from occurring.

1.1 Alzheimer's disease as a neuroinflammatory disorder

Alois Alzheimer first discovered clusters of abnormal protein built up in the cerebral cortex of a patient in 1906. Alzheimer described these clusters as "thick bundles [that] appear at the surface of the cell", noting specifically that neurons in the upper layers of tissue had "disappeared" [12]. These bundles were later identified as the two major hallmarks of AD, hyperphosphorylated tau and aggregated amyloid-beta (Aβ). Alzheimer also noted glial cells clustered around the plaques, concurrent with the theory of an immune response to the extracellular deposits of Aβ plaques and cellular death. In 2019, we are still no closer to mapping out the nature of this disease than Alois was in 1906, with the pathophysiology of the disease still debated: which came first, the tau or the plaques? There have been several hypotheses considered over the nature of the disease; however, the two major hallmarks remain the most probable causes.

To describe the basis of the two major hypotheses is easy; the amyloid cascade involves the cleavage of a transmembrane protein known as amyloid-precursor protein (APP) by the aspartic-acid protease beta-site amyloid precursor protein cleaving enzyme 1 (BACE1), which leads to the extracellular aggregation of a peptide called Aβ, whereas the neurofibrillary tangle (NFT) theory posits that AD is caused by the hyperphosphorylation of tau, a soluble microtubule-associated protein that can aggregate intracellularly into NFTs.

Before establishing the effects of a therapeutic for neuroprotection in AD, the causative agent of neuronal death needs to be identified. Examining both hypotheses in detail reveals that the deposition of Aβ plaques has more of an effect on NFT formation than hyperphosphorylation of tau has on amyloid build-up [13, 14]. Arguments for both options are common place in discussion about AD; however, there are some key facts on why Aβ plaques are crucial in the development of neurodegeneration, and therefore the symptoms of AD. In transgenic mouse models, it has been shown that NFT formation succeeds Aβ deposition extracellularly [15, 16]. As a causal agent, tau is seen in other diseases such as frontotemporal lobar degeneration, progressive supranuclear palsy and Pick's disease. All of which form tau aggregates without an onset of Aβ deposition. The distinct immune response from Aβ plaque deposition indicates that the amyloid cascade is the driving factor of neurodegeneration in AD [10]. From a neuroprotective standpoint, preventing the amyloid cascade from generating and depositing Aβ plaques seems the most probable option for prevention of neurodegeneration from chronic neuroinflammation.

2. Therapeutics for Alzheimer's disease: past, present and future

In a 20-year period from 1998 to 2017, a total of 146 drugs in clinical trials were halted or had not received approval by the FDA [17]. In that same time, four cognitive-enhancing therapeutics had been approved, giving some hope that there is a chance to identify a therapeutic for AD. Therapeutics in the AD clinical trial pipeline are split into two major classes of mechanism of action (MOA): symptomatic treatments and disease-modifying therapies (DMTs). Symptomatic treatments aim to alleviate symptoms that are present with the onset of the disease easing the burden on the affected individuals. There are currently five therapies that have been approved for use in patients that exhibit symptoms derived from neurotransmitter disturbance in mild to severe cases of AD. Suppressing symptoms such as memory loss and cognitive decline do not address the underlying nature of the disease [18]. Symptomatic treatments are beneficial for family and friends, demonstrating modest and consistent benefits for cognition. However, the underlying cause of the disease remains unchanged in these therapies where the disease progresses into a more severe state. DMTs are treatments that alter the pathology of the disease, changing the long-term course of the disease. A large proportion of DMTs targets the major hallmarks of AD, NFTs and Aβ formation. Other DMTs are present that target alternative aspects of the disease; however, these alternative targets are mostly downstream effects of NFTs or Aβ plaques. Of major interest are DMTs that target the amyloid cascade, their primary goal is to reduce plaque load, clear plaque depositions, or reduce inflammation. The nature of this MOA is of a neuroprotective stance, theoretically with the ability to reduce the amount of neurodegeneration that occurs due to chronic inflammation from Aβ seeding in the extracellular space.

As of February 2019, 132 therapeutics were in clinical trials for AD, 96 of those classed as DMTs presenting an increase of 25 DMTs from 2018 [19, 20]. Therapeutics labelled as neuroprotective, anti-inflammatory and anti-amyloid in the 2019 cohort of clinical trials will be described as neuroprotective DMTs as they all target the amyloid cascade as the priming step of neuroinflammation. Neuroprotective DMTs are described as either prophylactic treatments or disease-clearing treatments. Prophylactic treatment of AD aims at preventing the onset of the disease by targeting the steps prior to amyloid deposition aiming to prevent the activation of microglia and subsequent neuroinflammation. Disease-clearing therapeutics target plaques deposited into the extracellular space. They focus on removing plaques and debris to prevent chronic inflammation. There is no clear current trend in neuroprotective DMTs, with a broad selection of therapeutics covering different targets from amyloid clearance using antibodies or vaccines to mark areas for the immune system, anti-aggregation of Aβ fibrils, or preventing the production of Aβ fragments by targeting BACE1 or alpha secretase.

2.1 Lessons from previous clinical trials

With such a broad range of therapeutics in clinical trials, it would be easy to assume that we are close to finding a treatment for AD, but we are not. In the 20 years spanning 1998 to 2017, almost 150 therapeutics in clinical development had stopped or not received regulatory approval [17]. The FDA approved only four therapeutics in that time leaving a lot to learn from past failures. Neuroprotective DMTs made up 34% of the therapeutics discontinued in this time, leaving in their wake a plethora of lessons that can be applied to upcoming therapeutics [21]. A shift in development from the conventional small molecule drug (SMD) to a biological approach has shown benefits. Increased knowledge on the effects of more potent and specific therapeutics has led to the identification of new targets for therapeutic development, specifically the amyloid cascade. Of the therapeutics active in clinical trials in the 15 years from 2005 to 2019, 79 targeted the amyloid cascade in a disease-modifying mechanism (**Table 1**). Moreover, of the 79 clinical trials, 20 have been discontinued (**Table 1**).

2.1.1 Types of therapeutics

A shift in the type of therapeutic used in AD has given insights into how targets respond to certain molecules. A common issue encountered with amyloid targeting therapeutics is specificity, with off-target effects halting a few large-scale trials [22]. There are two major molecular classes present in amyloid targeting DMTs: small molecule, low molecular weight entities including chemical drugs and peptides, and biologics, larger structures such as proteins and antibodies.

2.1.1.1 Small molecular entities

Thought of as the traditional form of therapeutic, small molecular entities (SMEs) are typically chemical in nature and mostly target molecules with deep catalytic channels or clefts such as enzymes or receptors [23]. The nature of these SMDs is to bind to the target and exert its effect, doing so until there is no more target available for binding or the drug is cleared from the body. This overzealous technique of SMDs poses the risk of long-term modulation on the target, whether it be positively or negatively, regardless of whether the disease state improves or not [24].

The main target of an SME is commonly found in biological processes where a high amount of regulation is required, in the form of either enzymes or receptors [25]. The interaction that SMEs target is between an enzyme or receptor and its respective substrate, all of which are proteins. Referred to as protein–protein interactions (PPIs), they have gained popularity as a target for therapeutic intervention due to the control these interactions have on biological processes. Many PPIs have been identified as candidates targeting diseases similar to AD where a biological process has been altered resulting in disease [25].

NCT number	Drug name	Phase	Status	Start date	Completion date
NCT00303277	Simvastatin & Pravastatin	IV	C	08/2002	04/2005
NCT00479219	GSI-953	I	C	05/2007	10/2007
NCT00765115	LY450139	I	C	07/2006	09/2007
NCT0083808	LY2811376	I	C	12/2008	06/2009
NCT00733642	PF-04360365	I	A, NLR	08/2008	07/2009
NCT01125631	PF-04360365	I	C	05/2010	08/2011
NCT01148498	Solanezumab	II	C	08/2010	08/2012
NCT01482013	HPP854	I	D	10/2011	03/2012
NCT00464334	V950 and ISCOMATRIXTM	I	C	03/2007	01/2012
NCT00411580	CAD106	I	C	06/2005	12/2008
NCT00945672	PF-04360365	II	C	08/2009	06/2011
NCT01547169	Insulin detemir	II	C	03/2011	12/2012
NCT00500500	EGb 761	II	D	07/2005	04/2008
NCT00739037	PAZ-417	I	D	08/2008	12/2008
NCT01568086	Affitope AD03	I	D	12/2011	10/2013
NCT01661673	EVP 0962	II	C	11/2012	10/2013
NCT00812565	Immune Globulin	II	C	02/2009	09/2010
NCT00857506	Florbetapir F 18	II	C	01/2009	12/2011
NCT00397891	Bapineuzumab	I	C	10/2006	02/2010
NCT01035138	Semagacestat	III	C	12/2009	04/2011
NCT01669876	Anatabine	II	D	08/2012	02/2015
NCT01978548	Atabecestat	I	C	12/2013	04/2015
NCT02061878	Bexarotene	I	C	08/2014	11/2014
NCT00486044	Simvastatin	II	C	02/2005	06/2009
NCT00711321	Affitope AD02 & Aluminium hydroxide	I	C	11/2008	04/2010
NCT01093664	Affitope AD02 & Aluminium hydroxide	I	C	10/2009	07/2010
NCT01357629	Affitope AD02 & Aluminium hydroxide	I	D	07/2011	11/2013
NCT00633841	Affitope AD02 & Aluminium hydroxide	I	C	02/2008	09/2009
NCT01782742	Bexarotene	II	C	02/2013	12/2014
NCT02323334	LY3202626 & Itraconazole	I	C	12/2014	02/2016
NCT00722046	Ponezumab	II	C	12/2008	08/2011
NCT00956410	Amilomotide	II	C	09/2009	06/2011
NCT00762411	Semagacestat	III	C	09/2008	04/2011
NCT01097096	Amilomotide	II	C	03/2010	12/2012
NCT01928420	Pinitol	II	C	04/2007	06/2014
NCT00329082	Solanezumab	II	C	05/2006	05/2008

NCT number	Drug name	Phase	Status	Start date	Completion date
NCT01600859	Elenbecestat	I	C	07/2012	10/2013
NCT01297218	hMSC Therapy	I	C	02/2011	12/2011
NCT01193608	AAB 003	I	C	09/2010	10/2013
NCT02260674	Atabecestat	II	C	11/2014	06/2016
NCT02033668	GSK 933776	I	C	01/2014	07/2014
NCT01424436	GSK 933776	I	C	05/2010	12/2011
NCT02576639	Umibecestat	II	C	08/2015	03/2016
NCT00904683	Solanezumab	III	C	05/2009	06/2012
NCT02386306	GC 021109	I	C	02/2015	10/2015
NCT01595646	Insulin detemir	II	C	11/2011	03/2015
NCT01561430	LY 2886721	I/II	D	03/2012	Jun 2013
NCT02551809	UB 311	II	C	10/2015	08/2018
NCT03417986	Thiethylperazine	II	A, NLR	11/2017	07/2021
NCT01056965	Davunetide	I	C	01/2010	12/2012
NCT01428453	Rilapladib	II	C	07/2011	02/2013
NCT02036645	MEDI 1814	I	C	02/2014	09/2016
NCT01397578	Crenezumab	II	C	07/2011	04/2014
NCT01127633	Solanezumab	III	D	11/2010	02/2017
NCT02760602	Solanezumab	III	D	06/2016	05/2017
NCT01900665	Solanezumab	III	D	07/2013	02/2017
NCT02080364	Azeliragon	III	D	04/2015	06/2018
NCT01807026	LY 2886721	I	C	03/2013	05/2013
NCT02462161	Insulin aspart	I	C	03/2015	04/2019
NCT02899091	CB-AC 02	I/II	R	09/2016	12/2021
NCT02614131	LY 2599666 & Solanezumab	I	D	12/2015	12/2016
NCT02406027	Atabecestat	II	D	07/2015	06/2018
NCT02051608	Gantenerumab	III	A, NLR	03/2014	04/2021
NCT03114657	Crenezumab	III	D	03/2017	06/2019
NCT02565511	Amilomotide & Umibecestat	II/III	D	11/2015	03/2025
NCT01760005	Atabecestat & Gantenerumab & Solanezumab	II/III	D	12/2012	03/2021
NCT01224106	Gantenerumab	III	A, NLR	11/2010	08/2020
NCT01966666	TPI 287	I	A, NLR	11/2013	11/2019
NCT00594568	Semagacestat	III	C	03/2008	05/2011
NCT02719327	E-EPA	II/III	R	06/2017	11/2021
NCT02956486	Elenbecestat	III	D	10/2016	11/2023

NCT number	Drug name	Phase	Status	Start date	Completion date
NCT03036280	Elenbecestat	III	D	12/2016	11/2023
NCT02245737	Lanabecestat	II/III	D	09/2014	10/2018
NCT03443973	Gantenerumab	III	R	08/2018	03/2023
NCT03444870	Gantenerumab	III	R	06/2018	03/2023
NCT00299988	Immune Globulin	II	D	02/2006	04/2010
NCT02600130	hMSC Therapy-Longeveron	I	A, NLR	10/2016	09/2020
NCT03402659	Neflamapimod	II	C	12/2017	07/2019
NCT03117738	Adipose SC therapy-Anterogen	I/II	C	04/2017	06/2019

Abbreviations: A, Active; NLR, no longer recruiting; C, Completed; D, Discontinued. NOTE: 79 trials were identified as amyloid targeting as of January 9, 2020, according to https://adisinsight.springer.com.

Table 1.
Amyloid targeting clinical trials from 2005 to 2019.

Analysis of SMEs targeting PPIs has shown that they do not observe standard drug-like properties, specifically surrounding their size, hydrophobicity and specificity [26, 27]. These properties all show mild increases, compared to conventional SMDs, proving that the chemistry of PPIs requires molecules to be selected more carefully rather than selecting the molecule with the highest potency.

2.1.1.2 Biologics

Biologics fill the void of the upper end of the molecular weight scale, made up of antibodies, proteins and enzymes. Biological therapeutics like antibodies and vaccines aim to modulate the immune system to clear various threats from the body. Other therapies involve the replacement of an important molecule in a biological process, such as hormone replacement therapy (HRT) or lactose intolerance. Replacement therapies use therapeutics that mimic proteins in a healthy individual, usually using recombinant technology to produce the protein in different biological models.

The PPIs mentioned above have important regulatory roles in biological processes, keeping them in check as cell signalling molecules [28]. Biological intervention with molecules that mimic or stop these interactions enables control over biological pathways similar to SMDs, however, giving the pathway some control over feedback [24]. Antibodies are an excellent example of controlling the immune system in AD to remove the build-up of deposited plaques, while allowing the body to exert control over the reaction of the immune response to these antibodies. This shows the benefit of using biologics in the development of therapeutic options for AD and other diseases.

A common issue that has arisen in the therapeutic development of biologics is the bioavailability and half-life of the therapeutic. Biologics are not well known for high bioavailability, particularly where the oral route is concerned, an issue that can be overcome using other forms of administration [29]. Following administration, biologics are subjected to proteases and harsh conditions in the stomach or other accessory organs that reduces the half-life dramatically [30]. Intravenous and intramuscular administration has improved the half-life of biologics; however, modification to the structure of the therapeutic may be required to reach the target from the blood stream or the tissue at the site of injection. Although there are common issues regarding ideal therapeutic properties of biologics, new technology is improving every day allowing therapeutic development of biologics to overcome what seems to be simple obstacles.

2.1.2 Targets of the amyloid cascade

2.1.2.1 Inflammation

As the step preceding neurodegeneration, inflammation is a clear target for therapeutic intervention. Neuroinflammation has been a target in therapeutic development after the increasing recognition that glial activation is an important step in the process of neurodegeneration. Therapeutics targeting neuroinflammation have been evaluated in previous cohorts of clinical trials, all producing similar results of ineffectiveness at slowing cognitive decline [31]. The principle of anti-inflammatory targeting aims to prevent the off-target damage to neighbouring neurons, delaying the onset of neurodegeneration. However, without removing the stimulus causing neuroinflammation, therapeutics are fighting a losing battle. Factors such as rate of cognitive decline, severity of the neuroinflammatory response, and disease state play a role in anti-inflammatory and immunomodulatory drug discovery proving difficult as the timing of the intervention is critical [32]. Anti-inflammatory therapeutics made up 16% of therapeutics in clinical trials in 2019, many repurposed for AD [19]. As a sole therapeutic intervention for AD, anti-inflammatories are not ideal. Combined therapy using anti-inflammatories and a disease-clearing therapeutic will likely show a high rate of success in alleviating chronic inflammation caused by AD.

2.1.2.2 Amyloid-β

Aβ is an attractive target for neuroprotection, with many possible angles to approach the underlying cause of the disease. Two methods aimed at targeting Aβ plaques have been employed in clinical trials: immunotherapy, targeting the plaques for removal by the immune system using a vaccine or monoclonal antibodies (mAbs), and anti-aggregation, preventing the Aβ fragments from forming the plaques. In 2019, nine immunotherapies were part of clinical trials: three active immunotherapies (vaccines), CAD106, ABvac40 and GV1001, and six passive immunotherapies (mAbs), aducanumab, crenezumab, gantenerumab, solanezumab, LY3002813 and LY3372993 [19].

Thoroughly tested in animal models, Aβ vaccines exhibit the ability to prevent the formation of new Aβ plaques and contribute to the clearance of pre-deposited plaques [33]. Immunising an individual to Aβ grants the long-term effects of antibody production. However, immunisation can be difficult where adverse reactions in older individuals may occur due to inconsistent or lack of an immune system, as well as selecting a specific epitope that will not target similar structures [34]. Clinical trials into AN1792, an adjuvant vaccine of the full-length Aβ peptide and QS-21, were stopped due to development of meningoencephalitis in some patients [35]. Second-generation anti-Aβ vaccines such as CAD106 have proven to be efficacious in phase 2 clinical studies, eliciting Aβ-specific antibodies and showing long-term safety promising to be a valuable therapeutic option [36].

Passive immunotherapies have a major advantage over Aβ immunisation in that there is a consistent antibody titre [34]. Initial intravenous administration of immunoglobulin preparations containing high levels of human anti-Aβ42, which showed a significant improvement in cognition and lower levels of Aβ [33]. However, similar to the other discontinued anti-Aβ mAb therapies, large scale testing proved efficacy to be low or non-existent. A risk found in trials with Bapineuzumab was the presence of abnormalities after imaging the brain, identifying the onset of vasogenic oedema in 3 of the 10 participants. These abnormalities were coined as ARIA-E, amyloid-relating imaging abnormalities-vasogenic effusions, and are seen as a risk in large-scale studies of mAb therapies [37]. Many mAbs in 2019 are still plagued with these obstacles, presenting safety concerns surrounding ARIA-E, although some mAbs in Phase 2/3 or 3 trials are looking closer than ever at slowing the progression of AD.

As a target class, combined therapy of immunotherapeutics and anti-aggregates stand the highest chance of clearing deposited and newly generated Aβ fragments. Aggregation of Aβ monomers only make it more difficult to clear from the extracellular space with neuroprotective mechanisms naturally clearing monomers that build-up over time. From this perspective, Aβ is targeted as both monomers and plaques. Solanezumab targets Aβ monomers before they can aggregate. Targeting the causal feature of amyloid-based microglial activation, anti-aggregates prevent the conversion of Aβ monomers into oligomers or fibrils [38]. Many natural and synthetic compounds have been identified as potential anti-aggregates for Aβ; however, the only anti-aggregate for amyloidogenesis in clinical trials in 2019 is a combination therapy of polyphenol extract from grapeseeds and resveratrol [19]. The current cohort of anti-aggregates is not indicative of knowledge of the field, with other compounds such as epigallocatechin-3-gallate and curcumin showing promising results for both anti-aggregation and other purposes [39].

2.1.2.3 Secretase inhibitors

Modulating the upstream step of plaque formation provides an encouraging target as prevention of deposition of Aβ fragments may stop the neuroinflammatory response before it starts. A "one size fits all" therapy for secretase modulation is not possible as all three secretase enzymes play different roles in the generation of Aβ fragments, each requiring a different form of modulation specific to their role in the processing of APP.

2.1.2.3.1 Gamma secretase

Inhibitors of BACE1 and gamma secretase have thus far showed limited Aβ clearance in clinical trials, even after demonstration of excellent inhibition in preclinical animal models [40]. Studies into gamma secretase found that it was the last step in Aβ fragment generation and an ideal target to prevent the build-up of fragments and formation of plaques [41]. Semagacestat was identified as potential drug candidate for clinical trials in decreasing Aβ levels, only after Phase III in the IDENTITY trials was it found to have adverse effects on Notch signalling [42]. Identified as a drug with a higher selectivity for APP over Notch in preclinical studies, Avagacestat was another gamma secretase inhibitor that showed similar effects to Semagacestat forcing the discontinuation of the trials due to adverse dose-limiting effects [43]. The adverse effects and lack of efficacy had quashed further research into gamma secretase inhibitors; however, a new look into gamma secretase as a target has identified that it is available for modulation, specifically altering the cleavage site of the enzyme. NGP 555 is a promising SME gamma secretase modulator that has showed promising results *in vivo,* significantly lowering levels of $A\beta_{42}$ through a shift of cleavage site in gamma secretase [44].

2.1.2.3.2 Alpha secretases

Alpha secretase as a therapeutic target for AD offers a novel approach of upregulating cleavage of APP rather than preventing it. By cleaving APP within the Aβ domain, alpha secretase prevents the generation of Aβ fragments instead releasing non-toxic p3 peptide following gamma secretase cleavage [45]. Modulation of alpha secretase is expected to increase its activity and reduce levels of Aβ, potentially increasing the levels of a neuroprotective product of alpha secretase cleavage of APP, sAPPα [46]. Alpha secretases belong to the 'a disintegrin and metalloprotease' (ADAM) family, which are found to play roles in cell adhesion, migration, proteolysis and signalling [47]. ADAM10 was found to be the alpha secretase relevant to APP cleavage in neurons, making it the target of modulation in AD [48]. Two therapeutics that have undergone clinical trials showing potential as alpha secretases enhancers are etazolate (EHT-0202) and bryostatin-1. Both stimulate alpha secretase to increase generation of sAPPα [49]. The potential of alpha secretase enhancers as a therapeutic for AD is likely. However, studies into the effects of enhancers on the other substrates of ADAM10 are required to identify any possible adverse effects [50].

2.1.2.3.3 BACE1

Targeting BACE1 for therapeutic development in AD is ideal, as it is the determining step in the generation of Aβ fragments. Inhibition of BACE1 has shown to decrease levels of Aβ plaques. Studies in mouse models have proven that by removing BACE1 there is no generation of Aβ fragments, and subsequently no neurodegeneration and loss in cognitive abilities [51].

Since it was discovered to play a role in AD in 1999, BACE1 has been thoroughly researched as a potential target for AD. BACE1 has been an elusive target for inhibitors, its location in the brain, size of the active site, and similarity to other aspartic proteases making it difficult for the ideal therapeutic to be developed [52]. Initial inhibitors of BACE1 were non-cleavable peptide-based analogues, designed on the amino acid sequence of APP, which showed excellent inhibitory effects on BACE1. However, the size was too large to exhibit *in vivo* benefits, although ideal for the active site [53]. The development of SMEs for BACE1 renewed hope in the use of the aspartic protease as a target, hoping to increase blood–brain barrier (BBB) penetration and bioavailability that were identified as issues with the first-generation BACE1 inhibitors. From there, the hunt for a BACE1 inhibitor began with multiple classes of inhibitors being developed in an attempt to find the ideal therapeutic.

In a similar pattern to other amyloid therapies, BACE1 inhibitors in other trials were halted or discontinued due to lack of efficacy or off-target effects. Only two BACE1 inhibitors were in the 2019 cohort of clinical trials: CNP520, discontinued in July 2019 due to worsening of cognitive function, and E2609, discontinued in September 2019 due to unfavourable risk–benefit ratio [54, 55]. Both compounds joining the list of lessons learnt from BACE1 inhibitors, along with Lanabecestat, Atabecestat and Verubecestat. All of which proved excellent in reducing Aβ; however, translation into clinical trials was not as smooth, lacking efficacy or displaying off-target effects [56].

2.2 Improving therapeutics or target choice

With no current curative treatments for AD available, previous cohorts of clinical trials are missing something vital. The types of therapeutics used and targets available explained above show that therapeutic discovery is not a simple task, particularly in a disease as complex as AD. The ideal neuroprotective therapeutic for combating AD is one that targets the initiating steps of amyloid development with high specificity and potency, while not disrupting other biological processes. An attractive initiating step of amyloid development is BACE1, discussed above as a promising target to prevent the generation of Aβ fragments responsible for the activation of microglia and subsequent development of neurodegeneration. Previous attempts at inhibiting BACE1 have shown mixed and unfavourable responses of properties such as specificity, bioavailability and efficacy. Both biologicals and SMEs cannot fill the requirements of such a specific therapeutic, requiring a molecule that has the ideal properties of both. Such a molecule is already being explored in therapeutic development for AD although it is still in its infancy as a class of therapeutic molecule for AD. Peptides are becoming more attractive as a therapeutic to target BACE1 with new technology altering their structure to better fit the required properties. Such research promises to pave new and exciting ways to developing refined peptide inhibitors of BACE1 with high efficacy and specificity, and thus prepare novel reagents for the prophylactic treatment of AD in the near future.

3. New outlook for Alzheimer's disease

3.1 What are peptides?

Peptides are small molecular biologicals that play a major role in the body as signalling molecules. Naturally occurring peptides in humans are commonly called hormones, acting as messengers utilising the blood stream and other extracellular spaces to regulate the many biological processes that keep us going [57]. Two of the most well-known peptides are glucagon and insulin, both playing large roles in homeostasis of blood-glucose levels. These hormones act on blood-glucose levels by targeting accessory organs and stimulating glucose production or glycogen storage, respectively. The action of glucose and insulin is a classic example of how peptides work in the body with high specificity and rapid onset of effect. Although commonly linked to hormones, peptides are also used as neurotransmitters, anti-infectives and growth factors [58].

Peptides range in length from 10 to 50 amino acids long, and can have a mass of up to 5 kDa, putting them between SMEs and proteins in terms of size and weight. *In vivo*, natural peptides are highly efficacious and selective with limited off-target effects, transient at most for those that exist [59]. Their ability to act as signalling molecules both extracellularly and intracellularly displays the range of therapeutic opportunity that peptides exhibit. Following the discovery of peptides playing large roles in homeostasis in the body, research turned towards identifying and isolating certain peptides that were linked to diseases. To continue with the example of insulin, the development of insulin as a therapeutic comes from the identification of individuals lacking a "pancreatic secretion" in the early 1900s, where insulin was isolated from the pancreas of stray dogs and calves and used to treat a child with type I diabetes [57]. This discovery only fuelled the fire for further discovery and isolation of other natural peptides that were found to be involved in diseases, leading to the identification of over 7000 naturally occurring peptides. Although identified, not all can be used directly as a therapeutic due to unbeneficial properties such as poor bioavailability and short half-life [58].

3.2 Peptides as therapeutic options

The nature of tasks that peptides perform in the body makes them an enticing molecule, as an opportunity to control biological processes in a similar way that hormones and other natural peptides control everyday life. Many consider peptides to be the inferior option for therapeutic development as they display low oral bioavailability and a tendency to be metabolised by proteolytic enzymes in the local environment leading to a short half-life *in vivo* [57]. These unfavourable traits are mitigated in the body through close proximity of targets to the site of release, sometimes in high concentrations for when multiple targets exist. For peptides to be successful in therapeutic applications, an intense intravenous dosing regimen for the patient is required to maintain an adequate load of the therapeutic. Although hindered by poor bioavailability and short half-life, the biological nature of peptides offers plenty of properties that would make them an ideal therapeutic for complex diseases where specificity and toxicity are of concern [57].

The specific nature of peptides is due to their ability to cover a larger area of the target site compared to SMDs, decreasing the risk of off-target effects that have halted previous clinical trials into AD therapeutics [60]. A benefit of peptides over SMDs is the relative inability to build-up toxicity due to the metabolic instability of the amide bonds that hold the peptide together, resulting in the release of amino acids that can be utilised by various systems [61]. These qualities of peptides are what make them ideal therapeutics for most biological process disorders, specifically those found in the CNS. The delicate environment of the CNS requires therapeutics that are highly specific so as not to affect the normal functioning of the brain, but also produce minimal toxicity to prevent damage to nearby neurons.

3.3 Peptides approved for therapeutic use

In the 36 months that spanned 2016–2018, 8 peptide therapeutics were approved by the FDA making up just over 6% of the drugs approved in that time [62]. This can be looked at in both an optimistic and pessimistic view. However, looking at cumulative FDA approvals given since 1980, there is no denying that peptides have a place in therapeutic development. In 2018, there were over 70 peptides available for medical use in the United States, Europe and Japan, and more than 150 in clinical studies [63]. The most commonly used therapeutic peptides target biological processes in a similar way that biologics, such as proteins, do, replacing molecules that stimulate PPIs. Crucial hormones that were approved for therapeutic use are vasopressin, oxytocin, insulin, glucagon and corticotropin, all of which were approved last century yet still play a pivotal role in HRTs [63].

Currently approved peptides cover a large range of therapeutic areas, such as oncology, metabolic diseases, haematology, respiratory disorders and gastroenterology. Of the peptides approved by the FDA, only three are approved for CNS indications: corticotropin, approved for use in inflammatory diseases; glatiramer, approved for use in MS; and taltirelin, approved for use in spinocerebellar degeneration. After the discovery of taltirelin in 2000, no other peptides have been approved for CNS indications, even though there have been over 30 new peptides approved for other indications since [63]. This begs the question on whether research has moved away from peptides for CNS indications due to their difficulty passing through the BBB, or whether the technology is only now catching up.

3.4 Future considerations for peptide therapeutics for use in CNS indications

With a variety of unfavourable characteristics, peptides require modification prior to clinical testing. The field of peptide synthesis has improved in the past two decades contributing to a rise in more effective peptide therapeutics available for clinical trials [64]. Many traits of peptides that were initially unfavourable have been resolved with new techniques in peptide synthesis. However, there remains the large issue of bioavailability that is restricting the use of peptides as therapeutics for the CNS. The biological nature of peptides reduces their bioavailability, their size making it difficult to cross membrane barriers and the structure of their bonds increasing the rate of degradation in the gastrointestinal (GI) tract and plasma. Due to these features, most approved peptide therapeutics are parenterally administered, involving either intravenous or subcutaneous injections. Parenteral administration allows for the systemic distribution of a relatively large dose of the peptide providing high concentration of the therapeutic when it reaches its target, without having to cross any membrane barriers. The oral route does not allow for this as the conditions are acidic and tight mucosal barriers exist to protect the body from external threats [29].

Administration directly into the blood stream works for many indications where the target is easily reached through diffusion across capillary walls; however, CNS indications are protected from standard blood flow by the BBB. Peptides targeting the CNS endure this extra barrier that acts as a neuroprotective wall, preventing unwanted molecules from entering the sterile and sensitive environment [65]. Studies in transport of drugs across the BBB have shown that there are multiple ways that can be exploited to deliver drugs to the CNS, specifically using transporter pathways that shuttle hormones such as insulin into the CNS [66]. Delivery of previous therapeutics for AD in clinical trials involved either disruption of the BBB, increasing lipid solubility of the molecules or using pre-existing transport systems, with mouse model studies showing effectiveness of the latter two [67]. An alternative route through the olfactory pathway may provide hope for delivering peptides to the CNS; however, intranasal delivery has demonstrated limited progress in clinical settings. Offering an attractive opportunity to bypass the BBB, intranasal delivery presents similar patterns in degradation to other routes of delivery [68].

Although an issue present in the delivery of peptides to the CNS, transport into the CNS is secondary to proteolytic degradation in terms of bioavailability of peptides, with a large proportion of peptide load being degraded before it can reach the target site. Widely accepted as techniques that decrease degradation is conjugation or the production of peptidomimetics, techniques used in peptide synthesis today. The most common conjugate for increasing bioavailability of a peptide is polyethylene glycol (PEG), a molecule that has shown to help prevent clearance of therapeutics. PEG increases the overall size of peptide therapeutics, making it too large for renal clearance and hindering proteolytic cleavage in plasma [30]. Peptidomimetics are a modified form of the peptide that is biologically similar while containing unnatural amino acids or modified peptide bonds [69]. Through the addition of unnatural amino acids and altered peptide bonds, proteolytic enzymes are incapable of cleaving peptidomimetics due to the unnatural nature of the molecule. The process of screening the effects of multiple modifications to the structure of the peptide has improved with the development of simple screening assays, increasing the output of peptidomimetic therapeutics.

4. Conclusions

As a mechanism, neuroprotection in CNS indications where protein misfolding occurs is detrimental, exacerbating the disease by creating inflammation in the local area that leads to the degeneration of nearby neurons. In the case of AD, neuroinflammation occurs when Aβ plaques are recognised by circulating microglial cells, initiating an immune response and releasing pro-inflammatory molecules that lead to the neurodegeneration that is found in patients with AD. The neuroprotective response of microglia in effect begins the deterioration of the brain, calling for therapeutic intervention to aid in neuroprotection.

Current therapeutics used as therapy for AD are all neuromodulatory, addressing the symptoms related to the disease instead of the underlying mechanism. About 73% of the current cohort of therapeutics in clinical trials for AD is DMTs, indicating the need for a therapeutic that either slows or stops the progression of the disease. DMTs targeting the amyloid cascade are of particular interest from a neuroprotective standpoint due to Aβ plaques initiating neuroinflammation. Targeting inflammation and Aβ plaques and fragments will only slow the progression of the disease requiring a more robust target that can stop disease progression. The role of BACE1 in Aβ generation provides an ideal target for therapeutics although it has proved elusive in the past, with trials into SMD inhibitors for BACE1 being halted due to safety concerns from off-target effects.

To develop an ideal therapeutic for BACE1, a molecule that lies somewhere between SMEs and biologics is required. Peptides offer attractive properties from both classes of therapeutic specifically a relative lack of toxicity and great specificity, both of which are ideal for combating CNS indications. Although peptides are seen as inadequate for use as therapeutics, many approved peptide therapies have shown the ability of peptides to be modified, improving qualities that were lacking initially. With further advancements in the field of peptide synthesis and modifications, the number of peptide therapeutics in clinical trials, not just for AD but other indications, will likely increase. Similarly, the number of approved therapies, offering a promising outlook for diseases where therapeutic needs are currently unmet, is likely to increase.

Author details

Samuel King and Cenk Suphioglu*
NeuroAllergy Research Laboratory (NARL), School of Life and Environmental Sciences, Deakin University, Geelong, Victoria, Australia

*Address all correspondence to: cenk.suphiolgu@deakin.edu.au

References

[1] Barnham KJ, Masters CL, Bush AI. Neurodegenerative diseases and oxidative stress. Nature Reviews. Drug Discovery. 2004;**3**(3):205-214. DOI: 10.1038/nrd1330

[2] Nopoulos PC. Huntington disease: A single-gene degenerative disorder of the striatum. Dialogues in Clinical Neuroscience. 2016;**18**(1):91-98. Available from: https://www.ncbi.nlm.nih.gov/pubmed/27069383

[3] Jucker M, Walker LC. Pathogenic protein seeding in Alzheimer disease and other neurodegenerative disorders. Annals of Neurology. 2011;**70**(4):532-540. Available from: https://www.ncbi.nlm.nih.gov/pubmed/22028219

[4] Verma M, Vats A, Taneja V. Toxic species in amyloid disorders: Oligomers or mature fibrils. Annals of Indian Academy of Neurology. 2015;**18**(2):138-145. Available from: https://www.ncbi.nlm.nih.gov/pubmed/26019408

[5] Soto C. Unfolding the role of protein misfolding in neurodegenerative diseases. Nature Reviews Neuroscience. 2003;**4**(1):49-60. DOI: 10.1038/nrn1007

[6] Lucin KM, Wyss-Coray T. Immune activation in brain aging and neurodegeneration: Too much or too little? Neuron. 2009;**64**(1):110-122. Available from: https://www.ncbi.nlm.nih.gov/pubmed/19840553

[7] Venegas C, Heneka MT. Danger-associated molecular patterns in Alzheimer's disease. Journal of Leukocyte Biology. 2017;**101**(1):87-98. DOI: 10.1189/jlb.3MR0416-204R

[8] Van Eldik LJ, Carrillo MC, Cole PE, Feuerbach D, Greenberg BD, Hendrix JA, et al. The roles of inflammation and immune mechanisms in Alzheimer's disease. Alzheimer's & Dementia: Translational Research & Clinical Interventions. 2016;**2**(2):99-109. DOI: 10.1016/j.trci.2016.05.001

[9] Sarlus H, Heneka MT. Microglia in Alzheimer's disease. Journal of Clinical Investigation. 2017;**127**(9):3240-3249. DOI: 10.1172/JCI90606

[10] Kempuraj D, Thangavel R, Natteru PA, Selvakumar GP, Saeed D, Zahoor H, et al. Neuroinflammation Induces Neurodegeneration. Journal of Neurology, Neurosurgery and Spine. 2016;**1**(1):1003. Available from: https://www.ncbi.nlm.nih.gov/pubmed/28127589

[11] Lyman M, Lloyd DG, Ji X, Vizcaychipi MP, Ma D. Neuroinflammation: The role and consequences. Neuroscience Research. 2014;**79**:1-12

[12] Alzheimer A. Über eine eigenartige Erkrankung der Hirnrinde. Allgemeine Zeitschrift für Psychiatrie und psychisch-gerichtliche Medizin. 1907;**64**:146-148

[13] Stancu IC, Cremers N, Vanrusselt H, Couturier J, Vanoosthuyse A, Kessels S, et al. Aggregated Tau activates NLRP3–ASC inflammasome exacerbating exogenously seeded and non-exogenously seeded tau pathology in vivo. Acta Neuropathologica. 2019;**137**(4):599-617. DOI: 10.1007/s00401-018-01957-y

[14] Ising C, Venegas C, Zhang S, Scheiblich H, Schmidt SV, Vieira-Saecker A, et al. NLRP3 inflammasome activation drives tau pathology. Nature. 2019;**575**:669-673

[15] Götz J, Streffer JR, David D, Schild A, Hoerndli F, Pennanen L, et al. Transgenic animal models of Alzheimer's disease and related disorders:

Histopathology, behavior and therapy. Molecular Psychiatry. 2004;**9**(7):664-683. DOI: 10.1038/sj.mp.4001508

[16] Selenica M-LB, Brownlow M, Jimenez JP, Lee DC, Pena G, Dickey CA, et al. Amyloid oligomers exacerbate tau pathology in a mouse model of Tauopathy. Neurodegenerative Diseases. 2013;**11**(4):165-181. DOI: 10.1159/000337230

[17] Pharmaceutical Research and Manufacturer's of America. Alzheimer's Medicines: Setbacks and Stepping Stones [Internet]. 2018. Available from: https://www.phrma.org/en/Alzheimer-s-Medicines-Setbacks-and-Stepping-Stones

[18] Yiannopoulou KG, Papageorgiou SG. Current and future treatments for Alzheimer's disease. Therapeutic Advances in Neurological Disorders. 2013;**6**(1):19-33. Available from: https://www.ncbi.nlm.nih.gov/pubmed/23277790

[19] Cummings J, Lee G, Ritter A, Sabbagh M, Zhong K. Alzheimer's disease drug development pipeline: 2019. Alzheimer's & Dementia: Translational Research & Clinical Interventions. 2019;**5**:272-293. DOI: 10.1016/j.trci.2019.05.008

[20] Cummings J, Lee G, Ritter A, Zhong K. Alzheimer's disease drug development pipeline: 2018. Alzheimer's & Dementia: Translational Research & Clinical Interventions. 2018;**4**:195-214. DOI: 10.1016/j.trci.2018.03.009

[21] Kodamullil AT, Zekri F, Sood M, Hengerer B, Canard L, McHale D, et al. Tracing investment in drug development for Alzheimer disease. Nature Reviews Drug Discovery. 2017;**16**:819. DOI: 10.1038/nrd.2017.169

[22] Cummings JL, Morstorf T, Zhong K. Alzheimer's disease drug-development pipeline: Few candidates, frequent failures. Alzheimer's Research & Therapy. 2014;**6**(4):37. DOI: 10.1186/alzrt269

[23] Hopkins AL, Groom CR. The druggable genome. Nature Reviews Drug Discovery. 2002;**1**(9):727-730. DOI: 10.1038/nrd892

[24] Gurevich EV, Gurevich VV. In: Gurevich VV, editor. Therapeutic Potential of Small Molecules and Engineered Proteins BT - Arrestins - Pharmacology and Therapeutic Potential. Berlin, Heidelberg: Springer Berlin Heidelberg; 2014. pp. 1-12. DOI: 10.1007/978-3-642-41199-1_1

[25] Bosch J. PPI inhibitor and stabilizer development in human diseases. Drug Discovery Today: Technologies. 2017;**24**:3-9. Available from: http://www.sciencedirect.com/science/article/pii/S1740674917300100

[26] London N, Raveh B, Schueler-Furman O. Druggable protein–protein interactions – From hot spots to hot segments. Current Opinion in Chemical Biology. 2013;**17**(6):952-959. Available from: http://www.sciencedirect.com/science/article/pii/S1367593113001798

[27] Wells JA, McClendon CL. Reaching for high-hanging fruit in drug discovery at protein–protein interfaces. Nature. 2007;**450**(7172):1001-1009. DOI: 10.1038/nature06526

[28] Nero TL, Morton CJ, Holien JK, Wielens J, Parker MW. Oncogenic protein interfaces: Small molecules, big challenges. Nature Reviews Cancer. 2014;**14**:248. DOI: 10.1038/nrc3690

[29] Rekha MR, Sharma CP. Oral delivery of therapeutic protein/peptide for diabetes – Future perspectives. International Journal of Pharmaceutics. 2013;**440**(1):48-62. Available from:

http://www.sciencedirect.com/science/article/pii/S0378517312003249

[30] Werle M, Bernkop-Schnürch A. Strategies to improve plasma half life time of peptide and protein drugs. Amino Acids. 2006;**30**(4):351-367. DOI: 10.1007/s00726-005-0289-3

[31] Walker D, Lue L-F. Anti-inflammatory and immune therapy for Alzheimer's disease: Current status and future directions. Current Neuropharmacology. 2007;**5**(4):232-243. Available from: https://www.ncbi.nlm.nih.gov/pubmed/19305740

[32] Minter MR, Taylor JM, Crack PJ. The contribution of neuroinflammation to amyloid toxicity in Alzheimer's disease. Journal of Neurochemistry. 2016;**136**(3):457-474. DOI: 10.1111/jnc.13411

[33] Coman H, Nemeş B. New therapeutic targets in Alzheimer's disease. International Journal of Gerontology. 2017;**11**(1):2-6. Available from: http://www.sciencedirect.com/science/article/pii/S1873959817300224

[34] van Dyck CH. Anti-amyloid-β monoclonal antibodies for Alzheimer's disease: Pitfalls and promise. Biological Psychiatry. 2018;**83**(4):311-319. DOI: 10.1016/j.biopsych.2017.08.010

[35] Gilman S, Koller M, Black RS, Jenkins L, Griffith SG, Fox NC, et al. Clinical effects of Aβ immunization (AN1792) in patients with AD in AN interrupted trial. Neurology. 2005;**64**(9):1553 LP-1551562. Available from: http://n.neurology.org/content/64/9/1553.abstract

[36] Vandenberghe R, Riviere M-E, Caputo A, Sovago J, Maguire RP, Farlow M, et al. Active Aβ immunotherapy CAD106 in Alzheimer's disease: A phase 2b study. Alzheimer's & Dementia: Translational Research & Clinical Interventions. 2017;**3**(1):10-22. DOI: 10.1016/j.trci.2016.12.003

[37] Sperling RA, Jack CR Jr, Black SE, Frosch MP, Greenberg SM, Hyman BT, et al. Amyloid-related imaging abnormalities in amyloid-modifying therapeutic trials: Recommendations from the Alzheimer's association research roundtable workgroup. Alzheimers Dement. 2011;**7**(4):367-385. Available from: https://www.ncbi.nlm.nih.gov/pubmed/21784348

[38] Bu X-L, Rao PPN, Wang Y-J. Anti-amyloid aggregation activity of natural compounds: Implications for Alzheimer's drug discovery. Molecular Neurobiology. 2016;**53**(6):3565-3575. DOI: 10.1007/s12035-015-9301-4

[39] Cheng B, Gong H, Xiao H, Petersen RB, Zheng L, Huang K. Inhibiting toxic aggregation of amyloidogenic proteins: A therapeutic strategy for protein misfolding diseases. Biochimica et Biophysica Acta (BBA) - General Subjects. 2013;**1830**(10):4860-4871. Available from: http://www.sciencedirect.com/science/article/pii/S0304416513002894

[40] Toyn J. What lessons can be learned from failed Alzheimer's disease trials? Expert Review of Clinical Pharmacology. 2015;**8**(3):267-269. DOI: 10.1586/17512433.2015.1034690

[41] De Strooper B. Lessons from a failed γ-Secretase Alzheimer trial. Cell. 2014;**159**(4):721-726. DOI: 10.1016/j.cell.2014.10.016

[42] Henley DB, Sundell KL, Sethuraman G, Dowsett SA, May PC. Safety profile of semagacestat, a gamma-secretase inhibitor: IDENTITY trial findings. Current Medical Research and Opinion. 2014;**30**(10):2021-2032. DOI: 10.1185/03007995.2014.939167

[43] Coric V, Salloway S, van Dyck CH, Dubois B, Andreasen N, Brody M, et al. Targeting prodromal Alzheimer disease with avagacestat: A randomized clinical trial. JAMA Neurology. 2015;**72**(11):1324-1333. DOI: 10.1001/jamaneurol.2015.0607

[44] Kounnas MZ, Lane-Donovan C, Nowakowski DW, Herz J, Comer WT. NGP 555, a γ-secretase modulator, lowers the amyloid biomarker, Aβ42, in cerebrospinal fluid while preventing Alzheimer's disease cognitive decline in rodents. Alzheimer's & Dementia: Translational Research & Clinical Interventions. 2017;**3**(1):65-73. DOI: 10.1016/j.trci.2016.09.003

[45] Jean-Noel O, Nathalie P. Processing of amyloid precursor protein and amyloid peptide neurotoxicity. Current Alzheimer Research. 2008;**5**:92-99. Available from: http://www.eurekaselect.com/node/82425/article

[46] Lichtenthaler SF. Alpha-secretase in Alzheimer's disease: Molecular identity, regulation and therapeutic potential. Journal of Neurochemistry. 2011;**116**(1):10-21. DOI: 10.1111/j.1471-4159.2010.07081.x

[47] Edwards DR, Handsley MM, Pennington CJ. The ADAM metalloproteinases. Molecular Aspects of Medicine. 2008;**29**(5):258-289. Available from: http://www.sciencedirect.com/science/article/pii/S0098299708000551

[48] Kuhn P-H, Wang H, Dislich B, Colombo A, Zeitschel U, Ellwart JW, et al. ADAM10 is the physiologically relevant, constitutive alpha-secretase of the amyloid precursor protein in primary neurons. EMBO Journal. 2010;**29**(17):3020-3032. Available from: https://www.ncbi.nlm.nih.gov/pubmed/20676056

[49] Kumar D, Ganeshpurkar A, Kumar D, Modi G, Gupta SK, Singh SK. Secretase inhibitors for the treatment of Alzheimer's disease: Long road ahead. European Journal of Medicinal Chemistry. 2018;**148**:436-452. Available from: http://www.sciencedirect.com/science/article/pii/S022352341830165X

[50] MacLeod R, Hillert E-K, Cameron RT, Baillie GS, et al. The role and therapeutic targeting of α-, β- and γ-secretase in Alzheimer's disease. Future Science OA. 2015;**1**(3). DOI: 10.4155/fso.15.9

[51] Luo Y, Bolon B, Kahn S, Bennett BD, Babu-Khan S, Denis P, et al. Mice deficient in BACE1, the Alzheimer's β-secretase, have normal phenotype and abolished β-amyloid generation. Nature Neuroscience. 2001;**4**(3):231-232. DOI: 10.1038/85059

[52] Coimbra JRM, Marques DFF, Baptista SJ, Pereira CMF, Moreira PI, Dinis TCP, et al. Highlights in BACE1 inhibitors for Alzheimer's disease treatment [internet]. Frontiers in Chemistry. 2018;**6**:178. DOI: 10.3389/fchem.2018.00178

[53] Vassar R. BACE1 inhibition as a therapeutic strategy for Alzheimer's disease. Journal of Sport and Health Science. 2016;**5**(4):388-390. Available from: http://www.sciencedirect.com/science/article/pii/S2095254616300898

[54] Mullard A. Alzheimer prevention failure rattles field, anew. Nature Reviews. Drug Discovery. 2019;**18**:656

[55] Eisai. Eisai and Biogen to Discontinue Phase III Clinical Studies of BACE Inhibitor Elenbecestat in Early Alzheimer's Disease; 2019

[56] Parasrampuria DA, Benet LZ, Sharma A. Why drugs fail in late stages of development: Case study analyses from the last decade and

recommendations. The AAPS Journal. 2018;**20**(3):46. DOI: 10.1208/s12248-018-0204-y

[57] Wetzler M, Hamilton P. 8 - Peptides as therapeutics. In: Koutsopoulos S, editor. Biotechnology and Bioengineering SBT-PA in B. United Kingdom: Woodhead Publishing; 2018. pp. 215-230 Available from: http://www.sciencedirect.com/science/article/pii/B9780081007365000089

[58] Fosgerau K, Hoffmann T. Peptide therapeutics: Current status and future directions. Drug Discovery Today. 2015;**20**(1):122-128. Available from: http://www.sciencedirect.com/science/article/pii/S1359644614003997

[59] Haslam NJ, Shields DC. Peptide-binding domains: Are limp handshakes safest? Science Signaling. 2012;**5**(243):pe40. Available from: http://stke.sciencemag.org/content/5/243/pe40.abstract

[60] Hummel G, Reineke U, Reimer U. Translating peptides into small molecules. Molecular BioSystems. 2006;**2**(10):499-508. DOI: 10.1039/B611791K

[61] Loffet A. Peptides as drugs: Is there a market? Journal of Peptide Science. 2002;**8**(1):1-7. DOI: 10.1002/psc.366

[62] Al Shaer D, Al Musaimi O, Albericio F, de la Torre GB. 2018 FDA Tides Harvest. Vol. 12. Pharmaceuticals. Basel, Switzerland: MDPI; 2019

[63] Lau JL, Dunn MK. Therapeutic peptides: Historical perspectives, current development trends, and future directions. Bioorganic & Medicinal Chemistry. 2018;**26**(10):2700-2707. Available from: http://www.sciencedirect.com/science/article/pii/S0968089617310222

[64] Erak M, Bellmann-Sickert K, Els-Heindl S, Beck-Sickinger AG. Peptide chemistry toolbox – Transforming natural peptides into peptide therapeutics. Bioorganic & Medicinal Chemistry. 2018;**26**(10):2759-2765. Available from: http://www.sciencedirect.com/science/article/pii/S0968089617322277

[65] Stamatovic SM, Keep RF, Andjelkovic AV. Brain endothelial cell-cell junctions: How to "open" the blood brain barrier. Current Neuropharmacology. 2008 Sep;**6**(3):179-192. Available from: https://www.ncbi.nlm.nih.gov/pubmed/19506719

[66] Chen Y, Liu L. Modern methods for delivery of drugs across the blood–brain barrier. Advanced Drug Delivery Reviews. 2012;**64**(7):640-665. Available from: http://www.sciencedirect.com/science/article/pii/S0169409X11002900

[67] Banks WA. Drug delivery to the brain in Alzheimer's disease: Consideration of the blood–brain barrier. Advanced Drug Delivery Reviews. 2012;**64**(7):629-639. Available from: http://www.sciencedirect.com/science/article/pii/S0169409X11002997

[68] Khan AR, Liu M, Khan MW, Zhai G. Progress in brain targeting drug delivery system by nasal route. Journal of Controlled Release. 2017;**268**: 364-389. Available from: http://www.sciencedirect.com/science/article/pii/S0168365917308258

[69] Gentilucci L, Marco RD, Cerisoli L. Chemical modifications designed to improve peptide stability: Incorporation of non-natural amino acids, pseudo-peptide bonds, and cyclization. Current Pharmaceutical Design. 2010;**16**:3185-3203. Available from: http://www.eurekaselect.com/node/72674/article

Chapter 3

Polyphenols as Potential Therapeutic Drugs in Neurodegeneration

Patrizia Polverino de Laureto, Luana Palazzi and Laura Acquasaliente

Abstract

Several therapeutic approaches have been suggested so far for the treatment of neurodegenerative diseases, but to date, there are no approved therapies. The available ones are only symptomatic; they are employed to mitigate the disease manifestations and to improve the patient life quality. These diseases are characterized by the accumulation and aggregation of misfolded proteins in the nervous system, with different specific hallmarks. The onset mechanisms are not completely elucidated. Some promising approaches are focused on the inhibition of the amyloid aggregation of the proteins involved in the etiopathology of the disease, such as Aβ peptide, Tau, and α-synuclein, or on the increase of their clearance in order to avoid their aberrant accumulation. Here, we summarize traditional and new therapeutic approaches proposed for Alzheimer's and Parkinson's diseases and the recent technologies for brain delivery.

Keywords: Alzheimer's disease, Parkinson's disease, amyloidosis, protein fibrils and oligomers, polyphenols, brain delivery technologies

1. Introduction

Alzheimer's disease (AD) and Parkinson's disease (PD) are the most common neurodegenerative disorders. They are multifactorial, progressive, age-related, and influenced by genetic and environmental factors. Despite being public health problems and widely studied, there are no effective treatments. The therapies in use at the moment are only symptomatic and focused to ameliorate patients' life quality. Moreover, there are no diagnostic methods for the early detection of these diseases that, especially at the onset, share some pathological hallmarks. There are specific proteins associated with the diseases, but it is still unclear when and how they lose their functionality and become toxic. Several pathways of cellular dysfunction have been described to explain the toxicity associated with the disease, but the pathological role of proteins involved still remains controversial. Currently, the most promising therapeutic approaches are focused on personalized treatments and targeted drugs.

Here, we summarize some relevant features of the new proposed therapies for AD and PD. In the last decade, renewed interest rises toward alternative pharmacological treatments and products of natural origin, especially those associated with the Mediterranean diet, such as polyphenols. The unexpected benefits and the wide-range properties of polyphenols suggest deepening the study of these molecules for a more comprehensive understanding of their mechanism of action in order to use them in effective therapies.

2. Molecular aspects of Alzheimer's and Parkinson's diseases

2.1 Brief introduction to AD and PD

AD is characterized by the gradual decline in the cognitive function, memory loss, and behavior changes [1]. Typical features of the disease are a synaptic deficit in the neocortex and the limbic system, neuronal loss, white matter loss, astrogliosis, microglial cell proliferation, and oxidative stress [2]. The major areas of the human brain affected by AD are schematically represented in **Figure 1**. The pathological hallmarks of AD are the presence of intracellular flame-shaped neurofibrillary tangles and extracellular plaques in the brain. The tangles are especially present in the perinuclear cytoplasm and are prevalently formed by the Tau protein, in a hyperphosphorylated form. The plaques derive from the progressive accumulation of amyloid β-peptide (Aβ) in a filamentous form [3]. The neuritic plaques have a diameter ranging from 10 to more than 120 μm [2]. The methods used for the diagnosis of the pathology have been standardized. They refer to the density and the grade of compactness of the neuritis amyloid plaques and neurofibrillary tangles [4]. AD aggregates can be classified into positive and negative lesions as a function of their localization and level of progression [5]. Typical positive lesions are represented by amyloid plaques and neurofibrillary tangles, neuropil threads, and dystrophic neurites, essentially formed by hyperphosphorylated Tau [6]. The negative lesions provide loss of neurons and neuropil threads [7].

Clinically, PD typically manifests with motor symptoms, such as bradykinesia, rigidity, tremor at rest, and instability. Since there is no definitive test for the diagnosis of PD, the appearance of these clinical manifestations is important for the early treatment of the disease [8]. PD is characterized by the loss of dopaminergic neurons in the *Substantia nigra pars compacta* (**Figure 1**) and by the deposition of

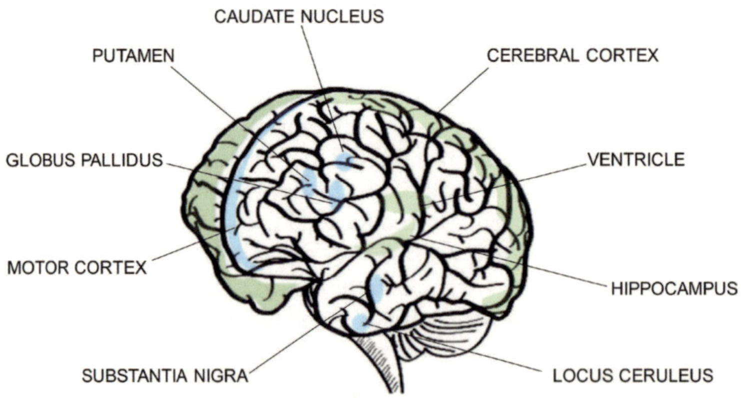

Figure 1.
Affected brain regions in AD and PD. Cross-section of human brain showing the principal districts affected by AD (green) and PD (blue). AD typically involves parts of the brain involved in memory, like hippocampus and ventricles, and the cerebral cortex responsible for language. In PD nerve cells of the motor cortex and in part of the basal ganglia (composed by substantia nigra, putamen, caudate nucleus, globus pallidus, and locus coeruleus) degenerate. As a result, the basal ganglia cannot control muscle movement as it normally does, leading to tremor, bradykinesia, and hypokinesia.

intraneuronal proteinaceous aggregates, mainly composed by α -synuclein (Syn), named Lewy bodies and Lewy neurites [9]. Syn was also found in the pathological inclusions of Lewy body variant of both AD and multiple system atrophy. Furthermore, Syn inclusions characterize other neurodegenerative diseases, defined as α-synucleinopathies, including Down's syndrome, progressive autonomic failure, and familial and sporadic AD [10]. In a very recent study, Shahmoradian and coll. have reported that Lewy bodies are not only formed by Syn deposit but also by clusters of lipid vesicles [11]. These important findings further correlate Syn-lipid interaction with neurodegeneration [12, 13].

AD and PD are generally sporadic and occur in individuals between ages 60 and 70, but the ~20% of patients have a genetically linked familial form. The onset of these forms occurs earlier, and it is associated with mutations in several genes [14]. The main mutations are listed in **Table 1**. The proteins involved in such neurodegenerative diseases, Aβ, tau, and Syn, are completely distinct in terms of structure and putative functions, most of which are not completely clarified. However, the formation of aggregated structures is a common feature among these macromolecules. Fibrils, which originate from the association of monomeric forms of the proteins, pass through intermediate species such as oligomers (**Figure 2**). Generally, they can cross the membrane and spread throughout the brain. Several evidences

Disease	Mutated protein	Phenotype	Notes	Refs
AD	APP	Abnormal production of Aβ	www.molgen.ua.ac.be/ADMutations	[15]
	ApoE	Increase of the density of Ab plaques High risk of AD, late onset of AD and Down syndrome	www.molgen.ua.ac.be/ADMutations	[16]
	Presenilin1	Increased the Aβ42/Aβ40, and reduced γ-secretase activity	>200 mutations	[17, 18]
	Presenilin2	Increased the Aβ42/Aβ40, and reduced γ-secretase activity	Rare, <40 mutations	[19]
PD	Syn	Familiar and early onset PD	A53T; A30P, E46K, G51D, H50Q, gene duplication and triplication	[20–25]
	Leucine-rich repeat kinase 2 (LRRK2)	Autosomal dominant PD; mid-to-late onset and slow progress	>20 mutations	[26, 27]
	E3 ubiquitin ligase Parkin	Early-onset PD and parkinsonism	>150 mutations, deletions, insertions	[28]
	PINK1	Sporadic early-onset Parkinsonism	>60 mutations	[29]
	DJ-1	Autosomal recessive PD	>10 mutation, deletions	[30]

Table 1.
Main mutations involved in familiar forms of AD and PD.

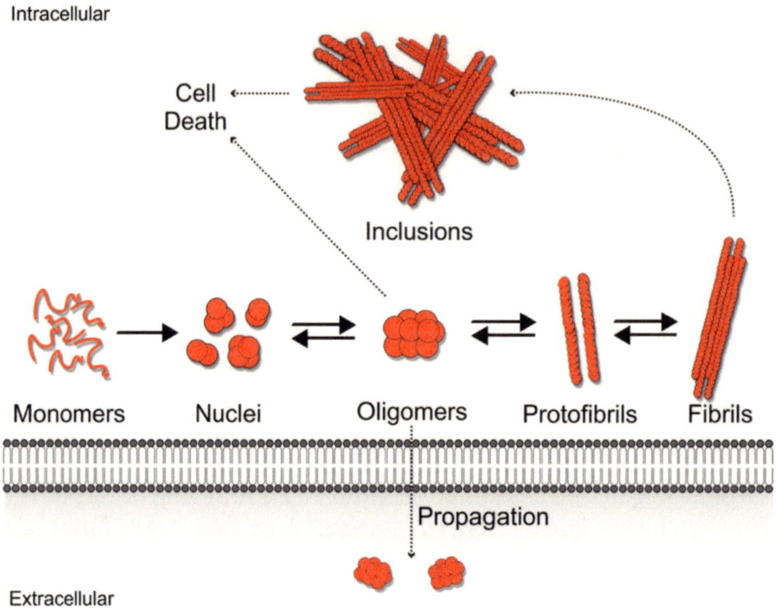

Figure 2.
Scheme of the aggregation process of amyloid proteins. The formation of fibrils occurs through a nucleation-dependent pathway starting from the monomeric form of the protein and leading to fibril elongation through intermediates (oligomers and protofibrils). The formation of the nucleus is the rate limiting step, and at this stage, the protein has acquired an aggregation-prone conformation. Fibrils are composed of a β-sheet structure in which hydrogen bonding occurs along the length of the fibril, and the β-strands run perpendicular to the fibril axis.

suggest that oligomers are the species responsible for the cytotoxicity. There are many proofs in support of this hypothesis, but unfortunately, due to the extreme heterogeneity in oligomer structures and their transient nature, a conclusive view has not been obtained yet [31–33]. The atomic structure of fibrils has been studied by several biophysical techniques. A quite accepted hypothesis agrees with the presence of a common molecular organization independent from the original structure of the involved protein: repetitive β-sheet units parallel to the fibril axis with their strands perpendicular to it [34, 35]. Amyloid fibrils can self-assemble *in vitro* from many structurally different proteins and peptides, not necessarily involved in diseases. It has been postulated that the cross-β structure represents a generic conformation, which represents another folding state for proteins [36, 37]. In addition to these characteristics, there are also some common aspects in the onset of the diseases. Several studies suggest possible interplays and synergistic activities between the involved proteins. Clinton et al. [38] provided evidence that Aβ, tau, and Syn could interact *in vivo* to promote their self-aggregation, thus accelerating the cognitive dysfunction [38]. High levels of Syn were found in patients suffering from AD [39]. Aβ stimulates Syn fibril formation in the transgenic mouse model through a seed mechanism [40]. In another study, Syn seems to inhibit the deposition of Aβ into the amyloid plaques [41].

2.2 Key proteins in neurodegeneration

2.2.1 Aβ peptide

The Aβ peptide was found in the amyloid plaques in 1984 [3]. Aβ represents a group of peptides constituted by 37–49 residues (**Figure 3A**), derived from the proteolytic processing of the amyloid precursor protein (APP) [42, 43] (**Figure 4**).

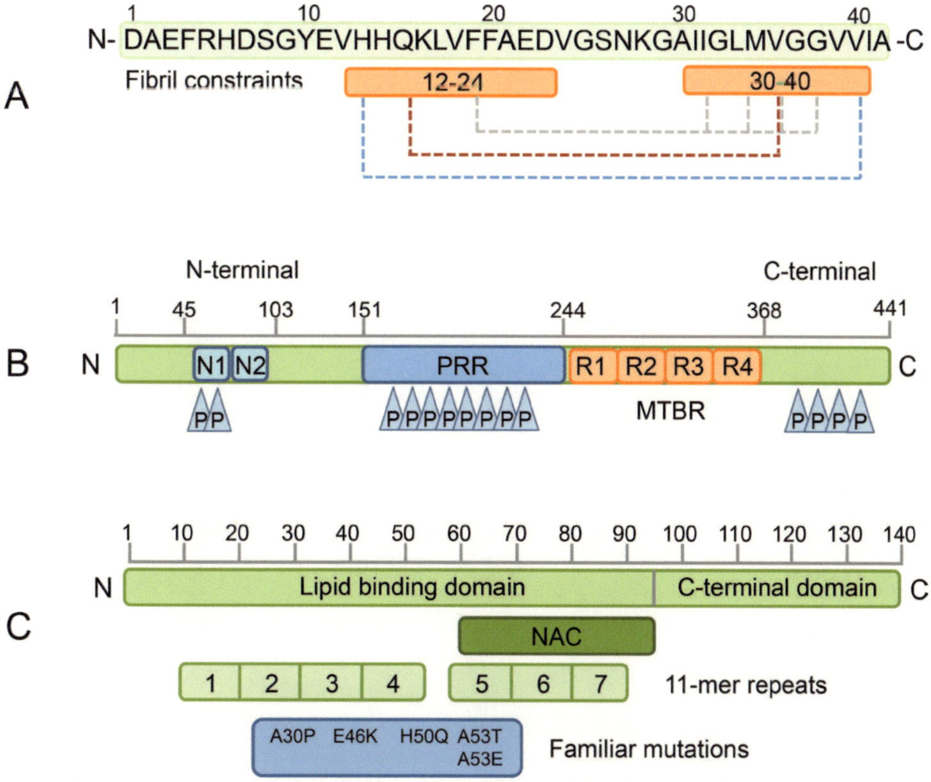

Figure 3.
Sequence and structural domain organization for Aβ (A), tau (B), and Syn (C). For Aβ, the residues 12–24 and 30–40 involved in the formation of a cross-β fibril structure are highlighted and connected by dashed lines. In (B), the longest isoform (441 residues) of tau is shown, where N indicates the possible N-terminal insertion defining other isoform, PRR, the proline-rich region, target of phosphorylation (P), and MTBR, the microtubule binding region that can contain three or four repeats (R), and other phosphorylations (P) occur at the C-terminal. In the case of Syn (C), the N- and C-terminals and NAC domains are shown, as well as the position of the mutations responsible for familiar form of PD. Residues 1–95 form the lipid-binding region.

APP is a single membrane-spanning domain protein, containing a large extracellular glycosylated N-terminus and a shorter cytoplasmic C-terminus. The enzymatic processes responsible for the release of Aβ from APP are to date well elucidated [2]. Specifically, APP undergoes several proteolytic cleavages. The processing by α-secretase results in the release of the large fragment sAPPα in the lumen, and the C-terminal fragment (CTF83) remains in the membrane. Two membrane endoproteases β- and γ-secretase sequentially hydrolyze APP. Firstly, APP releases sAPPβ by the action of β-secretase in the extracellular space. A fragment of 99 amino acids, CTFβ, remains bound to the membrane. CTFβ is successively and rapidly processed by γ-secretase generating Aβ. A precise cleavage site was not defined; therefore, Aβ is characterized by heterogeneity at the C-terminal and the peptide can end at position 40 (Aβ40) with a high frequency of occurrence (~80–90%) or at position 42 (Aβ42, ~5–10%). It is well established that Aβ42 generally generates fibrils more quickly than Aβ40 [44]. The production of Aβ is a normal metabolic event; in fact, these species are found in the cerebrospinal fluid and the plasma in healthy subjects [45]. Their abnormal accumulation, deriving from an imbalance between the production and clearance of these peptides, is associated with the pathogenesis of AD. Monomer, oligomer, and fibril forms of Aβ are differently involved in the onset of AD. The most common hypothesis is the Aβ-amyloid cascade [46]. The overproduction or the reduced clearance of Aβ leads to the deposition of fibrillar Aβ in the

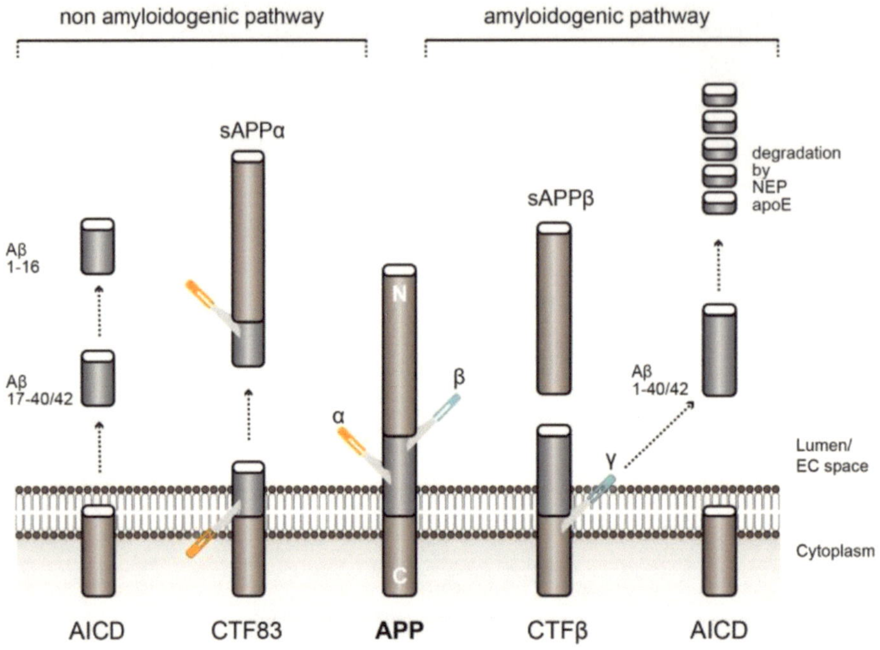

Figure 4.
Scheme of metabolism of APP and accumulation of the Aβ peptide. Aβ1–40/42 peptides are released from APP by the action of two membrane endoprotease β- and γ-secretases. Firstly, APP releases sAPPβ by the action of β-secretase in the extracellular space, and a fragment of 99 amino acids, CTFβ, remains bound to the membrane. CTFβ is successively and rapidly processed by γ-secretase generating Aβ peptides. Under physiological conditions, Aβ1–40/42 are degraded by enzymatic clearance processes. The proteolytic pathway mediated by α-secretase is also shown.

brain, determining synaptic and neuronal toxicity and thus neurodegeneration. There are many evidences in support of the so-called Aβ-amyloid oligomer hypothesis [31]. The proteolytic degradation of Aβ is a major route of clearance. Neprilysin (NEP) is considered one of the most important endopeptidase for the control of cerebral Aβ levels [47, 48] and for the degradation of some vasoactive peptides including natriuretic peptides and neuropeptides. Aβ clearance is mediated by other proteolytic enzymes such as apolipoprotein E (apoE) [49] and by autophagy [50]. Reduced activity of the clearance enzymes, which could be caused by aging, can contribute to AD development by promoting Aβ accumulation.

The secondary and tertiary structure of Aβ in solution has been studied by several biophysical techniques. These conformational studies are difficult for the protein high tendency to aggregate in solution. However, Aβ seems to populate distinct states in solution and to adopt a collapsed-coil structure, as deduced by NMR studies [51, 52]. Aβ preferentially binds to negatively charged lipids and acquires α-helical structure in the presence of membranes, membrane-like systems, and fluorinated alcohols [53, 54]. In the presence of phospholipids, Aβ undergoes conformational transition and forms β-sheets [55, 56]. Oligomeric Aβ binds to membranes with high affinity. Upon interaction, a membrane damage can occur as causative of the cellular toxicity [57]. It seems that especially oligomeric Aβ can disrupt the membrane bilayer by a detergent mechanism [58].

2.2.2 Tau

Tau is a neuronal protein associated with the microtubules [59]. Six Tau isoforms, which differ only in their primary structure, were detected in the human brain and central nervous system (**Figure 3B**), while in the peripheral nervous system other Tau isoforms were also found [60]. The longest isoform contains 441 residues and the shortest 352 residues [61]. Depending on the isoform, the N-terminal can contain 0, 1, or 2 inserts (N). The protein appears largely post-translational modified, especially in terms of phosphorylation (P). Other modifications are acetylation, deamidation, methylation, glycosylation, or ubiquitination [59]. Tau proteins are also subjected to proteolytic degradation that seems to be correlated with AD [62]. The region PRR (proline-rich region) contains the main sites of phosphorylation. Although all the post-translational modifications seem to contribute to the physiological and pathological properties of Tau, the signaling cascades and the effect on protein kinases and phosphatases are not completely clarified yet. The region 244–369 (microtubule binding region, MTBR) is responsible for the binding to the microtubule and contains three or four repeats (R1-R4). Physiologically, Tau stabilizes the microtubule through MTBR, and such binding is modulated by the coordinated actions of kinases and phosphatases. Structurally, Tau belongs to the intrinsically disordered proteins, lacking a well-defined secondary and tertiary structure [59] and can interact with several other proteins. Upon aggregation, Tau can form dimers, oligomers, and larger polymers. In such aggregates, cysteine residues may play an important role [63]. Similarly, to other proteins involved in neurodegeneration, the oligomeric forms have a cytotoxic effect and might be involved in the Tau-related pathogeneses [64]. In neurofibrillary tangles, Tau forms the so-called paired helical filaments (PHFs) and straight filaments (SFs) [65, 66]. In PHF, Tau is ~three to four-fold more hyperphosphorylated than in the normal brain. The Tau filaments exhibit the typical cross-β structure found in other types of fibrils [67].

2.2.3 α-Synuclein (Syn)

Syn is a small protein (14.4 kDa) mainly expressed in pre-synaptic nerve terminals of the central nervous system and very abundant in erythrocytes and platelets [68]. Despite the intensive investigation and the discovery that the protein plays a central role in synaptic transmission and vesicle recycling [69], the complete Syn biological function remains still elusive. Syn may control the neurotransmitter release, promoting the formation and assembly of the SNARE complex [70, 71]. Syn structure could be divided into three main domains: N-, central, and C-terminals (**Figure 3C**). The N-terminal region (amino acids 1–60) contains seven imperfect repeats, with a hexameric consensus motif (KTKGEV). All the known missense mutations of Syn, responsible for the familiar forms of PD, are located in this region (**Table 1**). The central hydrophobic domain (amino acids 61–95) is known as the non-amyloid-β component of AD amyloid plaques (NAC). It is responsible for Syn amyloid aggregation [72]. N-terminal and NAC domains together (amino acids 1–95) mediate the interaction of Syn with lipids, membranes, and fatty acids [73]. The C-terminal domain (amino acids 96–140) is an acidic, negatively charged, highly soluble, and disordered tail, target of post-translational modifications. This region plays a series of important roles, modulates Syn binding to membrane and metals, Syn aggregation and its protein-protein interaction properties. The deletion of this domain increases the aggregation rate of Syn *in vitro* and in cells [74].

Syn is the prototype of the natively unfolded proteins, but adopts a stable secondary structure as a function of the environment [75]. Multiple studies have demonstrated that Syn is more compact than expected for a random coil due to long-range interactions between the C-terminal tail and the NAC domain as well as electrostatic interactions between the N terminus and the C terminus [76]. Syn is supposed to populate different conformers in solution and can undergo conformational transition as a function of the environment and/or upon binding. The extreme Syn conformational flexibility is responsible for its multifunctional properties, its capability to adopt different conformations, and to interact with different systems and other proteins [77]. For example, the interaction of Syn with negatively charged membranes, vesicles, bilayers, and lipids in general has important physiological consequences [78, 79], corroborating the hypothesis that Syn functions are correlated with lipids [80].

3. Overview of recent therapeutic approaches in Alzheimer's and Parkinson's diseases

3.1 Traditional ongoing therapies

Current pharmacological therapies (**Table 2**) for neurodegenerative diseases focus to ameliorate the life conditions of patients and are generally only palliative. Since in many cases, the aberrant deposition of the protein strongly contributes to the toxicity associated with the diseases, some treatments are currently thought to target such specific proteins (i.e., Syn and Aβ) in order to restore their correct physiological levels *in vivo.* Given the complexity in the onset and progression of these diseases, treatments should be customized and tailored to the individual needs of the patients.

In the case of AD, a therapy based on the use of cholinesterase inhibitors (ChEIs) and the N-methyl-d-aspartate (NMDA) antagonist is currently available and Food and Drug Administration (FDA)-approved. In particular, three ChEIs are used: donepezil, rivastigmine, and galantamine [81]. The aim is to increase the levels of acetylcholine, a neurotransmitter responsible for memory and cognitive function, by reducing its enzymatic breakdown. Another class is represented by NMDA receptor antagonists, such as memantine, a noncompetitive antagonist, capable to block the effects of the excitatory neurotransmitter glutamate [82]. There are

DISEASE	CLASS	DRUG	MECHANISM of ACTION
AD	cholinesterase inhibitors	donepezil	selective reversible non-competitive inhibitor
		rivastigmine	pseudo irreversible inhibitor
		galantamine	reversible inhibitor
	NMDA antagonist	memantine dimebolin	non-competitive antagonists
	antidepressants	escitalopram	selective serotonin reuptake inhibitor
		mirtazapine	antihistamine, α2-antagonist
	anticonvulsants	carbamazepine	Na^+Ca^{2+}channels inhibitor, adenosine receptor antagonist
		levetiracetam	Ca^{2+}channel inhibitor, binder of synaptic vesicle glycoprotein SV2A
	mood stabilizer	lithium	Na^+K^+ATPasi inhibitor, neurotransmitter modulator
	stimulant	methylphenidate	norepinephrine and dopamine reuptake inhibitor
PD	dopaminergic drugs	levodopa	dopamine precursor
	dopamine agonists	ropinirole	non-ergoline agonist
		rotigotine	
	monoamino oxidase B inhibitors	rasagiline	irreversible inhibitor
		selegiline	
	catechol-O methyl-transferase inhibitors	entacapone	reversible inhibitor

Table 2.
Current available drugs for the treatment of AD and PD.

a series of molecules under study referred to as "disease-modifying" drugs. They should interfere with key steps in AD development, including the deposition of Aβ plaques and neurofibrillary tangle formation, inflammation, oxidative damage, iron deregulation, and cholesterol metabolism. Many drugs are proposed for their ability to alleviate behavioral symptoms of AD. A few examples include antidepressants, such as escitalopram and mirtazapine, anticonvulsants, that is, carbamazepine and levetiracetam, mood stabilizers, and stimulants, such as methylphenidate [83]. The treatments for PD are still based on dopaminergic drugs, such as levodopa, the precursor of dopamine [84]. Long-term use of levodopa determines the development of motor problems. In association with levodopa, a decarboxylase inhibitor is administered to prevent some side effects. PD therapy involves the use of dopamine agonists, such as ropinirole or rotigotine, monoamino oxidase B inhibitors, such as rasagiline and selegiline, and catechol-O-methyltransferase (COMT) inhibitors, which can reduce the metabolism of endogenous dopamine.

3.2 New generation therapies

Novel experimental approaches are under investigation and the most promising have as a target the protein involved in the diseases. The stages of intervention could be at the level of the protein synthesis or clearance and at the level of protein aggregation or propagation of the toxic species or their precursors (**Figure 5**).

1. *Control of the protein concentration in vivo*. To reduce the production of Aβ, Tau, and Syn, the RNA interference approach is to date quite attractive [85–87]. It is based on the idea to inhibit specific protein expression by activating a sequence-specific RNA degradation process. This technology results useful to study gene function, investigate the mechanism of the disease, and validate drug targets. Of course, the suppression of the target protein might have

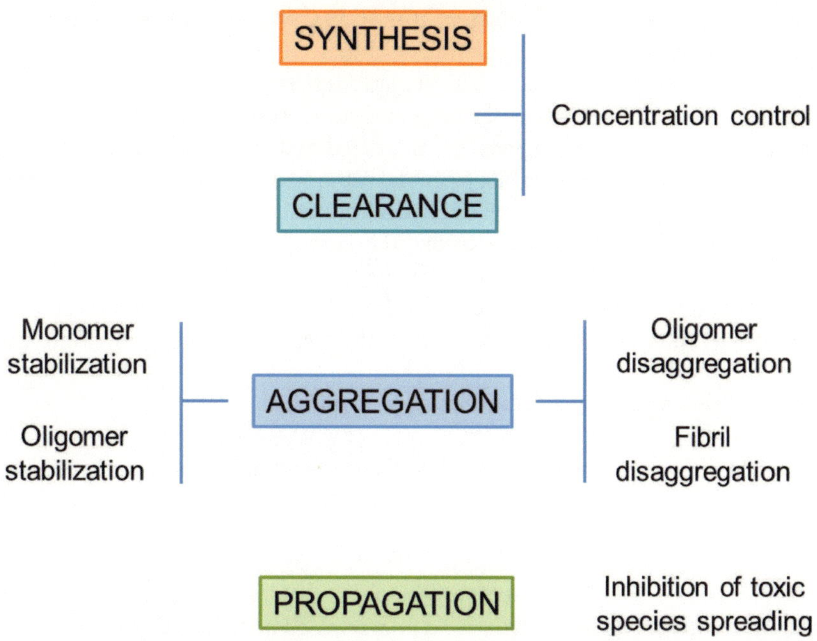

Figure 5.
New generation therapies in AD and PD. Potential levels of intervention to counteract the abnormal accumulation of the amyloidogenic proteins and restore their physiological concentration, which results from a balance between the rates of synthesis, clearance, aggregation, and propagation.

negative implications, due to the alteration of its physiological equilibrium. Additionally, the transcription of the gene can be reduced. Clenbuterol was shown to be efficient in reducing Syn expression by 35% in neuroblastoma cell lines [88]. Some AD therapies based on the modulation of AD gene expression are proposed on the basis of the important progresses made in the understanding of the transcriptional regulation of some enzymes such as beta-secretase 1 (BACE1), apolipoprotein E (apoE), APP amyloid precursor protein (APP), and presenilin (PSEN) promoters [89]. Alternatively, to reduce the level of the active protein *in vivo*, its clearance can be enhanced. This can be obtained by increasing the intracellular degradation *via* autophagy or *via* the ubiquitin system. This topic is excellently reviewed by Boland et al. [90].

2. *Protein aggregation inhibitors*. An attractive approach would be the use of small molecules able to bind the monomeric form of the protein preventing its assembly into potentially toxic aggregates. Unfortunately, it remains still unclear which conformation of these proteins must be targeted, since all of them are natively unfolded, and multiple and concurrent events contribute to their conversion in oligomers and fibrils [91]. In this ambit, the use of polyphenols is quite promising, and, as described below, these compounds exhibit in some cases the ability to disaggregate preformed oligomers and fibrils [92].

4. Effect of polyphenol compounds in neurodegeneration

4.1 Natural polyphenol products

Polyphenols are natural compounds, generally secondary metabolites, produced by plants and found mainly in fruits, vegetables, and cereals and in their derivatives. Some of them are synthetized during the normal development of the plant while others are produced in response to stress stimuli [93, 94]. They exert their function acting during the phase of development, reproduction, nutrition, growth, and communication with other plants, as well as in plant defense mechanisms like resistance to microbial pathogens, herbivore, insects, and protection to UV-light radiation [95]. More than 8.000 polyphenols have been identified in different plant species. They all derive from common precursors like phenylalanine and shikimic acid [96]. Often, they are linked with a sugar through the hydroxyl moiety, directly to the aromatic ring or conjugated with other compounds [97]. Polyphenols are characterized by a minimal hydroxyphenyl structure, and despite the multitude of existing polyphenols, they are grouped into different classes according to the number of phenol rings. The main groups are phenolic acids, flavonoids, stilbenes, and lignans [98] (**Figure 6**).

4.2 Potential therapeutic applications of polyphenols

Several epidemiological studies have been reported concerning the potentiality of polyphenols compounds in disease treatment and prevention [99, 100]. Polyphenols exert a positive role in cardiovascular disease [101–103], diabetes [104, 105], cancer [106, 107], aging, and neurodegeneration [108, 109]. One of the main activities of polyphenol resides is their antioxidant properties. Indeed, they are capable to protect cells and macromolecules from oxidative damage which in turn leads to degenerative age-associated diseases [110, 111]. Nevertheless, polyphenol function is also bound to its action on enzymes, immune defense, inflammation, cell signaling, and other pathways critical for the onset of the disease [112]. All these properties make the polyphenols potential drugs for preventing and treating neurodegenerative diseases, in particular

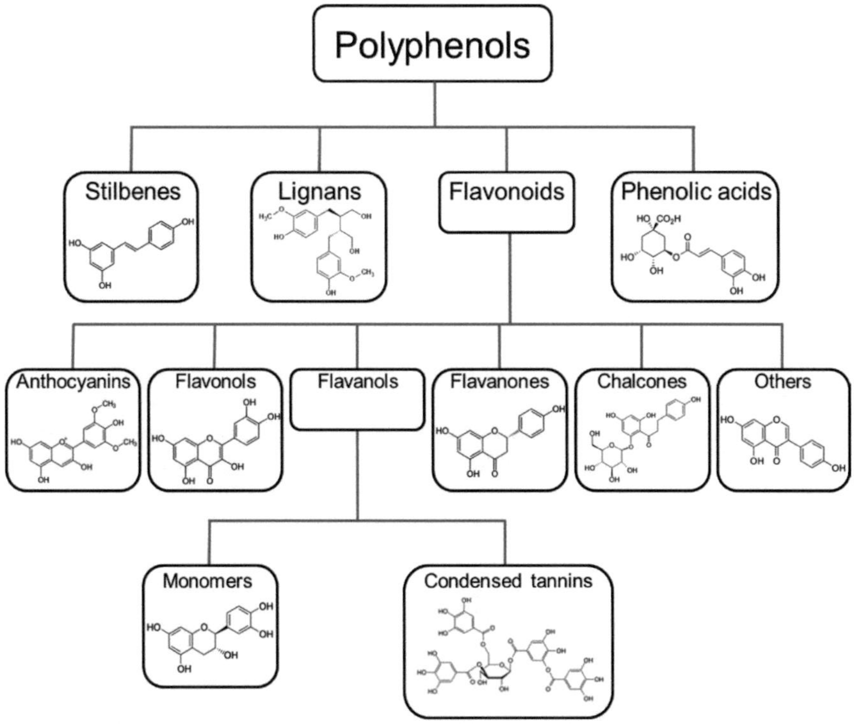

Figure 6.
Scheme of the main polyphenols and their chemical structures. Polyphenols are grouped into four principal classes: stilbenes, lignans, phenolic acids, and flavonoids. The last one is organized into six subclasses: anthocyanins, flavonols, flavanols, flavanones, chalcones, and others.

AD and PD. Actually, these compounds have shown to be effective in epidemiological, *in vitro*, and pre-clinical studies, but not in the early phase of the disease.

4.3 Polyphenols in Alzheimer's and Parkinson's disease

The effects of polyphenols on AD and PD can be divided into two main categories: the effects on nonamyloidogenic pathways (i.e., anti-oxidation pathway, interaction with cell signaling events, and interactions with enzymes) and the effects on amyloidogenic pathways. Below, the main beneficial effects shown by polyphenols on AD and PD are analyzed.

1. *Effects on memory*. One of the hallmarks of AD is the memory impairment. This can be due to deficiency of factors, such as the brain-derived neurotrophic factor (BDNF) and the accumulation of formaldehyde. Polyphenols have been shown to improve the long-term memory by increasing BDNF concentration *in vivo* and decreasing the accumulation of formaldehyde [113–115].

2. *Effects on inflammation pathway*. Inflammation plays an important role in the development of neurodegeneration. It is demonstrated that there is a correlation between the microglia activation and the neuroinflammatory response [116, 117]. Upon microglia activation, the transcription factor NF-kB (nuclear factor k-light-chain-enhancer of activated B cells) moves from cytoplasm to nucleus, inducing the expression of interleukins (i.e., IL-1β, IL-6, IL-12, and IL-23), other factors (i.e., TNF-α and iNOS), and cyclooxygenase 2 (COX-2). In this scenario, polyphenols can interact with certain types of kinases (including the mitogen-activated protein (MAP) kinase) preventing the activation of

proinflammatory mediators [118, 119]. Polyphenol compounds are able to protect cells from inflammation by acting on reactive oxygen species (ROS), decreasing the secretion of prostaglandin E2 [120–123] and increasing the amount of the regulatory enzyme sirtuin1 over sirtuin2, unbalanced after accumulation of Aβ [20]. Cell and PD-mouse model studies demonstrated that these compounds decrease the expression of NF-kB and other inflammatory factors [124–126].

3. *Effects on oxidative pathway, cell death and mitochondrial dysfunction*. In neurodegeneration, there is an uncontrolled production of free radicals and ROS that are not detoxified by the dedicated systems [127]. This leads to macromolecule damage and progressively to cell death [128]. Polyphenols lower the amount of ROS, increase the expression of enzymes, like glutathione, dedicated to scavenger the free radicals and prevent the disruption of mitochondrial membranes [129]. In addition, these compounds seem to prevent the lipid peroxidation [130]. These effects indirectly influence the fibrillation process of Syn, affected by some byproducts of lipid oxidation and peroxidation [131], as demonstrated in PD-animal model studies [132]. Moreover, polyphenols inhibit the cell death by acting on proteins involved in the apoptosis mechanism like Bcl/Bax, caspase 3, and protein kinases and by decreasing the accumulation of Aβ fibrils that exert cytotoxic effects [133, 134]. Another important scenario affected by polyphenols is the mitochondrial dysfunction (MD) that becomes increasingly important in the onset of PD [135]. Different factors play a pivotal role in MD: the presence of neurotoxin, Complex 1 deficiency (involved in mitochondrial electron transport), and penetration of mitochondrial membrane by amyloid aggregates [136, 137]. Polyphenol compounds exert their activity restoring membrane potential, increasing the expression and activity of the Complex 1 and scavenging the ROS, free radicals, and metals [138–141].

4. *Effects on acetylcholinesterase activity*. Nearly 30 years ago, dysfunction in the cholinergic system was found correlated with AD and cognitive impairment [142]. This dysfunction can be originated by a reduction in acetylcholine synthesis, reduced levels of choline acetyltransferase, reduced choline uptake, or cholinergic neurons degeneration [143]. The use of acetylcholinesterase inhibitors to restore the cholinergic pathway has proved to alleviate the cognitive dysfunction in neurodegenerative diseases [144]. Polyphenol compounds have shown to inhibit acetylcholinesterase, improving memory, learning, and cognitive functions [145].

5. *Effects on Aβ formation*. Polyphenol compounds act on the enzyme responsible for Aβ formation, decreasing the cleavage of APP into the peptide. They interact with and inhibit β-secretase [146]. In addition, they are able to restore the normal levels of γ-secretase, another enzyme involved in APP processing [147].

6. *Effects on the amyloidogenic pathways*. Polyphenols can act on Aβ monomer preventing its fibrillation, through the stabilization of the monomer and/or to the formation of an off-pathway oligomer. This can be due to the interaction of polyphenols with metal ions that promote the Aβ aggregation or to the non-covalent interaction with the peptide [148]. They are also able to disaggregate oligomers and fibrils, interacting with the β-sheet structure. This has been confirmed by *in vivo* studies where polyphenol intake reduces the amyloid deposit in the mouse brain [149, 150]. Polyphenols exert their anti-amyloidogenic action by interfering also with the aggregation of Tau [151–153], inhibiting Tau phosphorylation *in vitro* [154] and *in vivo* [155]. Several polyphenols have been tested for their anti-fibrillogenic properties *in vitro* and in PD-animal models.

Their main activity regards the interaction with Syn monomers leading to protein stabilization and fibrillation prevention [92]. Another factor concerns the formation of not toxic off-pathway oligomers that do not form fibrils nor interact with the membrane [156, 157]. Some polyphenols are also able to interact with oligomeric and fibrillar species, leading to their destabilization [65, 92]. The major effect of polyphenols is due to the noncovalent interaction with the Syn C-terminal domain. In addition, these compounds can chemically modify the lysine residues, present mainly in the N-terminal region, through Michael addition and Schiff-base formation [158]. This reduces the conformational plasticity of Syn and its tendency to be converted into fibrils. Moreover, structure-activity relationship studies indicate that the differences in polyphenols activities reside in the number and position of OH groups in the phenyl ring [159].

5. Polyphenols as a drug in the brain delivery system

5.1 Blood-brain barrier and neurodegeneration

The human brain comprises more than 600 km of blood vessels that guarantee oxygen, energy metabolites, and nutrients to brain cells and remove carbon dioxide and toxic metabolic products from the brain to the systemic circulation. A highly selective semipermeable border, called blood-brain barrier (BBB), separates the circulating blood from the central nervous system (CNS), regulating CNS homeostasis. Brain microvascular endothelia cells, neurons, astrocyte, pericytes, tight junctions, and basal membrane constitute tight brain capillaries in the BBB [160, 161]. It follows that BBB does not have fenestrations or other physical fissures for diffusion of small molecules. In fact, ions, solutes, and hormones can pass the BBB by passive diffusion through the paracellular pathway between adjacent cells. Hydrophilic biomolecules (i.e., proteins and peptides) can cross the BBB within specific and saturable receptor-mediated transport mechanisms [162]. The components of BBB constantly adapt in response to various physiological and pathological modifications into the brain [163, 164]. Loss of BBB integrity is correlated with vascular permeability increase, cerebral blood flow impairs, and hemodynamic response alteration [165]. In neurodegenerative disorders, endothelia degeneration leads to loss of tight junctions [166, 167], brain capillary leakages [168, 169], pericyte degeneration [170], endothelial cell remodeling [164], cellular infiltration [171, 172], and aberrant angiogenesis [173, 174]. All these BBB disruptions let different blood proteins (i.e., fibrinogen, plasminogen, and thrombin), water, and electrolytes to accumulate in different zones of CNS, enhancing the on progress of PD and AD [165]. Consequently, to project effective drugs for neurodegeneration, it is necessary to understand in detail BBB pathological aberrations.

Due to their safeness and tolerance [175–177], polyphenols are currently studied as neuroprotectors. It is important to point out that for exerting their action, polyphenols must accumulate in the brain in an active form and in sufficient concentration. The limiting step is choosing the right administration route. In most of the clinical studies, the oral administration is the preferred way, but recently the nasal delivery is taken into consideration for the easiness to bypass the BBB [178], the increased bioavailability, the decreased metabolism, and peripheral side effects [179, 180]. The major problem of oral administration relies on poor absorbance of the modified form of polyphenols (i.e., glycosides and ester polymers) in the upper portion of the gut leading to the passage in the colon in which polyphenols are converted by gut-microbiota in the aglycone form or other substances able to be better absorbed [181, 182]. Once absorbed, they can be further modified by enzymes and eliminated [183, 184] or adsorbed to plasmatic proteins (i.e., albumin) and then accumulated in different districts [185].

5.2 Nanotechnology-based delivery system: An innovative strategy

Nanotechnology is a new branch of science involving the formulation, synthesis, and characterization of small particles, with diameters ranging from 1 to 1000 nm [186], which become key players in innovative drug delivery and cell targeting. Recent studies suggest that nanoparticle-based delivery systems represent innovative and promising approaches to improve drug solubility, prevent acid-degradation, minimize toxic side effects, and increase blood availability [187, 188]. Considering the low bioavailability of polyphenols, different strategies have been developed in order to enhance their chemical stability, solubility, and cell-membrane permeability. These goals have been achieved by adding chemical agents to preserve the structure [189], enzyme inhibitors to contrast biotransformation [190], and lipids or proteins to increase the solubility [191]. Recently, nanoparticle-mediated delivery system is emerged as the most promising approach. Using biodegradable and biocompatible polymers, polyphenols can be encapsulated in different nanostructures and then possibly administrated *via* intravenous, transdermal, nasal, and oral route. As describe above, this aspect is fundamental in neurological diseases, in which polyphenols must cross the BBB, with the opportune grade of lipophilicity [162, 192, 193] and reach the brain tissue in sufficient quantities for therapeutic use. These new delivery systems are represented by nanospheres, nanocapsules, nanoemulsions, solid lipid nanoparticles, cyclodextrins, liposomes, and micelles (**Figure 7**).

Nanospheres (10–200 nm) [194] are homogeneous solid matrix particles characterized by a hydrophobic portion in the inner part and hydrophilic chains anchored on the surface. In nanospheres, the drug is dissolved, entrapped, encapsulated, or attached to the matrix of the polymer, so protected from chemical and enzymatic degradation. Various kinds of polymers are used to prepare nanospheres: polylactic acid (PLA), poly-glycolic acid (PGA), poly-lactic-co-glycolic acid (PLGA), polyethylene glycol (PEG), poly ε-caprolactone (PCL), and chitosan (CS) [195, 196].

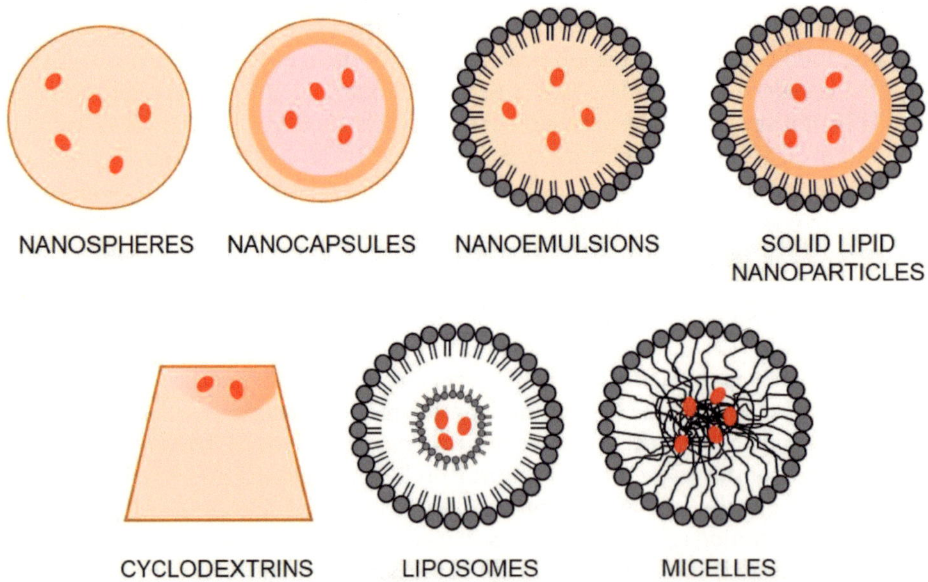

Figure 7.
Schematic representation of nanosized delivery systems for polyphenols. Nanoparticles can enhance polyphenol bioavailability, enhancing their adsorption across intestinal epithelium, increasing their concentration in the bloodstream, and improving their ability to cross the blood-brain barrier.

Nanocapsules (10–1000 nm) have a similar chemical composition but comprise an oily or aqueous core, which is surrounded by a thin polymer membrane [197, 198]. The cavity can contain the drug in liquid or solid form. Furthermore, the medication can be carried on nanovector surface or absorbed in the polymeric membrane [198–200].

Nanoemulsions are oil-in-water or water-in-oil emulsions stabilized by one or more surfactants (i.e., phosphatidylcholine, sodium deoxycholate, sorbitan monolaurate, poloxamers, sodium dodecyl sulfate, and poly(ethylene glycol)) delivered in droplets of small dimensions (100–300 nm) [191]. The strategy allows having a higher surface area and a long-term chemical and physical stability [201, 202]. Nanoemulsions represent an innovative formulation to deliver polyphenols directly into the brain through the intranasal route. In fact, mucoadesive polymers, such as CS, can be added to slow down nasal clearance [191].

Solid lipid nanoparticles (50–1000 nm) [194] are composed of high melting point lipid, organized in a solid core, coated by aqueous surfactants (i.e., sphingomyelins, bile salts, and sterols) [198]. Even though these nanoparticles present high biocompatibility, bioavailability and physical stability, the common undesirable disadvantages are particle growth, arbitrary gelation tendency, and unpredicted dynamic of polymorphic transitions [198].

Cyclodextrins (1–2 nm) [194] are a group of structurally related natural products formed from the bacterial digestion of cellulose. Cyclodextrins are cyclic oligosaccharides consisting of (α-1,4)-linked α-D-glucopyranose units with a lipophilic central cavity and a hydrophilic outer surface [203]. The hydroxyl functions are orientated to the exterior, while the central cavity is wrinkled by the skeletal carbons and ethereal oxygens of the glucose residues. Natural cyclodextrins are classified by the number of glucopyranose units in α-(six units), β-(seven units), and γ-(eight units) [204]. Recently, cyclodextrins containing from 9 to 13 glucopyranose units have been reported. These carriers are useful for increasing the solubility and the stability of poorly water-soluble drugs. Moreover, cyclodextrins can be derivatized with hydroxypropyl, methyl, and sulfobutyl-ether additives [203]. So, drugs can be allocated into the cavity *via* van der Waals forces, hydrophobic interactions, or hydrogen bonds [205].

Liposomes (30–2000 nm) [194] are phospholipid vesicles containing one or more concentric lipid bilayers enclosing an aqueous space. Liposomes can assemble spontaneously by hydration of lipid-derivate powder (i.e., cholesterol, glycolipids, sphingolipids, long chain fatty acids, and membrane proteins) in aqueous buffer [195]. Due to their ability to capture hydrophilic and lipophilic substances, in the aqueous space or into the lipid bilayer membrane, respectively, they can protect drugs from early inactivation, degradation, and loss [206].

Micelles (5–100 nm) are colloidal dispersions, consisting of amphiphilic copolymers (i.e., PEG, PLGA, and PCL) that assemble naturally in water at a specific concentration and temperature [207]. When polymer concentration is greater than the critical micelle concentration, micelles start to be assembled: hydrophobic fragments of amphiphilic reagents form the core, whereas hydrophilic portion form the shells [208]. Micelles are characterized by high stability, biocompatibility, and ability to keep in solution poorly soluble drugs.

5.3 Nanotechnology as an innovative delivery system of polyphenols

The use of biodegradable and biocompatible polymers allows rationalizing the design of innovative nanostructures able to encapsulate polyphenols that can cross the BBB, improving the limitations associated with conventional administrations. In this scenario, curcumin is the most studied drug candidate, due to the prominent results obtained in the animal model of neurodegenerative diseases [209–211].

In fact, the efficacy of curcumin is so far limited by the poor aqueous solubility, low adsorption in the gastrointestinal tract, and rapid metabolism. Nanosphere of PGLA containing curcumin can be the right strategy for crossing BBB. Recent studies indicated how curcumin-PGLA nanoparticles can interfere with Aβ aggregation and improve the brain self-repair mechanism, increasing the neural stem cell proliferation and neuronal differentiation [212]. In the same way, liposomes loaded with curcumin can efficiently inhibit the *in vitro* formation of Aβ fibrils and deposition in the brain [213]. Curcumin-solid lipid nanoparticles seem to be effective for MD and central oxidative stress [214]. In addition, curcumin and piperine co-loaded glycerol mono-oleate nanoparticles can interfere with Syn aggregation, reducing oxidative damage and apoptosis [215]. Curcumin was also taken in consideration for intranasal delivery to the central nervous system by nanoemulsions. In the presence of CS, nanoemulsions of curcumin (added in the oil phase) can effectively cross the mucosa without showing cytotoxicity [209].

Another good candidate is resveratrol. It is known for its ability to induce the degradation of APP and to remove Aβ [216]. But, due to its rapid and extensive metabolism, resveratrol is subjected to a *person-to-person* bioavailability. PEG-PCL and PGLA nanoparticles loaded with resveratrol let a controlled release profile of the drug, essential for prolonging its plasmatic level and the antioxidant activity [217, 218]. A promising approach is the oil-in-water nanoemulsion [219]. Adding Vitamin E and other surfactants, this formulation can reach the brain *via* the nasal route, with encouraging efficacy [220]. Furthermore, the co-encapsulation of curcumin and resveratrol (1:1 weight ratio) in mucoadhesive nanoemulsions protects the active substances from degradation and preserves their antioxidant properties. Notably, *in vivo* quantification in animal brain indicated an increase of the amount of the two polyphenols after 6 hours [221]. Unfortunately, these systems have not yet reached clinical trials, but the results accumulated so far encourage new original therapeutic approaches.

Acknowledgements

This project was supported by Progetti di Ateneo-University of Padova 2017-N. C93C1800002600 and by MIUR-PNRA (Programma Nazionale Ricerche in Antartide) (PNRA16_00068). We thank Samuele Cesaro and Ferdinando Polverino de Laureto for the elaboration of the images.

Author details

Patrizia Polverino de Laureto*, Luana Palazzi and Laura Acquasaliente
Protein Chemistry Unit, Department of Pharmaceutical and Pharmacological Sciences, University of Padova, Padova, Italy

*Address all correspondence to: patrizia.polverinodelaureto@unipd.it

References

[1] Katzman R. Alzheimer's disease. The New England Journal of Medicine. 1986;**314**(15):964-973

[2] Selkoe DJ. Alzheimer's disease: Genes, proteins, and therapy. Physiological Reviews. 2001;**81**(2):741-766

[3] Glenner GG, Wong CW. Alzheimer's disease: Initial report of the purification and characterization of a novel cerebrovascular amyloid protein. Biochemical and Biophysical Research Communications. 1984;**120**(3):885-890

[4] Lee VM, Goedert M, Trojanowski JQ. Neurodegenerative tauopathies. Annual Review of Neuroscience. 2001;**24**:1121-1159

[5] Serrano-Pozo A, Frosch MP, Masliah E, Hyman BT. Neuropathological alterations in Alzheimer disease. Cold Spring Harbor Perspectives in Medicine. 2011;**1**(1):a006189

[6] Trojanowski JQ, Lee VM. "Fatal attractions" of proteins. A comprehensive hypothetical mechanism underlying Alzheimer's disease and other neurodegenerative disorders. Annals of the New York Academy of Sciences. 2000;**924**:62-67

[7] Masliah E, Miller A, Terry RD. The synaptic organization of the neocortex in Alzheimer's disease. Medical Hypotheses. 1993;**41**(4):334-340

[8] Jankovic J. Parkinson's disease: Clinical features and diagnosis. Journal of Neurology, Neurosurgery, and Psychiatry. 2008;**79**(4):368-376

[9] Spillantini MG, Schmidt ML, Lee VM, Trojanowski JQ, Jakes R, Goedert M. Alpha-synuclein in Lewy bodies. Nature. 1997;**388**(6645):839-840

[10] Goedert M. Alpha-synuclein and neurodegenerative diseases. Nature Reviews. Neuroscience. 2001;**2**(7):492-501

[11] Shahmoradian SH, Lewis AJ, Genoud C, Hench J, Moors TE, Navarro PP, et al. Lewy pathology in Parkinson's disease consists of crowded organelles and lipid membranes. Nature Neuroscience. 2019;**22**(7):1099-1109

[12] Ruiperez V, Darios F, Davletov B. Alpha-synuclein, lipids and Parkinson's disease. Progress in Lipid Research. 2010;**49**(4):420-428

[13] Fecchio C, Palazzi L, Polverino de Laureto P. Alpha-synuclein and polyunsaturated fatty acids: Molecular basis of the interaction and implication in neurodegeneration. Molecules. 2018;**23**(7):1531-1551

[14] Bekris LM, Yu CE, Bird TD, Tsuang DW. Genetics of Alzheimer disease. Journal of Geriatric Psychiatry and Neurology. 2010;**23**(4):213-227

[15] Goate A, Chartier-Harlin MC, Mullan M, Brown J, Crawford F, Fidani L, et al. Segregation of a missense mutation in the amyloid precursor protein gene with familial Alzheimer's disease. Nature. 1991;**349**(6311):704-706

[16] Corder EH, Saunders AM, Strittmatter WJ, Schmechel DE, Gaskell PC, Small GW, et al. Gene dose of apolipoprotein E type 4 allele and the risk of Alzheimer's disease in late onset families. Science. 1993;**261**(5123):921-923

[17] Citron M, Westaway D, Xia W, Carlson G, Diehl T, Levesque G, et al. Mutant presenilins of Alzheimer's disease increase production of 42-residue amyloid beta-protein in both transfected cells and transgenic mice. Nature Medicine. 1997;**3**(1):67-72

[18] Kelleher RJ 3rd, Shen J. Presenilin-1 mutations and Alzheimer's disease. Proceedings of the National Academy of Sciences of the United States of America. 2017;**114**(4):629-631

[19] Scheuner D, Eckman C, Jensen M, Song X, Citron M, Suzuki N, et al. Secreted amyloid beta-protein similar to that in the senile plaques of Alzheimer's disease is increased in vivo by the presenilin 1 and 2 and APP mutations linked to familial Alzheimer's disease. Nature Medicine. 1996;**2**(8):864-870

[20] Porquet D, Casadesus G, Bayod S, Vicente A, Canudas AM, Vilaplana J, et al. Dietary resveratrol prevents Alzheimer's markers and increases life span in SAMP8. Age (Dordrecht, Netherlands). 2013;**35**(5):1851-1865

[21] Kruger R, Kuhn W, Muller T, Woitalla D, Graeber M, Kosel S, et al. Ala30Pro mutation in the gene encoding alpha-synuclein in Parkinson's disease. Nature Genetics. 1998;**18**(2):106-108

[22] Lesage S, Anheim M, Letournel F, Bousset L, Honore A, Rozas N, et al. G51D alpha-synuclein mutation causes a novel parkinsonian-pyramidal syndrome. Annals of Neurology. 2013;**73**(4):459-471

[23] Polymeropoulos MH, Higgins JJ, Golbe LI, Johnson WG, Ide SE, Di Iorio G, et al. Mapping of a gene for Parkinson's disease to chromosome 4q21-q23. Science. 1996;**274**(5290):1197-1199

[24] Singleton AB, Farrer M, Johnson J, Singleton A, Hague S, Kachergus J, et al. Alpha-Synuclein locus triplication causes Parkinson's disease. Science. 2003;**302**(5646):841

[25] Zarranz JJ, Alegre J, Gomez-Esteban JC, Lezcano E, Ros R, Ampuero I, et al. The new mutation, E46K, of alpha-synuclein causes Parkinson and Lewy body dementia. Annals of Neurology. 2004;**55**(2):164-173

[26] Nuytemans K, Theuns J, Cruts M, Van Broeckhoven C. Genetic etiology of Parkinson disease associated with mutations in the SNCA, PARK2, PINK1, PARK7, and LRRK2 genes: A mutation update. Human Mutation. 2010;**31**(7):763-780

[27] Kumari U, Tan EK. LRRK2 in Parkinson's disease: Genetic and clinical studies from patients. The FEBS Journal. 2009;**276**(22):6455-6463

[28] Dawson TM, Dawson VL. The role of parkin in familial and sporadic Parkinson's disease. Movement Disorders. 2010;**25**(Suppl 1):S32-S39

[29] Valente EM, Abou-Sleiman PM, Caputo V, Muqit MM, Harvey K, Gispert S, et al. Hereditary early-onset Parkinson's disease caused by mutations in PINK1. Science. 2004;**304**(5674): 1158-1160

[30] Cookson MR. Parkinsonism due to mutations in PINK1, parkin, and DJ-1 and oxidative stress and mitochondrial pathways. Cold Spring Harbor Perspectives in Medicine. 2012;**2**(9):a009415

[31] Cline EN, Bicca MA, Viola KL, Klein WL. The amyloid-beta oligomer hypothesis: Beginning of the third decade. Journal of Alzheimer's Disease. 2018;**64**(s1):S567-s610

[32] Serpell LC. Alzheimer's amyloid fibrils: Structure and assembly. Biochimica et Biophysica Acta. 2000;**1502**(1):16-30

[33] Petkova AT, Ishii Y, Balbach JJ, Antzutkin ON, Leapman RD, Delaglio F, et al. A structural model for Alzheimer's beta -amyloid fibrils based on experimental constraints from solid state NMR. Proceedings of the National Academy of Sciences

of the United States of America. 2002;**99**(26):16742-16747

[34] Nelson R, Sawaya MR, Balbirnie M, Madsen AO, Riekel C, Grothe R, et al. Structure of the cross-beta spine of amyloid-like fibrils. Nature. 2005;**435**(7043):773-778

[35] Makin OS, Atkins E, Sikorski P, Johansson J, Serpell LC. Molecular basis for amyloid fibril formation and stability. Proceedings of the National Academy of Sciences of the United States of America. 2005;**102**(2):315-320

[36] Fitzpatrick AW, Debelouchina GT, Bayro MJ, Clare DK, Caporini MA, Bajaj VS, et al. Atomic structure and hierarchical assembly of a cross-beta amyloid fibril. Proceedings of the National Academy of Sciences of the United States of America. 2013;**110**(14):5468-5473

[37] Dobson CM. The structural basis of protein folding and its links with human disease. Philosophical Transactions of the Royal Society of London. Series B, Biological Sciences. 2001;**356**(1406):133-145

[38] Clinton LK, Blurton-Jones M, Myczek K, Trojanowski JQ, LaFerla FM. Synergistic interactions between Abeta, tau, and alpha-synuclein: Acceleration of neuropathology and cognitive decline. The Journal of Neuroscience. 2010;**30**(21):7281-7289

[39] Larson ME, Sherman MA, Greimel S, Kuskowski M, Schneider JA, Bennett DA, et al. Soluble alpha-synuclein is a novel modulator of Alzheimer's disease pathophysiology. The Journal of Neuroscience. 2012;**32**(30):10253-10266

[40] Masliah E, Rockenstein E, Veinbergs I, Sagara Y, Mallory M, Hashimoto M, et al. Beta-amyloid peptides enhance alpha-synuclein accumulation and neuronal deficits in a transgenic mouse model linking Alzheimer's disease and Parkinson's disease. Proceedings of the National Academy of Sciences of the United States of America. 2001;**98**(21):12245-12250

[41] Bachhuber T, Katzmarski N, McCarter JF, Loreth D, Tahirovic S, Kamp F, et al. Inhibition of amyloid-beta plaque formation by alpha-synuclein. Nature Medicine. 2015;**21**(7):802-807

[42] Haass C, Selkoe DJ. Cellular processing of beta-amyloid precursor protein and the genesis of amyloid beta-peptide. Cell. 1993;**75**(6):1039-1042

[43] Nunan J, Small DH. Regulation of APP cleavage by alpha-, beta- and gamma-secretases. FEBS Letters. 2000;**483**(1):6-10

[44] Kim W, Hecht MH. Sequence determinants of enhanced amyloidogenicity of Alzheimer a{beta}42 peptide relative to a{beta}40. The Journal of Biological Chemistry. 2005;**280**(41):35069-35076

[45] Shoji M, Golde TE, Ghiso J, Cheung TT, Estus S, Shaffer LM, et al. Production of the Alzheimer amyloid beta protein by normal proteolytic processing. Science. 1992;**258**(5079):126-129

[46] Selkoe DJ. Amyloid beta protein precursor and the pathogenesis of Alzheimer's disease. Cell. 1989;**58**(4):611-612

[47] Iwata N, Tsubuki S, Takaki Y, Shirotani K, Lu B, Gerard NP, et al. Metabolic regulation of brain Abeta by neprilysin. Science. 2001;**292**(5521):1550-1552

[48] Turner RT 3rd, Koelsch G, Hong L, Castanheira P, Ermolieff J, Ghosh AK, et al. Subsite specificity of memapsin

2 (beta-secretase): Implications for inhibitor design. Biochemistry. 2001;**40**(34):10001-10006

[49] Kim J, Basak JM, Holtzman DM. The role of apolipoprotein E in Alzheimer's disease. Neuron. 2009;**63**(3):287-303

[50] Bendiske J, Bahr BA. Lysosomal activation is a compensatory response against protein accumulation and associated synaptopathogenesis--an approach for slowing Alzheimer disease? Journal of Neuropathology and Experimental Neurology. 2003;**62**(5):451-463

[51] Zhang S, Iwata K, Lachenmann MJ, Peng JW, Li S, Stimson ER, et al. The Alzheimer's peptide a beta adopts a collapsed coil structure in water. Journal of Structural Biology. 2000;**130**(2-3):130-141

[52] Sgourakis NG, Yan Y, McCallum SA, Wang C, Garcia AE. The Alzheimer's peptides Abeta40 and 42 adopt distinct conformations in water: A combined MD/NMR study. Journal of Molecular Biology. 2007;**368**(5):1448-1457

[53] D'Ursi AM, Armenante MR, Guerrini R, Salvadori S, Sorrentino G, Picone D. Solution structure of amyloid beta-peptide (25-35) in different media. Journal of Medicinal Chemistry. 2004;**47**(17):4231-4238

[54] Crescenzi O, Tomaselli S, Guerrini R, Salvadori S, D'Ursi AM, Temussi PA, et al. Solution structure of the Alzheimer amyloid beta-peptide (1-42) in an apolar microenvironment. Similarity with a virus fusion domain. European Journal of Biochemistry. 2002;**269**(22):5642-5648

[55] McLaurin J, Chakrabartty A. Characterization of the interactions of Alzheimer beta-amyloid peptides with phospholipid membranes. European Journal of Biochemistry. 1997;**245**(2):355-363

[56] Williams TL, Serpell LC. Membrane and surface interactions of Alzheimer's Abeta peptide–insights into the mechanism of cytotoxicity. The FEBS Journal. 2011;**278**(20):3905-3917

[57] Butterfield SM, Lashuel HA. Amyloidogenic protein-membrane interactions: Mechanistic insight from model systems. Angewandte Chemie (International Ed. in English). 2010;**49**(33):5628-5654

[58] Bode DC, Freeley M, Nield J, Palma M, Viles JH. Amyloid-beta oligomers have a profound detergent-like effect on lipid membrane bilayers, imaged by atomic force and electron microscopy. The Journal of Biological Chemistry. 2019;**294**(19):7566-7572

[59] Avila J, Jimenez JS, Sayas CL, Bolos M, Zabala JC, Rivas G, et al. Tau Structures. Frontiers in Aging Neuroscience. 2016;**8**:262

[60] Goedert M, Spillantini MG, Cairns NJ, Crowther RA. Tau proteins of Alzheimer paired helical filaments: Abnormal phosphorylation of all six brain isoforms. Neuron. 1992;**8**(1):159-168

[61] Goedert M, Spillantini MG, Jakes R, Rutherford D, Crowther RA. Multiple isoforms of human microtubule-associated protein tau: Sequences and localization in neurofibrillary tangles of Alzheimer's disease. Neuron. 1989;**3**(4):519-526

[62] Zhang Z, Song M, Liu X, Kang SS, Kwon IS, Duong DM, et al. Cleavage of tau by asparagine endopeptidase mediates the neurofibrillary pathology in Alzheimer's disease. Nature Medicine. 2014;**20**(11):1254-1262

[63] Soeda Y, Yoshikawa M, Almeida OF, Sumioka A, Maeda S, Osada H, et al. Toxic tau oligomer formation blocked by capping of cysteine residues with

1,2-dihydroxybenzene groups. Nature Communications. 2015;**6**:10216

[64] Gerson JE, Sengupta U, Lasagna-Reeves CA, Guerrero-Munoz MJ, Troncoso J, Kayed R. Characterization of tau oligomeric seeds in progressive supranuclear palsy. Acta Neuropathologica Communications. 2014;**2**:73

[65] Ahsan N, Mishra S, Jain MK, Surolia A, Gupta S. Curcumin Pyrazole and its derivative N-(3-Nitrophenylpyrazole) Curcumin inhibit aggregation, disrupt fibrils and modulate toxicity of wild type and mutant alpha-Synuclein. Scientific Reports. 2015;**5**:9862

[66] Grundke-Iqbal I, Iqbal K, Quinlan M, Tung YC, Zaidi MS, Wisniewski HM. Microtubule-associated protein tau. A component of Alzheimer paired helical filaments. The Journal of Biological Chemistry. 1986;**261**(13):6084-6089

[67] Fitzpatrick AWP, Falcon B, He S, Murzin AG, Murshudov G, Garringer HJ, et al. Cryo-EM structures of tau filaments from Alzheimer's disease. Nature. 2017;**547**(7662):185-190

[68] Barbour R, Kling K, Anderson JP, Banducci K, Cole T, Diep L, et al. Red blood cells are the major source of alpha-synuclein in blood. Neurodegenerative Diseases. 2008;**5**(2):55-59

[69] Pineda A, Burre J. Modulating membrane binding of alpha-synuclein as a therapeutic strategy. Proceedings of the National Academy of Sciences of the United States of America. 2017;**114**(6):1223-1225

[70] Chandra S, Gallardo G, Fernandez-Chacon R, Schluter OM, Sudhof TC. Alpha-synuclein cooperates with CSPalpha in preventing neurodegeneration. Cell. 2005;**123**(3):383-396

[71] Burre J, Sharma M, Tsetsenis T, Buchman V, Etherton MR, Sudhof TC. Alpha-synuclein promotes SNARE-complex assembly in vivo and in vitro. Science. 2010;**329**(5999):1663-1667

[72] Ueda K, Fukushima H, Masliah E, Xia Y, Iwai A, Yoshimoto M, et al. Molecular cloning of cDNA encoding an unrecognized component of amyloid in Alzheimer disease. Proceedings of the National Academy of Sciences of the United States of America. 1993;**90**(23):11282-11286

[73] Eliezer D, Kutluay E, Bussell R Jr, Browne G. Conformational properties of alpha-synuclein in its free and lipid-associated states. Journal of Molecular Biology. 2001;**307**(4):1061-1073

[74] Hoyer W, Cherny D, Subramaniam V, Jovin TM. Impact of the acidic C-terminal region comprising amino acids 109-140 on alpha-synuclein aggregation in vitro. Biochemistry. 2004;**43**(51):16233-16242

[75] Uversky VN, Eliezer D. Biophysics of Parkinson's disease: Structure and aggregation of alpha-synuclein. Current Protein & Peptide Science. 2009;**10**(5):483-499

[76] Dedmon MM, Lindorff-Larsen K, Christodoulou J, Vendruscolo M, Dobson CM. Mapping long-range interactions in alpha-synuclein using spin-label NMR and ensemble molecular dynamics simulations. Journal of the American Chemical Society. 2005;**127**(2):476-477

[77] Davidson WS, Jonas A, Clayton DF, George JM. Stabilization of alpha-synuclein secondary structure upon binding to synthetic membranes. The Journal of Biological Chemistry. 1998;**273**(16):9443-9449

[78] Madine J, Doig AJ, Middleton DA. A study of the regional effects of

alpha-synuclein on the organization and stability of phospholipid bilayers. Biochemistry. 2006;**45**(18): 5783-5792

[79] Kamp F, Beyer K. Binding of alpha-synuclein affects the lipid packing in bilayers of small vesicles. The Journal of Biological Chemistry. 2006;**281**(14):9251-9259

[80] Galvagnion C. The role of lipids interacting with alpha-synuclein in the pathogenesis of Parkinson's disease. Journal of Parkinson's Disease. 2017;**7**(3):433-450

[81] Hansen RA, Gartlehner G, Webb AP, Morgan LC, Moore CG, Jonas DE. Efficacy and safety of donepezil, galantamine, and rivastigmine for the treatment of Alzheimer's disease: A systematic review and meta-analysis. Clinical Interventions in Aging. 2008;**3**(2):211-225

[82] van Marum RJ. Update on the use of memantine in Alzheimer's disease. Neuropsychiatric Disease and Treatment. 2009;**5**:237-247

[83] Baazaoui N, Iqbal K. A novel therapeutic approach to treat Alzheimer's disease by neurotrophic support during the period of synaptic compensation. Journal of Alzheimer's Disease. 2018;**62**(3):1211-1218

[84] Jankovic J, Aguilar LG. Current approaches to the treatment of Parkinson's disease. Neuropsychiatric Disease and Treatment. 2008;**4**(4):743-757

[85] Chen S, Ge X, Chen Y, Lv N, Liu Z, Yuan W. Advances with RNA interference in Alzheimer's disease research. Drug Design, Development and Therapy. 2013;**7**:117-125

[86] Sapru MK, Yates JW, Hogan S, Jiang L, Halter J, Bohn MC. Silencing of human alpha-synuclein in vitro and in rat brain using lentiviral-mediated RNAi. Experimental Neurology. 2006;**198**(2):382-390

[87] Lewis PA. Emerging pathways in genetic Parkinson's disease. The FEBS Journal. 2008;**275**(23):5747

[88] Mittal S, Bjornevik K, Im DS, Flierl A, Dong X, Locascio JJ, et al. beta2-Adrenoreceptor is a regulator of the alpha-synuclein gene driving risk of Parkinson's disease. Science. 2017;**357**(6354):891-898

[89] Chen XF, Zhang YW, Xu H, Bu G. Transcriptional regulation and its misregulation in Alzheimer's disease. Molecular Brain. 2013;**6**:44

[90] Boland B, Yu WH, Corti O, Mollereau B, Henriques A, Bezard E, et al. Promoting the clearance of neurotoxic proteins in neurodegenerative disorders of ageing. Nature Reviews. Drug Discovery. 2018;**17**(9):660-688

[91] Brundin P, Dave KD, Kordower JH. Therapeutic approaches to target alpha-synuclein pathology. Experimental Neurology. 2017;**298**(Pt B):225-235

[92] Palazzi L, Bruzzone E, Bisello G, Leri M, Stefani M, Bucciantini M, et al. Oleuropein aglycone stabilizes the monomeric alpha-synuclein and favours the growth of non-toxic aggregates. Scientific Reports. 2018;**8**(1):8337-8354

[93] Harborne JB. Introduction to Ecological Biochemistry. 2nd ed. New York: Academic Press; 1982

[94] Nicholson R, Hammerschmidt R. Phenolic compounds and their role in disease resistance. Annual Review of Phytopathology. 1992;**30**:369-389

[95] Lattanzio V, Cardinali A, Ruta C, Morone Fortunato I, Lattanzio VM, Linsalata V, et al. Relationship of secondary metabolism to growth in oregano (*Origanum vulgare* L.) shoot

cultures under nutritional stress. Environmental and Experimental Botany. 2009;**65**(1):54-62

[96] Andersen ØM, Markham KR. Flavonoids, chemistry, biochemistry and applications. Journal of Natural Products. 2007;**70**:1-1256

[97] Kondratyuk TP, Pezzuto JM. Natural product polyphenols of relevance to human health. Pharmaceutical Biology. 2004;**42**:46-63

[98] Spencer JP, Abd El Mohsen MM, Minihane AM, Mathers JC. Biomarkers of the intake of dietary polyphenols: Strengths, limitations and application in nutrition research. The British Journal of Nutrition. 2008;**99**(1):12-22

[99] Arts IC, Hollman PC. Polyphenols and disease risk in epidemiologic studies. The American Journal of Clinical Nutrition. 2005;**81**(1 Suppl):317s-325s

[100] Scalbert A, Manach C, Morand C, Remesy C, Jimenez L. Dietary polyphenols and the prevention of diseases. Critical Reviews in Food Science and Nutrition. 2005;**45**(4):287-306

[101] Nardini M, Natella F, Scaccini C. Role of dietary polyphenols in platelet aggregation. A review of the supplementation studies. Platelets. 2007;**18**(3):224-243

[102] Renaud S, de Lorgeril M. Wine, alcohol, platelets, and the French paradox for coronary heart disease. Lancet. 1992;**339**(8808):1523-1526

[103] Dubick MA, Omaye ST. Evidence for grape, wine and tea polyphenols as modulators of atherosclerosis and ischemic heart disease in humans. Journal of Nutraceuticals, Functional & Medical Foods. 2001;**3**:67-93

[104] Rizvi SI, Zaid MA. Insulin-like effect of (−)epicatechin on erythrocyte membrane acetylcholinesterase activity in type 2 diabetes mellitus. Clinical and Experimental Pharmacology & Physiology. 2001;**28**(9):776-778

[105] Rizvi SI, Zaid MA, Anis R, Mishra N. Protective role of tea catechins against oxidation-induced damage of type 2 diabetic erythrocytes. Clinical and Experimental Pharmacology & Physiology. 2005;**32**(1-2):70-75

[106] Yang CS, Landau JM, Huang MT, Newmark HL. Inhibition of carcinogenesis by dietary polyphenolic compounds. Annual Review of Nutrition. 2001;**21**:381-406

[107] Johnson IT, Williamson G, Musk SR. Anticarcinogenic factors in plant foods: A new class of nutrients? Nutrition Research Reviews. 1994;7(1):175-204

[108] Cao G, Booth SL, Sadowski JA, Prior RL. Increases in human plasma antioxidant capacity after consumption of controlled diets high in fruit and vegetables. The American Journal of Clinical Nutrition. 1998;**68**(5):1081-1087

[109] Letenneur L, Proust-Lima C, Le Gouge A, Dartigues JF, Barberger-Gateau P. Flavonoid intake and cognitive decline over a 10-year period. American Journal of Epidemiology. 2007;**165**(12): 1364-1371

[110] Luqman S, Rizvi SI. Protection of lipid peroxidation and carbonyl formation in proteins by capsaicin in human erythrocytes subjected to oxidative stress. Phytotherapy Research. 2006;**20**(4):303-306

[111] Pandey KB, Rizvi SI. Plant polyphenols as dietary antioxidants in human health and disease. Oxidative Medicine and Cellular Longevity. 2009;**2**(5):270-278

[112] Garcia-Lafuente A, Guillamon E, Villares A, Rostagno MA, Martinez JA. Flavonoids as anti-inflammatory agents: Implications in cancer and cardiovascular disease. Inflammation Research. 2009;**58**(9):537-552

[113] Zhao YN, Li WF, Li F, Zhang Z, Dai YD, Xu AL, et al. Resveratrol improves learning and memory in normally aged mice through microRNA-CREB pathway. Biochemical and Biophysical Research Communications. 2013;**435**(4):597-602

[114] Mei Y, Jiang C, Wan Y, Lv J, Jia J, Wang X, et al. Aging-associated formaldehyde-induced norepinephrine deficiency contributes to age-related memory decline. Aging Cell. 2015;**14**(4):659-668

[115] Moorthi P, Premkumar P, Priyanka R, Jayachandran KS, Anusuyadevi M. Pathological changes in hippocampal neuronal circuits underlie age-associated neurodegeneration and memory loss: Positive clue toward SAD. Neuroscience. 2015;**301**:90-105

[116] Imamura K, Hishikawa N, Sawada M, Nagatsu T, Yoshida M, Hashizume Y. Distribution of major histocompatibility complex class II-positive microglia and cytokine profile of Parkinson's disease brains. Acta Neuropathologica. 2003;**106**(6):518-526

[117] Beach TG, Sue LI, Walker DG, Lue LF, Connor DJ, Caviness JN, et al. Marked microglial reaction in normal aging human substantia nigra: Correlation with extraneuronal neuromelanin pigment deposits. Acta Neuropathologica. 2007;**114**(4):419-424

[118] Chen X, Yang X, Liu T, Guan M, Feng X, Dong W, et al. Kaempferol regulates MAPKs and NF-kappaB signaling pathways to attenuate LPS-induced acute lung injury in mice. International Immunopharmacology. 2012;**14**(2):209-216

[119] Choi JS, Islam MN, Ali MY, Kim EJ, Kim YM, Jung HA. Effects of C-glycosylation on anti-diabetic, anti-Alzheimer's disease and anti-inflammatory potential of apigenin. Food and Chemical Toxicology. 2014;**64**:27-33

[120] Yao Y, Li J, Niu Y, Yu JQ, Yan L, Miao ZH, et al. Resveratrol inhibits oligomeric Abeta-induced microglial activation via NADPH oxidase. Molecular Medicine Reports. 2015;**12**(4):6133-6139

[121] Wight RD, Tull CA, Deel MW, Stroope BL, Eubanks AG, Chavis JA, et al. Resveratrol effects on astrocyte function: Relevance to neurodegenerative diseases. Biochemical and Biophysical Research Communications. 2012;**426**(1):112-115

[122] Kim YA, Lim SY, Rhee SH, Park KY, Kim CH, Choi BT, et al. Resveratrol inhibits inducible nitric oxide synthase and cyclooxygenase-2 expression in beta-amyloid-treated C6 glioma cells. International Journal of Molecular Medicine. 2006;**17**(6):1069-1075

[123] Cheng X, Wang Q, Li N, Zhao H. Effects of resveratrol on hippocampal astrocytes and expression of TNF-alpha in Alzheimer's disease model rate. Wei Sheng Yan Jiu. 2015;**44**(4):610-614

[124] Raza SS, Khan MM, Ahmad A, Ashafaq M, Islam F, Wagner AP, et al. Neuroprotective effect of naringenin is mediated through suppression of NF-kappaB signaling pathway in experimental stroke. Neuroscience. 2013;**230**:157-171

[125] Jia Z, Babu PV, Si H, Nallasamy P, Zhu H, Zhen W, et al. Genistein inhibits TNF-alpha-induced endothelial inflammation through the protein kinase pathway a and improves vascular

inflammation in C57BL/6 mice. International Journal of Cardiology. 2013;**168**(3):2637-2645

[126] Qureshi AA, Guan XQ, Reis JC, Papasian CJ, Jabre S, Morrison DC, et al. Inhibition of nitric oxide and inflammatory cytokines in LPS-stimulated murine macrophages by resveratrol, a potent proteasome inhibitor. Lipids in Health and Disease. 2012;**11**:76

[127] Kumar H, Lim HW, More SV, Kim BW, Koppula S, Kim IS, et al. The role of free radicals in the aging brain and Parkinson's disease: Convergence and parallelism. International Journal of Molecular Sciences. 2012;**13**(8):10478-10504

[128] Floyd RA, Carney JM. Free radical damage to protein and DNA: Mechanisms involved and relevant observations on brain undergoing oxidative stress. Annals of Neurology. 1992;**32**(Suppl):S22-S27

[129] Kwon KJ, Kim HJ, Shin CY, Han SH. Melatonin potentiates the neuroprotective properties of resveratrol against beta-amyloid-induced neurodegeneration by modulating AMP-activated protein kinase pathways. Journal of Clinical Neurology. 2010;**6**(3):127-137

[130] Schinella G, Mosca S, Cienfuegos-Jovellanos E, Ángeles Pasamar M, Muguerza B, Ramón D, et al. Antioxidant properties of polyphenol-rich cocoa products industrially processed. Food Research International. 2010;**43**(6):1614-1623

[131] Xiang W, Schlachetzki JC, Helling S, Bussmann JC, Berlinghof M, Schaffer TE, et al. Oxidative stress-induced posttranslational modifications of alpha-synuclein: Specific modification of alpha-synuclein by 4-hydroxy-2-nonenal increases dopaminergic toxicity. Molecular and Cellular Neurosciences. 2013;**54**:71-83

[132] Frei B, Higdon JV. Antioxidant activity of tea polyphenols in vivo: Evidence from animal studies. The Journal of Nutrition. 2003;**133**(10):3275s-3284s

[133] Bastianetto S, Krantic S, Chabot JG, Quirion R. Possible involvement of programmed cell death pathways in the neuroprotective action of polyphenols. Current Alzheimer Research. 2011;**8**(5):445-451

[134] Zhang K, Ma Z, Wang J, Xie A, Xie J. Myricetin attenuated MPP(+)-induced cytotoxicity by anti-oxidation and inhibition of MKK4 and JNK activation in MES23.5 cells. Neuropharmacology. 2011;**61**(1-2):329-335

[135] van Loo G, Saelens X, van Gurp M, MacFarlane M, Martin SJ, Vandenabeele P. The role of mitochondrial factors in apoptosis: A Russian roulette with more than one bullet. Cell Death and Differentiation. 2002;**9**(10):1031-1042

[136] Lev N, Melamed E, Offen D. Apoptosis and Parkinson's disease. Progress in Neuro-Psychopharmacology & Biological Psychiatry. 2003;**27**(2):245-250

[137] Camilleri A, Zarb C, Caruana M, Ostermeier U, Ghio S, Hogen T, et al. Mitochondrial membrane permeabilisation by amyloid aggregates and protection by polyphenols. Biochimica et Biophysica Acta. 2013;**1828**(11):2532-2543

[138] Kumar A, Prakash A, Dogra S. Naringin alleviates cognitive impairment, mitochondrial dysfunction and oxidative stress induced by D-galactose in mice. Food and Chemical Toxicology. 2010;**48**(2):626-632

[139] Gao QG, Xie JX, Wong MS, Chen WF. IGF-I receptor signaling pathway is involved in the neuroprotective effect of genistein in the neuroblastoma SK-N-SH cells. European Journal of Pharmacology. 2012;**677**(1-3):39-46

[140] Jeon SM, Bok SH, Jang MK, Lee MK, Nam KT, Park YB, et al. Antioxidative activity of naringin and lovastatin in high cholesterol-fed rabbits. Life Sciences. 2001;**69**(24):2855-2866

[141] Renault TT, Teijido O, Antonsson B, Dejean LM, Manon S. Regulation of Bax mitochondrial localization by Bcl-2 and Bcl-x(L): Keep your friends close but your enemies closer. The International Journal of Biochemistry & Cell Biology. 2013;**45**(1):64-67

[142] Perry EK, Tomlinson BE, Blessed G, Bergmann K, Gibson PH, Perry RH. Correlation of cholinergic abnormalities with senile plaques and mental test scores in senile dementia. British Medical Journal. 1978;**2**(6150):1457-1459

[143] Fisher A. Cholinergic treatments with emphasis on m1 muscarinic agonists as potential disease-modifying agents for Alzheimer's disease. Neurotherapeutics. 2008;**5**(3):433-442

[144] Lahiri DK, Rogers JT, Greig NH, Sambamurti K. Rationale for the development of cholinesterase inhibitors as anti-Alzheimer agents. Current Pharmaceutical Design. 2004;**10**(25):3111-3119

[145] Zhang L, Cao H, Wen J, Xu M. Green tea polyphenol (−)-epigallocatechin-3-gallate enhances the inhibitory effect of huperzine a on acetylcholinesterase by increasing the affinity with serum albumin. Nutritional Neuroscience. 2009;**12**(4):142-148

[146] Zaky A, Mohammad B, Moftah M, Kandeel KM, Bassiouny AR. Apurinic/apyrimidinic endonuclease 1 is a key modulator of aluminum-induced neuroinflammation. BMC Neuroscience. 2013;**14**:26

[147] Ohta K, Mizuno A, Ueda M, Li S, Suzuki Y, Hida Y, et al. Autophagy impairment stimulates PS1 expression and gamma-secretase activity. Autophagy. 2010;**6**(3):345-352

[148] Toni M, Massimino ML, De Mario A, Angiulli E, Spisni E. Metal dyshomeostasis and their pathological role in prion and prion-like diseases: The basis for a nutritional approach. Frontiers in Neuroscience. 2017;**11**:3

[149] Yang F, Lim GP, Begum AN, Ubeda OJ, Simmons MR, Ambegaokar SS, et al. Curcumin inhibits formation of amyloid beta oligomers and fibrils, binds plaques, and reduces amyloid in vivo. The Journal of Biological Chemistry. 2005;**280**(7):5892-5901

[150] Garcia-Alloza M, Borrelli LA, Rozkalne A, Hyman BT, Bacskai BJ. Curcumin labels amyloid pathology in vivo, disrupts existing plaques, and partially restores distorted neurites in an Alzheimer mouse model. Journal of Neurochemistry. 2007;**102**(4):1095-1104

[151] Cornejo A, Aguilar Sandoval F, Caballero L, Machuca L, Munoz P, Caballero J, et al. Rosmarinic acid prevents fibrillization and diminishes vibrational modes associated to beta sheet in tau protein linked to Alzheimer's disease. Journal of Enzyme Inhibition and Medicinal Chemistry. 2017;**32**(1):945-953

[152] Duff K, Kuret J, Congdon EE. Disaggregation of tau as a therapeutic approach to tauopathies. Current Alzheimer Research. 2010;**7**(3):235-240

[153] Wang J, Santa-Maria I, Ho L, Ksiezak-Reding H, Ono K, Teplow DB, et al. Grape derived polyphenols attenuate tau neuropathology in a mouse

model of Alzheimer's disease. Journal of Alzheimer's Disease. 2010;**22**(2):653-661

[154] Gueroux M, Fleau C, Slozeck M, Laguerre M, Pianet I. Epigallocatechin 3-Gallate as an inhibitor of tau phosphorylation and aggregation: A molecular and structural insight. The Journal of Prevention of Alzheimer's Disease. 2017;**4**(4):218-225

[155] Rezai-Zadeh K, Shytle D, Sun N, Mori T, Hou H, Jeanniton D, et al. Green tea epigallocatechin-3-gallate (EGCG) modulates amyloid precursor protein cleavage and reduces cerebral amyloidosis in Alzheimer transgenic mice. The Journal of Neuroscience. 2005;**25**(38):8807-8814

[156] Ehrnhoefer DE, Bieschke J, Boeddrich A, Herbst M, Masino L, Lurz R, et al. EGCG redirects amyloidogenic polypeptides into unstructured, off-pathway oligomers. Nature Structural & Molecular Biology. 2008;**15**(6):558-566

[157] Yang JE, Rhoo KY, Lee S, Lee JT, Park JH, Bhak G, et al. EGCG-mediated protection of the membrane disruption and cytotoxicity caused by the 'Active Oligomer' of alpha-synuclein. Scientific Reports. 2017;7(1):17945

[158] Palhano FL, Lee J, Grimster NP, Kelly JW. Toward the molecular mechanism(s) by which EGCG treatment remodels mature amyloid fibrils. Journal of the American Chemical Society. 2013;**135**(20):7503-7510

[159] Ardah MT, Paleologou KE, Lv G, Abul Khair SB, Kazim AS, Minhas ST, et al. Structure activity relationship of phenolic acid inhibitors of alpha-synuclein fibril formation and toxicity. Frontiers in Aging Neuroscience. 2014;**6**:197

[160] Pehlivan SB. Nanotechnology-based drug delivery systems for targeting, imaging and diagnosis of neurodegenerative diseases. Pharmaceutical Research. 2013;**30**(10):2499-2511

[161] Guerra M, Blazquez JL, Rodriguez EM. Blood-brain barrier and foetal-onset hydrocephalus, with a view on potential novel treatments beyond managing CSF flow. Fluids Barriers CNS. 2017;**14**(1):19

[162] Ballabh P, Braun A, Nedergaard M. The blood-brain barrier: An overview: Structure, regulation, and clinical implications. Neurobiology of Disease. 2004;**16**(1):1-13

[163] Banks WA. From blood-brain barrier to blood-brain interface: New opportunities for CNS drug delivery. Nature Reviews. Drug Discovery. 2016;**15**(4):275-292

[164] Komarova YA, Kruse K, Mehta D, Malik AB. Protein interactions at endothelial junctions and signaling mechanisms regulating endothelial permeability. Circulation Research. 2017;**120**(1):179-206

[165] Sweeney MD, Sagare AP, Zlokovic BV. Blood-brain barrier breakdown in Alzheimer disease and other neurodegenerative disorders. Nature Reviews. Neurology. 2018;**14**(3):133-150

[166] Zlokovic BV. Neurovascular pathways to neurodegeneration in Alzheimer's disease and other disorders. Nature Reviews. Neuroscience. 2011;**12**(12):723-738

[167] Zhao Z, Nelson AR, Betsholtz C, Zlokovic BV. Establishment and dysfunction of the blood-brain barrier. Cell. 2015;**163**(5):1064-1078

[168] Hultman K, Strickland S, Norris EH. The APOE varepsilon4/varepsilon4 genotype potentiates vascular fibrin(ogen) deposition in amyloid-laden vessels in the brains of

Alzheimer's disease patients. Journal of Cerebral Blood Flow and Metabolism. 2013;**33**(8):1251-1258

[169] Pienaar IS, Lee CH, Elson JL, McGuinness L, Gentleman SM, Kalaria RN, et al. Deep-brain stimulation associates with improved microvascular integrity in the subthalamic nucleus in Parkinson's disease. Neurobiology of Disease. 2015;**74**:392-405

[170] Sweeney MD, Ayyadurai S, Zlokovic BV. Pericytes of the neurovascular unit: Key functions and signaling pathways. Nature Neuroscience. 2016;**19**(6):771-783

[171] Cullen KM, Kocsi Z, Stone J. Pericapillary haem-rich deposits: Evidence for microhaemorrhages in aging human cerebral cortex. Journal of Cerebral Blood Flow and Metabolism. 2005;**25**(12):1656-1667

[172] Gray MT, Woulfe JM. Striatal blood-brain barrier permeability in Parkinson's disease. Journal of Cerebral Blood Flow and Metabolism. 2015;**35**(5):747-750

[173] Wada K, Arai H, Takanashi M, Fukae J, Oizumi H, Yasuda T, et al. Expression levels of vascular endothelial growth factor and its receptors in Parkinson's disease. Neuroreport. 2006;**17**(7):705-709

[174] Desai Bradaric B, Patel A, Schneider JA, Carvey PM, Hendey B. Evidence for angiogenesis in Parkinson's disease, incidental Lewy body disease, and progressive supranuclear palsy. Journal of Neural Transmission (Vienna). 2012;**119**(1):59-71

[175] Boocock DJ, Faust GE, Patel KR, Schinas AM, Brown VA, Ducharme MP, et al. Phase I dose escalation pharmacokinetic study in healthy volunteers of resveratrol, a potential cancer chemopreventive agent. Cancer Epidemiology, Biomarkers & Prevention. 2007;**16**(6):1246-1252

[176] Almeida L, Vaz-da-Silva M, Falcao A, Soares E, Costa R, Loureiro AI, et al. Pharmacokinetic and safety profile of trans-resveratrol in a rising multiple-dose study in healthy volunteers. Molecular Nutrition & Food Research. 2009;**53**(Suppl 1):S7-S15

[177] Ringman JM, Frautschy SA, Teng E, Begum AN, Bardens J, Beigi M, et al. Oral curcumin for Alzheimer's disease: Tolerability and efficacy in a 24-week randomized, double blind, placebo-controlled study. Alzheimer's Research & Therapy. 2012;**4**(5):43

[178] Crowe TP, Greenlee MHW, Kanthasamy AG, Hsu WH. Mechanism of intranasal drug delivery directly to the brain. Life Sciences. 2018;**195**:44-52

[179] Hanson LR, Frey WH 2nd. Intranasal delivery bypasses the blood-brain barrier to target therapeutic agents to the central nervous system and treat neurodegenerative disease. BMC Neuroscience. 2008;**9**(Suppl. 3):S5

[180] Chapman CD, Frey WH 2nd, Craft S, Danielyan L, Hallschmid M, Schioth HB, et al. Intranasal treatment of central nervous system dysfunction in humans. Pharmaceutical Research. 2013;**30**(10):2475-2484

[181] Aura AM, O'Leary KA, Williamson G, Ojala M, Bailey M, Puupponen-Pimia R, et al. Quercetin derivatives are deconjugated and converted to hydroxyphenylacetic acids but not methylated by human fecal flora in vitro. Journal of Agricultural and Food Chemistry. 2002;**50**(6):1725-1730

[182] Shortt C, Hasselwander O, Meynier A, Nauta A, Fernandez EN, Putz P, et al. Systematic review of the effects of the intestinal microbiota on selected nutrients and non-nutrients.

European Journal of Nutrition. 2018;**57**(1):25-49

[183] El-Mohsen MA, Bayele H, Kuhnle G, Gibson G, Debnam E, Srai SK, et al. Distribution of [3H] trans-resveratrol in rat tissues following oral administration. The British Journal of Nutrition. 2006;**96**(1):62-70

[184] Wenzel E, Somoza V. Metabolism and bioavailability of trans-resveratrol. Molecular Nutrition & Food Research. 2005;**49**(5):472-481

[185] Delmas D, Aires V, Limagne E, Dutartre P, Mazue F, Ghiringhelli F, et al. Transport, stability, and biological activity of resveratrol. Annals of the New York Academy of Sciences. 2011;**1215**:48-59

[186] Hu B, Liu X, Zhang C, Zeng X. Food macromolecule based nanodelivery systems for enhancing the bioavailability of polyphenols. Journal of Food and Drug Analysis. 2017;**25**(1):3-15

[187] Aqil F, Munagala R, Jeyabalan J, Vadhanam MV. Bioavailability of phytochemicals and its enhancement by drug delivery systems. Cancer Letters. 2013;**334**(1):133-141

[188] Irimie AI, Sonea L, Jurj A, Mehterov N, Zimta AA, Budisan L, et al. Future trends and emerging issues for nanodelivery systems in oral and oropharyngeal cancer. International Journal of Nanomedicine. 2017;**12**:4593-4606

[189] Ader P, Wessmann A, Wolffram S. Bioavailability and metabolism of the flavonol quercetin in the pig. Free Radical Biology & Medicine. 2000;**28**(7):1056-1067

[190] Brand W, Padilla B, van Bladeren PJ, Williamson G, Rietjens IM. The effect of co-administered flavonoids on the metabolism of hesperetin and the disposition of its metabolites in Caco-2 cell monolayers. Molecular Nutrition & Food Research. 2010;**54**(6):851-860

[191] Bonferoni MC, Rossi S, Sandri G, Ferrari F, Gavini E, Rassu G, et al. Nanoemulsions for "nose-to-brain" drug delivery. Pharmaceutics. 2019;**11**(2):1-17

[192] Squillaro T, Schettino C, Sampaolo S, Galderisi U, Di Iorio G, Giordano A, et al. Adult-onset brain tumors and neurodegeneration: Are polyphenols protective? Journal of Cellular Physiology. 2018;**233**(5):3955-3967

[193] Figueira I, Garcia G, Pimpao RC, Terrasso AP, Costa I, Almeida AF, et al. Polyphenols journey through blood-brain barrier towards neuronal protection. Scientific Reports. 2017;7(1):11456

[194] Squillaro T, Cimini A, Peluso G, Giordano A, Melone MAB. Nano-delivery systems for encapsulation of dietary polyphenols: An experimental approach for neurodegenerative diseases and brain tumors. Biochemical Pharmacology. 2018;**154**:303-317

[195] Conte R. Polyphenols Nanoencapsulation for therapeutic applications. Journal of Biomolecular Research & Therapeutics. 2019;5:2

[196] Shive MS, Anderson JM. Biodegradation and biocompatibility of PLA and PLGA microspheres. Advanced Drug Delivery Reviews. 1997;**28**(1):5-24

[197] Anton N, Benoit JP, Saulnier P. Design and production of nanoparticles formulated from nano-emulsion templates-a review. Journal of Controlled Release. 2008;**128**(3):185-199

[198] Mora-Huertas CE, Fessi H, Elaissari A. Polymer-based nanocapsules for drug delivery. International Journal of Pharmaceutics. 2010;**385**(1-2):113-142

[199] Radtchenko I, Sukhorukov G, Mohwald H. A novel method for encapsulation of poorly water-soluble drugs: Precipitation in polyelectrolyte multilayer shells. International Journal of Pharmaceutics. 2002;**242**(1-2):219-223

[200] Khoee S, Yaghoobian M. An investigation into the role of surfactants in controlling particle size of polymeric nanocapsules containing penicillin-G in double emulsion. European Journal of Medicinal Chemistry. 2009;**44**(6):2392-2399

[201] Comfort C, Garrastazu G, Pozzoli M, Sonvico F. Opportunities and challenges for the nasal administration of nanoemulsions. Current Topics in Medicinal Chemistry. 2015;**15**(4):356-368

[202] Mahajan HS, Mahajan MS, Nerkar PP, Agrawal A. Nanoemulsion-based intranasal drug delivery system of saquinavir mesylate for brain targeting. Drug Delivery. 2014;**21**(2):148-154

[203] Tiwari G, Tiwari R, Rai AK. Cyclodextrins in delivery systems: Applications. Journal of Pharmacy & Bioallied Sciences. 2010;**2**(2):72-79

[204] Szejtli J. Introduction and general overview of cyclodextrin chemistry. Chemical Reviews. 1998;**98**(5):1743-1754

[205] Stella VJ, He Q. Cyclodextrins. Toxicologic Pathology. 2008;**36**(1):30-42

[206] Sercombe L, Veerati T, Moheimani F, Wu SY, Sood AK, Hua S. Advances and challenges of liposome assisted drug delivery. Frontiers in Pharmacology. 2015;**6**:286

[207] Torchilin VP. Structure and design of polymeric surfactant-based drug delivery systems. Journal of Controlled Release. 2001;**73**(2-3):137-172

[208] Chen Y, Zhang X, Lu J, Huang Y, Li J, Li S. Targeted delivery of curcumin to tumors via PEG-derivatized FTS-based micellar system. The AAPS Journal. 2014;**16**(3):600-608

[209] Sood S, Jain K, Gowthamarajan K. Optimization of curcumin nanoemulsion for intranasal delivery using design of experiment and its toxicity assessment. Colloids and Surfaces. B, Biointerfaces. 2014;**113**:330-337

[210] Ono K, Hasegawa K, Naiki H, Yamada M. Curcumin has potent anti-amyloidogenic effects for Alzheimer's beta-amyloid fibrils in vitro. Journal of Neuroscience Research. 2004;**75**(6):742-750

[211] Agrawal R, Mishra B, Tyagi E, Nath C, Shukla R. Effect of curcumin on brain insulin receptors and memory functions in STZ (ICV) induced dementia model of rat. Pharmacological Research. 2010;**61**(3):247-252

[212] Tiwari SK, Agarwal S, Seth B, Yadav A, Nair S, Bhatnagar P, et al. Curcumin-loaded nanoparticles potently induce adult neurogenesis and reverse cognitive deficits in Alzheimer's disease model via canonical Wnt/beta-catenin pathway. ACS Nano. 2014;**8**(1):76-103

[213] Taylor M, Moore S, Mourtas S, Niarakis A, Re F, Zona C, et al. Effect of curcumin-associated and lipid ligand-functionalized nanoliposomes on aggregation of the Alzheimer's Abeta peptide. Nanomedicine. 2011;**7**(5):541-550

[214] Sandhir R, Yadav A, Mehrotra A, Sunkaria A, Singh A, Sharma S. Curcumin nanoparticles attenuate neurochemical and neurobehavioral deficits in experimental model of Huntington's disease. Neuromolecular Medicine. 2014;**16**(1):106-118

[215] Kundu P, Das M, Tripathy K, Sahoo SK. Delivery of dual drug loaded lipid based nanoparticles across the blood-brain barrier impart enhanced neuroprotection in a rotenone induced mouse model of Parkinson's disease. ACS Chemical Neuroscience. 2016;**7**(12):1658-1670

[216] Braidy N, Jugder BE, Poljak A, Jayasena T, Mansour H, Nabavi SM, et al. Resveratrol as a potential therapeutic candidate for the treatment and management of Alzheimer's disease. Current Topics in Medicinal Chemistry. 2016;**16**(17):1951-1960

[217] Singh G, Pai RS. Optimized PLGA nanoparticle platform for orally dosed trans-resveratrol with enhanced bioavailability potential. Expert Opinion on Drug Delivery. 2014;**11**(5):647-659

[218] Shao J, Li X, Lu X, Jiang C, Hu Y, Li Q, et al. Enhanced growth inhibition effect of resveratrol incorporated into biodegradable nanoparticles against glioma cells is mediated by the induction of intracellular reactive oxygen species levels. Colloids and Surfaces. B, Biointerfaces. 2009;**72**(1):40-47

[219] Pangeni R, Sharma S, Mustafa G, Ali J, Baboota S. Vitamin E loaded resveratrol nanoemulsion for brain targeting for the treatment of Parkinson's disease by reducing oxidative stress. Nanotechnology. 2014;**25**(48):485102

[220] Chongtham A, Agrawal N. Curcumin modulates cell death and is protective in Huntington's disease model. Scientific Reports. 2016;**6**:18736

[221] Nasr M. Development of an optimized hyaluronic acid-based lipidic nanoemulsion co-encapsulating two polyphenols for nose to brain delivery. Drug Delivery. 2016;**23**(4):1444-1452

Chapter 4

Extracts and Essential Oils from Medicinal Plants and Their Neuroprotective Effect

Ianara Mendonça da Costa,
Elaine Cristina Gurgel Andrade Pedrosa,
Ana Paula de Carvalho Bezerra,
Luciana Cristina Borges Fernandes,
José Rodolfo Lopes de Paiva Cavalcanti,
Marco Aurélio Moura Freire, Dayane Pessoa de Araújo,
Amália Cinthia Meneses do Rego, Irami Araujo Filho,
Francisco Irochima Pinheiro and Fausto Pierdoná Guzen

Abstract

Current therapies for neurodegenerative diseases offer only limited benefits to their clinical symptoms and do not prevent the degeneration of neuronal cells. Neurological diseases affect millions of people around the world, and the economic impact of treatment is high, given that health care resources are scarce. Thus, many therapeutic strategies to delay or prevent neurodegeneration have been the subject of research for treatment. One strategy for this is the use of herbal and essential oils of different species of medicinal plants because they have several bioactive compounds and phytochemicals with neuroprotective capacity. In addition, they respond positively to neurological disorders, such as dementia, oxidative stress, anxiety, cerebral ischemia, and oxidative toxicity, suggesting their use as complementary treatment agents in the treatment of neurological disorders.

Keywords: neuroprotection, herbal medicines, neurological disorders, oxidative stress

1. Introduction

A number of complementary treatment are currently being investigated to provide neuroprotection or to treat neurodegenerative diseases. Some therapies are known to provide limited benefits because, despite their treating the clinical symptoms, they are not effective in preventing neuronal cell degeneration.

The economic impact of treating neurodegenerative disorders is also high with disproportionately scarce neurological services and resources that patient survival may depend on. Studies have shown that over 80% of natural deaths in low- and middle-income countries may be attributed to stroke [1]. In the United States alone, the combined annual costs of neurological diseases total nearly $ 800 billion, expected to increase in the coming years due to an aging population, resulting in a severe economic burden to the health system [2].

Recent advances in understanding the pathophysiological mechanisms of neurological disorders have led to new strategies in drug development. Animal models have contributed considerably to these advances, as they play an important role in evaluating potential drugs that can alleviate these conditions and also delay their processes [3].

Interest in natural products has increased significantly, resulting in the increasing use of herbal medicines [4]. In a recent review, Izzo et al. report a 6.8% increase in US herbal and food supplement sales in 2014, with an estimated over $ 6.4 billion in total sales [5].

The clinical and social repercussions of neuropathologies reveal an important theme of study and commitment to structure strategies that can contribute to the quality of life of society. Scientific research has explored which stimuli and substances can contribute to neural cell plasticity, resulting in improved quality of life for people with depression, Alzheimer's Disease (AD), Parkinson's Disease (PD), among other nervous system-related disorders [6].

Increased neurogenesis and the facilitating effects of plasticity can be produced by a variety of treatments, including enriched environment, physical activity or drug action [7]. A complementary treatment proposed is the use of herbal medicines, which have scientific relevance in the treatment of neurological diseases because they contain multiple compounds and phytochemicals that can have neuroprotective effect, with a consequent beneficial action for health in different neuropsychiatric and neurodegenerative disorders [8].

2. Neuroprotective effect of extracts

Studies have investigated therapies that can alleviate the symptoms of neurodegenerative disorders and also avoid the multiple pathogenic factors involved in these diseases. One promising approach is the use of herbal extracts and their isolated bioactive compounds for the treatment of conditions such as Parkinson's, Alzheimer's, cerebral ischemia. Behavioral analysis has shown them to have neurochemical activity and symptom reduction [9].

Recent advances in understanding the pathophysiological mechanisms related to neurodegenerative diseases point to new strategies in drug development [10]. Animal models have contributed considerably to these advances and play an even greater role in evaluating possible drugs with therapeutic potential, not only to alleviate these pathologies, but also to modify the disease process [3]. Rodents are suitable models for these studies because of their well-characterized brain organization and the magnitude of information focused on altered states of the nervous system [11, 12].

Phytotherapics have scientific relevance in the treatment of neurological diseases, as they contain multiple compounds and phytochemicals that can have neuroprotective effects, with consequent beneficial health action between different neuropsychiatric and neurodegenerative disorders [8–10]. Several extracts that have shown beneficial action in these disorders as will be addressed in this paper.

2.1 Alzheimer's disease

Alzheimer's disease (AD) is a neurodegenerative pathology that results in progressive loss of cell function, structure and number, leading to widespread brain atrophy and profound cognitive and behavioral deficit [13]. Histopathologically, it is characterized by accumulation of beta-amyloid peptide (ßA), which can initiate a cascade of oxidative events and chronic inflammation leading to neuronal death [14].

Several studies have investigated the action of *Piper methysticum* in experimental models of neurodegenerative diseases, specifically in AD, demonstrating the neuroprotective effect of this herbal medicine [15–17].

Piper methysticum is popularly known as Kava or Kava-kava, a perennial shrub belonging to the Pacific Ocean pepper family (Piperaceae) with historical and cultural significance is described in the literature as a compound that has neuroprotective action and anxiolytic effects and is used in sedatives, and analgesics, being anti-inflammatory, anticonvulsant and anti-ischemic. Most of these pharmacological effects have been attributed to six kavalactones isolated from kava extracts, including yangonin, kawain and methysticin, dihydromethysticin, dihydrokavain and desmethoxyyangonin [18].

Recent studies, such as Fragoulis et al. have shown that one of the possible explanations for the action of piper mechanism in AD is associated with the activation of the erythroid2-related nuclear factor (NrF2) [15].

Nrf2 is the major regulator of phase II detoxifying/antioxidant enzymes, including heme oxygenase 1 (HO-1). Transcription factor Nrf2 binds to ARE (antioxidant response element), transcribing a battery of genes involved in redox status, anti-inflammatory response and detoxification [19]. A study by Lobota et al. reports that Nrf2 activation and HO-1 induction are involved in the regulation of inflammation [20].

Another study developed to find agents that activate the Nrf2 factor was performed and three analytically pure kavalactones - Methysticin, Yangonin and Kavain - were researched. The effects of kavalactones on the protection of neural cells against beta-amyloid peptide (ßA)-induced neurotoxicity were evaluated using the ARE-luciferase and Western blot assay. The results indicated that kavalactones Methysticin, Yangonin and Kavain activate time and dose-dependent Nrf2/ARE in astroglial PC-12 and C6 neural C6 cells and thus up-regulate cytoprotective genes. At the same time, viability and cytotoxicity assays have shown that Nrf2 activation is able to protect neuronal cells from neurotoxicity by attenuating neuronal cell death caused by β amyloid [14].

Taken together, it is understood that the Nrf2/ARE signaling pathway is an attractive therapeutic target for neurodegenerative diseases and that chemically modified kavalactones as well as naturally occurring kavalactones can attenuate neurological damage by reducing oxidative stress and neuroinflammation.

Some herbal medicines have shown neuroprotective effects, such as curcumin, which is the main polyphenol found in turmeric (*Curcuma longa*), belonging to the Zingiberaceae family, native to South Asia and cultivated in the tropics [21]. It has been reported that this compound has properties that can prevent or ameliorate pathological processes related to neurodegenerative diseases such as cognitive decline, dementia and mood disorders [22]. In addition, curcumin has been investigated for experimental models of treatment for Parkinson's disease and has shown hopeful results [9].

Saffron compounds have been linked to beneficial biological properties such as anti-inflammatory, pro-apoptotic, antiproliferative, anti-amyloidogenic, antioxidant, antiviral, and antidiabetic [23, 24]. Saffron's most bioactive constituents are curcuminoids, including curcumin and its derivatives such as demethoxycurcumin and bisdemetoxycurcumin [25, 26].

The features attributed to curcumin, such as inhibition of amyloid pathology, protection against inflammation and oxidative stress, inhibition of beta amyloid plaque aggregation and tau protein hyperphosphorylation, suggest that this compound may prevent or improve pathological processes related to cognitive decline and dementia, as occur in the symptomatology of AD patients [27, 28].

A systematic review study showed that curcumin has a positive action on AD symptoms, both when assessing biochemical and behavioral symptoms. The proposed mechanisms of its action in AD show that it is able to act by preventing the formation and aggregation of β-amyloid protein and tau protein hispanphosphorylation [10], in addition curcumin has also been shown to prevent neural damage, mitochondrial disorders, cellular stress and glial hyperactivation, as shown in **Figure 1**.

Another compound that represents a promising approach is *astragaloside IV* (AS-IV), a triterpenoid saponin present in the root of *Astragalus membranaceus* (Fisch.) Bge. It is part of Chinese traditional culture [29], first described in the Chinese book Shen Nong Ben Cao Jing in 200 AD with a number of beneficial effects and no toxicity.

The biological and pharmacological properties of AS-IV include its protective effect on pathologies due to its wide range of beneficial actions, such as antioxidant, antibacterial, antiviral [30, 31], anti-inflammatory, anti-asthmatic, antidiabetic, antifibrotic, immunoregulatory and antimicrobial, and cardioprotective effects, preventing myocardial insufficiency in rats [29–32], able to improve the immune system, digestion and promote wound healing [33].

Astragalus action can be understood based on the regulation of the release of caspases and cytochrome c (both being inducers of apoptosis), since cytochrome binds to Apaf-1 and Procaspase-9c when released into cytosol, forming a functional apoptosome and subsequently triggering the sequential activation of caspase-3 and 9 [34]. Several stimuli that induce apoptosis, leading to the release of mitochondrial cytochrome c which plays a key role in a common pathway of caspase activation [34, 35]. In addition, caspase-3 activation has been shown to be a fundamental step in the apoptosis process and its inhibition may block cellular apoptosis.

In addition, Chang et al. evaluated the action of AS-IV on the cerebral cortex after Aβ infusion, showing that i.p. Administration of 40 mg/kg/day of the herbal compound once daily for 14 days reduced the levels of mitochondrial dysfunction apoptosis in cortical cells blocked by inhibition of phosphoinositol 3-kinase (PI3K) protein kinase, known as AKT [36].

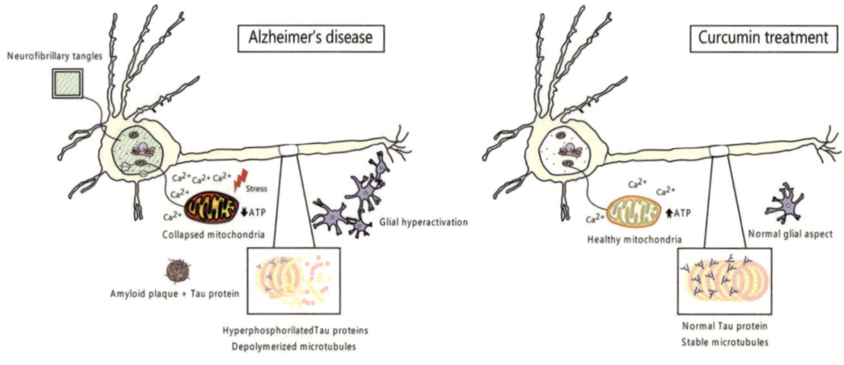

Figure 1.
Active curcumin mechanisms after experimental treatment in AD models. Curcumin acts by preventing the formation and aggregation of β-amyloid protein and hyperphosphorylation of tau protein, stabilizing microtubules and preventing the formation of neurofibrillary tangles that occur due to deposition of this protein. It has also been shown to prevent mitochondrial damage favoring the increase of cellular ATP and the healthy maintenance of mitochondria, avoiding excessive Ca^{2+} intake. Curcumin is also able to counteract cellular stress and glial overactivation.

The beneficial effects of AS-IV administration in experimental models of neurodegenerative diseases proved to be effective in both in vivo and in vitro models, such as PD and AD, cerebral ischemia and encephalomyelitis by characterizing the antioxidant, antiapoptotic and anti-inflammatory action of this bioactive compound on the various neurochemical substances and behavioral mechanisms. This suggests that the mechanisms presented by AS-IV offer a possible future complementary treatment for the potential treatment of these pathologies [10].

2.2 Parkinson's disease

Parkinson's disease (PD) is a condition that causes progressive neurodegeneration of dopaminergic neurons with the consequent reduction of dopamine content in the substantia nigra. The 6-hydroxydopamine neurotoxin (6-OHDA) is widely used to mimic the neuropathology of PD [37].

There are reports in the literature analyzing the effect of supplementation, including Chinese herbs and herbal extracts that have shown clinical potential to attenuate the progression of PD in humans. In addition, plant extracts act on the neurochemical or motor profile in isolation [38]. It is known, however, that this pathology involves symptomatology related to both characteristics.

A recently published systematic review study discussed studies showing neuroprotective properties of medicinal plants and their bioactive compounds. These included *Amburana cearenses* (Amburoside A), *Camellia sinensis* (Catechins and Polyphenols), *Gynostemma pentaphyllum* (Saponin Extract), *Pueraria lobata* (Puerarin), *Alpinia oxyphylla* (Protocatechuic Acid), *Cistanches salsa* (Glycosides or Phenylethanoids), *Spirulina platensis* (Polysaccharide), and *Astragalus Membranaceus* - AS IV Tetracillic Saponin Triterpenoid [9].

As previously mentioned, Astragaloside showed a neuroprotective effect on several AD models. In addition, studies have shown the positive action of AS-IV in PD models. One of the studies induced Parkinson by the action of 6-OHDA, where AS IV attenuated the loss of dopaminergic neurons and the treated group presented intact germination, neurite growth and increased immunoreactive TH and NOS. In addition, when the pathology was induced in SH-SY5Y cell culture by MPP + (DP inducing drug) action, it also significantly reversed cell loss, nuclear condensation, intracellular generation of reactive oxygen species and pathway inhibition *as m*ediated by Bax; these effects, however, were related only to neurochemical analysis. Behavioral findings were not reported [39].

One legume that has become the target of scientific research for its neuroprotective properties is *Mucuna pruriens*. Behavioral analysis studies have been carried out with *Mucuna pruriens* (Alkaloids, coumarins, flavonoids, triterpenes, saponins, carotenoids) and Baicalein (Flavonoids) for PD, but no neurochemical evaluation has been performed. There are also publications demonstrating in vivo behavioral effects and in vitro neurochemical analyses, such as a recent publication showing the effect of *Ligusticum officinale* (Makino) on MPTP (1-methyl-4-phenyl-1,2,3,6)-induced with an animal model and tetrahydropyridine, a neurotoxin capable of permanently causing symptoms of Parkinson's disease by destroying the dopaminergic neurons of the substantia nigra. This drug has been used to study the disease in experiments with animals; the treatment restored behavior when compared to the control group. In this study, *Withania somnifera* (Ashwagandha) extract also showed improvement in all these physiological anomalies [9, 40–43].

Another study investigated the ability of guanosine to protect neuronal PC12 cells from toxicity induced by 1-methyl-4-phenylpyridinium (MPP), the active metabolite of 1-methyl-4-phenyl-1, 2, 3, 6-tetrahydropyridine (MPTP), which mediates selective damage to dopaminergic neurons and causes irreversible

Parkinson-like symptoms in humans and primates. The results demonstrated that MPP-induced apoptosis of PC12 cells (cell line derived from a rat adrenal membrane pheochromocytoma) was significantly prevented by guanosine pretreatment for 3 h. In addition, guanosine attenuated the collapse of the MPP-induced mitochondrial transmembrane potential and prevented subsequent activation of caspase-3, thus protecting dopaminergic neurons against mitochondrial stress-induced damage [44].

Other studies have shown plants with neuroprotective properties capable of protecting from PD damage. These include plants such as *Amburana Cearenses* (Amburoside A) [5], *Myracrodruon urundeuva* (tannins and chalcones) [45], *Camellia sinensis* (catechins and polyphenols) [46], *Gynostemma pentaphyllum* (saponin extract) [47], *Pueraria lobata* (Puerarin) [48], *Alpinia oxyphylla* (protocatecholic citric acid) [49], parsley *Cistanches salsa* (phenylethane glycosides) [50, 51], *Spirulina platensis* (polysaccharide) [22] and *Astragalus membranaceus* (triterpenoid saponin), as mentioned in a review study [9, 39].

Current PD medications treat symptoms; none prevent or retard the degeneration of dopaminergic neurons. It is understood that the above-mentioned herbal medicines have neuroprotective properties.

2.3 Neurological disorders/cerebrovascular diseases/brain dysfunctions

Stroke is the second leading cause of death in industrialized countries and the leading medical cause of acquired adult disability [52].

Piper methysticum is cited as a multi-potent phytopharmaceutical due to its numerous pharmacological effects including anxiolytic, sedative, anticonvulsant, anti-ischemic, local anesthetic, anti-inflammatory and analgesic activities. The use of Kava in brain dysfunctions has clinical and financial advantages, acting as an adjunct or complementary treatment to existing medications [53].

Chang et al. [9] have shown that the use of combined glucose and oxygen administration of guanosine (100 μM) significantly reduced the proportion of apoptosis. To determine whether guanosine was also neuroprotective in vivo, middle cerebral artery occlusion (CoA) was performed in male Wistar rats and guanosine (8 mg/kg) intraperitoneally or saline (control vehicle) was administered daily for 7 days. Guanosine prolongs survival and decreased neurological deficits and tissue damage resulting from CoA. These data are the first to demonstrate that guanosine is neuroprotective in stroke.

Through an experimental study developed by Backhauss and Krieglstein [55] that induced focal cerebral ischemia in rodents, through left middle cerebral artery (MCA) microbipolar coagulation, with the objective of evaluating whether kava extract and its constituents, kawain, dihydrokawain, Methysticin, dihydromethysticin and yangonin, are capable of reducing the size of a heart attack zone in rats and mice, providing protection against ischemic brain damage. Compounds were administered ip, except kava extract, which was administered orally. The results demonstrated that Kava extract decreased the infarct area in mouse brains and the infarct volume in rat brains. Methysticin and dihydromethysticin significantly reduced the infarct area in mouse brain, thus evidencing neuroprotective activity of the mice. Kava extract works by the action of its constituent's methysticin and dihydromethysticin. The other Kavapyronas could not produce a beneficial effect on the infarct area.

The study by Deng et al. examined whether late administration of GUO (guanosine) improved long-term functional recovery after stroke. Late administration of GUO improved functional recovery from day 14 after stroke when compared with the vehicle group [56].

Gerbatin et al. evaluated the effect of guanosine on TBI-induced neurological damage. The findings showed that a single dose of guanosine (7.5 mg/kg), intraperitoneally (i.p) injected 40 min after fluid percussion injury (IPF) in rats protected them from locomotor and exploratory impairment, observed 8 h after injury, guanosine protected against neuronal death and activation of caspase 3 (protein responsible for cleaving genetic material.) This study suggests that guanosine plays a neuroprotective role in TBI and can be explored as a new pharmacological strategy [57].

Experimental models of ischemic stroke help our understanding of the events that occur in the ischemic and reperfused brain. One of the main developments in the treatment of acute ischemic stroke is neuroprotection.

2.4 Psychological disorders/anxiety/depression

Depression and stress-related disorders affect approximately 17% of the population, resulting in enormous personal suffering as well as social and economic burdens [58].

Guanosine is a nucleoside that has a neuroprotective effect. Current studies have analyzed the action of guanosine as an antidepressant. One study investigated the effects of guanosine on the tail suspension test (TT), open field test and adult hippocampal neurogenesis. The results suggest that the antidepressant effect of chronic guanosine use causes an increase in neuronal differentiation, suggesting that this nucleoside may be an endogenous mood modulator [59].

The ability of this nucleoside to nullify acute stress-induced behavioral and biochemical changes has not been evaluated in female mice, given that depression has a greater impact on women. A study aimed at investigating the protective effect of this nucleoside against oxidative damage and stress response evaluated this using the FST (forced swimming test). The Acute Containment Stress Protocol (ARS) has been proposed as a model that triggers biochemical changes in the rat brain that may be detrimental to CNS (central nervous system) function, implicated in several psychiatric disorders, including major depression [60].

Considering that the hippocampus plays a key role in mood regulation, numerous studies have evaluated whether adult hippocampal neurogenesis is altered in psychiatric disorders. Stress is a risk factor for depression that can manifest itself years after the stressful event [54].

Behavioral studies have shown that guanosine produces anxiolytic substances and amnesic effects. Other analyses have shown that reductions induced by hippocampal stress, cell proliferation and/or neuronal differentiation cause depressive symptoms. Deng et al. explain that hippocampal neurogenesis in humans is affected by various neurological disorders, including depression [56].

According to Duman et al. chronic administration of an antidepressant regulates neurogenesis in the hippocampus of adult rodents. Overregulation of neurogenesis could block or reverse the effects of stress on hippocampal neurons, which include downregulation of neurogenesis as well as atrophy. The possibility that the cAMP signal transduction cascade contributes to antidepressant regulation of neurogenesis is supported by previous studies and recent work [61].

Disturbances in hippocampal neurogenesis may be involved in the pathophysiology of depression. It has been argued that an increase in the generation of new hippocampal nerve cells is involved in the mechanism of action of antidepressants. This study, using adult Wistar rats given fluoxetine, showed that a significant behavioral effect occurred. It also pointed out that chronic antidepressant treatment increases cell proliferation as well as neurogenesis in the dentate gyrus.

Neurogenesis may serve as an important parameter for examining the efficacy and mechanism of action of new drugs [61].

Anxiety is a diffuse mental condition manifested through unpleasant feelings of fear and apprehension without specific cause [62].

Currently, the psychotherapeutic complementary treatment chosen to treat patients is through antidepressant drugs such as selective serotonin and serotonin-norepinephrine reuptake inhibitors (SSRIs), tricyclic antidepressants and benzodiazepines [63]. Due to the undesirable and destructive side effects of these drugs, including drowsiness, cognitive impairment, and symptoms of dependence and withdrawal, many patients prefer herbal remedies. Several plants with anxiolytic activity have been studied in clinical trials, and Kava (*Piper methysticum*) has been shown to be effective and is mentioned as a nonadditive, nonhypnotic anxiolytic with phytotherapeutic potential to act as an adjuvant or complementary treatment to anxiolytic drugs [64, 65].

A meta-analysis review by Pittler et al. evaluated the efficacy and safety of kava extract versus placebo for treating anxiety. Seven randomized controlled trials using *Piper methysticum* indicated that kava extract is superior to placebo and relatively safe as a treatment option for anxiety [66].

Another recent meta-analysis, conducted by Ooi et al., revealed similar results, mentioning that there is promising evidence from well-designed clinical studies suggesting Kava, particularly aqueous extracts, as an effective treatment for generalized anxiety disorder (GAD) [67]. The authors add that the effect of Kava is comparable to commonly prescribed pharmacological drugs (buspirone and opipramol), but with fewer adverse consequences.

It is suggested that the progression of new treatments for psychological disorders is described in the identification of neural substrates and mechanisms underlying their etiology and pathophysiology. Adult hippocampal neurogenesis is a candidate mechanism for the etiology of depression and may be used as a substrate for antidepressant action, as it may also be important for some of the behavioral effects of antidepressants [68].

The therapeutic properties of kava are supported by the six major kavalactones (dihydromethysticin, kavain, dihydrokavain, methysticin, yangonin and desmethoxyyangonin), of which kawain and dihydrokawain have more intense anxiolytic activity [69].

3. Neuroprotective effect of essential oils

In recent years, growing interest in research on medicinal plants and the effects of essential oils (EOs), especially for the treatment of neuropathologies, has emerged [70]. EOs (also called volatile or ethereal oils) are odorous and volatile compounds found only in 10% of the plant kingdom [71–76].

Secondary metabolites present in SOs have been widely used as antibacterial, antifungal and insecticidal agents. Their chemical and biological properties, especially antioxidants, have been considered important tools for the management of various neurological disorders [76].

Natural antioxidants derived from herbaceous plants have demonstrated in vitro cytoprotective properties and have a long history of providing benefits to human health [70]. Evidence of oxidative stress in neuronal damage and the benefits of antioxidant therapy have elucidated the importance of eliminating free radicals as a fundamental principle for the prevention and treatment of neurological disorders [77]. In addition, OEs derived antioxidants have been considered as a complementary treatment against neuronal loss as they have the ability to counteract the activity of free radicals responsible for neurodegeneration [78], protecting against cellular stress, as outlined in **Figure 2**.

Neural cells suffer functional or sensory loss due to neurological disorders and, in addition to other environmental or genetic factors that contribute to this loss, oxidative stress is a major contributor to neurodegeneration. Therefore, excess reactive

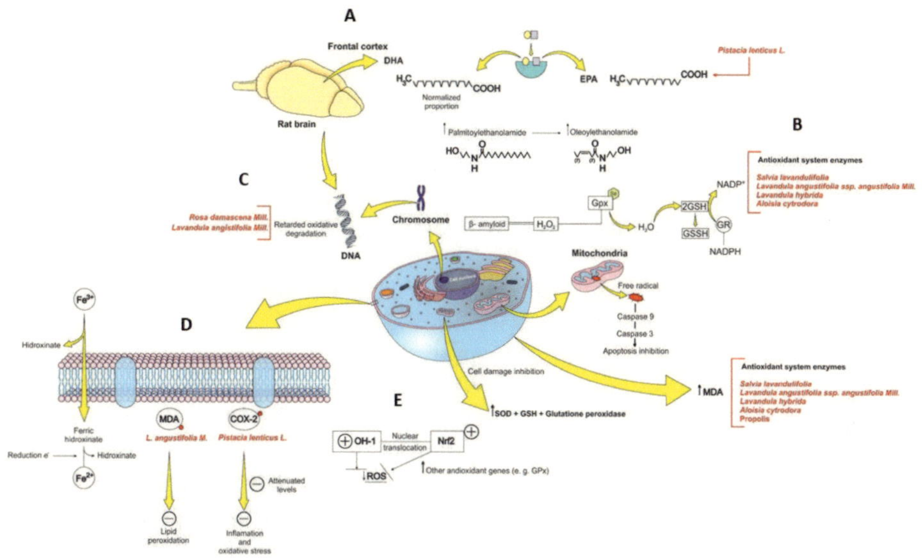

Figure 2.
Main identified mechanisms for the action of medicinal plant essential oils in experimental models of neurological disorders. In step A: In an experimental model of cerebral ischemia after occlusion of the common carotid artery followed by reperfusion (BCCAO/R), it was observed that occlusion in the frontal cortex caused a decrease in docosahexaenoic acid (DHA). with Pistacia lentiscus L. *showing positive plasma levels in the proportion of DHA-for its precursor, eicosapentaenoic acid (EPA) and levels of palmitoylethanolamide (PEA) and oleoylethanolamine (OAS), reversing its reduction, consequently decreasing the susceptibility to oxidation. In step B: essential oils from different medicinal plants demonstrated positive effect on the cellular antioxidant system.* Salvia lavandulifolia Vahl, Lavandula angustifolia SSP. mill *and* Lavandula hybrida *acted by increasing the multiple enzyme system (Cat, SOD, GPX, GSH and GSSG), Salvia l. (GR) and propolis (SOD) after induction of oxidative stress induced by different oxidants. Salvia essential oil reduced the expression of malondialdehyde (MDA), a marker of lipid peroxidation, thus inhibiting effector caspase-3 by preventing cellular apoptosis and preventing mitochondrial damage. The essential oil of* Lavandula angustifolia ssp. angustifolia Mill *also potentiated the described antioxidant enzyme system, reversing the scopolamine-induced damage (simulating a dementia model) as well as decreasing MDA levels.* Aloysia citrodora *acted upon damage in an experimental model of H_2O_2 and B-amyloid induced AD and its ability to act on the antioxidant system was observed due to the ability of its compounds to act as free radical scavengers or hydrogen donors. Increasing the antioxidant defense system through the action of these essential oils assists in reducing hydrogen peroxide (H_2O_2) to H_20 and O_2. Essential oils from other medicinal plants also regulated MDA (*Lavandula hybrida, Aloysia citrodora *and Propolis) levels. In step C:* Lavandula A. Mill. *and* Lavandula hybrida *demonstrated effects on DNA fragmentation (cleavage patterns were absent in the treated groups suggesting their antiapoptotic activity), similar effects were also observed in* Rosa damascena mill *treatment. Which also slowed the oxidative degradation of DNA, lipids and proteins due to the presence of phenols in their composition. In step D:* Aloysia citrodora *essential oils acted on the cell membrane, helping to increase iron chelation in vitro through Fe_3 + to Fe_2 + hydroximation, an important mechanism because the transition metal ions contribute to the oxidative damage in Neurodegenerative disorders, thus the chelation of transition metals, prevent catalysis of hydrogen peroxide decomposition via Fenton-type reaction.* L. angustifolia Mill, *acting on MDA levels and in the formation of reactive oxygen species (ROS), which are oxidative markers, consequently also prevents lipid peroxidation (determined by MDA level) in rat temporal lobe homogenates. Pistacia lenticus also acts by attenuating the levels of the enzyme Cox-2 cyclooxygenase 2, consequently decreasing the inflammation and oxidative stress observed in untreated groups. In step E: The essential oils of* S. lavandulifolia *are capable of activating the transcription factor Nrf2 - Nuclear factor (erythroid-derived 2) -like 2, a regulator of antioxidant genes, since protein expression and enzyme activity CAT, SOD, GR, GPx and HO-1 is markedly reduced, correlating with a decrease in nuclear Nrf2 protein. After treatment with* S. lavandulifolia, *regulation of Nrf2 was identified with a concomitant increase in antioxidant enzymes and HO-1, avoiding the formation of ROS, oxidation and decreased cell viability.*

oxygen species and an unbalanced metabolism lead to a number of neurological disorders, such as Alzheimer's disease (AD) and Parkinson's disease (PD) [78].

3.1 Alzheimer's disease

Alzheimer's disease (AD) is an age related neurodegenerative disease of the brain and this disease is characterized by a progressive deterioration of cognitive functions [79]. Oxidative stress, a detrimental factor during aging and pathologies, is involved in various neurodegenerative disorders [80, 81].

Studies suggest that caspase activation and apoptosis play important roles in AD neuropathogenesis [82]. Thus, SOs have been considered multi-potent agents against neurological disorders, being able to improve cognitive performance [83].

Lavender EO has several protective properties for the nervous system, as evidenced by its effectiveness in controlling depression, anxiety, stress, and cerebral ischemia [84, 85]. Some experimental models of AD have confirmed the neuroprotective effect and cognitive improvement of lavender OS, whose properties have been attributed to its antioxidant activity [86, 87].

EO (100 mg/kg) presented significant protection in the cognitive deficits evaluated, where the mechanism involved seems to be by a protection against decrease in the cellular antioxidant defense system, thus avoiding the reduction of the activity of superoxide dismutase, glutathione peroxidase and protection of the increase acetylcholinesterase malondialdehyde activity. The authors also demonstrated that lavender EO and its active component linalool protect against oxidative stress, cholinergic function and Nrf2/HO-1 pathway protein expression and synaptic plasticity. Therefore, it is suggested that linalool extracted from lavender OS may be a potential agent for improving cognitive impairment, especially in AD [88].

3.2 Oxidative stress

Oxidative stress occurs when the balance between antioxidants and reactive oxygen species (ROS) occurs negatively due to the depletion of antioxidants or the accumulation of ROS (Reactive Oxygen Species) [89]. Hydrogen peroxide (H_2O_2) is a major ROS and is involved in most cellular oxidative stresses [90, 91]. Several plants are considered a rich source of antioxidants because they inhibit or retard ROS-induced oxidative degradation [92–94].

Porres-Martínez et al. demonstrated that *Salvia lavandulifolia* E.O has neuroprotective activity against H_2O_2-induced oxidative stress in PC12 cells [93]. These effects appear to be related to Salvia lavandulifolia EO's ability to activate the transcription factor Nrf2. Therefore, pretreatments with S. lavandulifolia EO resulted in decreased lipid peroxidation, ROS levels and caspase-3 activity, showing cell viability and morphological recovery.

Natural antioxidants present in some herbal plants are responsible for inhibiting or preventing oxidative stress, one of the agents that acts in AD, due to their ability to eliminate free radicals. The neuroprotective effect of *A. citrodora* has been attributed to its chelating activity. As described in the literature, an important mechanism of antioxidant effect is the chelation of transition metals, thus avoiding the catalysis of hydrogen peroxide decomposition via the Fenton type reaction [95]. The main proposed mechanisms regarding the action of *A. citrodora* and *Salvia lavandulifolia* OE in vitro models of neurological disorders.

A pioneering study by Abuhamdah et al. showed that *Aloysia citrodora* EO provides complete and partial protection from oxidative stress in an experimental model with H_2O_2-induced Alzheimer's disease and β-amyloid-induced neurotoxicity using neuroblastoma cells. This study showed that 250 μm H_2O_2 could not trigger its neurotoxic effect when in the presence of 0.01 and 0.001 mg/mL O. citrodora EO, exhibiting neuroprotective activity at both concentrations [70].

Chelating agents have been reported to be effective as secondary antioxidants because they reduce the redox potential of transition metals, thereby stabilizing the oxidized form of the metal ion [96]. This seems to be one of the mechanisms involved in the antioxidant activity of some essential oils, as some of them were able to effectively chelate iron (II).

3.3 Brain ischemia

Cerebral ischemia consists in decreased blood flow in specific areas of the brain, causing hypoxia, which leads to an insufficient supply of glucose and oxygen, the magnitude of which disturbs the development of normal brain functions [97].

Currently, treatments that minimize neuronal damage after cerebral ischemia are limited, thus leading to the search for new complementary treatment therapies [98]. Terpenoids present in some essential oils constitute the largest group of secondary metabolites with neurological properties, including sedative, antidepressant and antinociceptive activities [99].

Another metabolite with neuroprotective function is linalool, a monoterpene present in volatile lavender oil, responsible for important therapeutic properties [100]; its activity on nerve disorders is well documented [101, 102]. Vakili et al. demonstrated that *Lavandula angustifolia* had a protective effect on focal cerebral ischemia in Wistar rats, especially when the treatment was performed with *Lavandula angustifolia* EO at 200 and 400 mg/kg. The results of the administration of this EO were an avoidance of a total antioxidant defense, reduced cerebral edema, and reduced infarct size. In addition, it improved functional performance after cerebral ischemia [103].

4. Concluding remarks

Neurodegenerative and neuropsychiatric diseases have multiple etiology. Multiple studies have been developed to clarify which approaches might be promising in prevention and treatment. We have targeted studies that present a neuroprotective perspective, herbal medicines and essential oils from different species of medicinal plants. These have various bioactive and phytochemical compounds with neuroprotective capacity, and also have given positive responses in studies on neurological disorders such as dementia, oxidative stress, anxiety, cerebral ischemia and oxidative toxicity. We suggest that these present a potential as agents in the treatment of neurological disorders.

Acknowledgements

The English text of this paper has been revised by Sidney Pratt, Canadian, MAT (The Johns Hopkins University), RSAdip - TESL (Cambridge University).

Author details

Ianara Mendonça da Costa[1*], Elaine Cristina Gurgel Andrade Pedrosa[1], Ana Paula de Carvalho Bezerra[1], Luciana Cristina Borges Fernandes[1,3], José Rodolfo Lopes de Paiva Cavalcanti[1], Marco Aurélio Moura Freire[1], Dayane Pessoa de Araújo[1], Amália Cinthia Meneses do Rego[2], Irami Araujo Filho[2], Francisco Irochima Pinheiro[2] and Fausto Pierdoná Guzen[1,2]

1 Department of Biomedical Sciences, Laboratory of Experimental Neurology, Health Science Center, University of the State of Rio Grande do Norte (UERN), Mossoró, RN, Brazil

2 School of Health, Potiguar University (UnP), Natal, RN, Brazil

3 Federal Rural University of the Semi Arid (UFERSA), Mossoró, RN, Brazil

*Address all correspondence to: ianara.nutricao@gmail.com

References

[1] World Health Organization. Neurological Disorders: Public Health Challenges. Geneva: WHO; 2006. Available from: http://www.who.int/mental_health/neurology/neurodiso/en/. [Accessed: 18 May 2018]

[2] Shaw G. The economic burden of neurologic disease—$800 billion annually in the US. Neurology Today. 2017;**17**(12):1-14. DOI: 10.1097/01.NT.0000521169.52982.7f

[3] Van Dam D, De Deyn PP. Drug discovery in dementia: The role of rodent models. Nature Reviews. Drug Discovery. 2006;**5**:956-970. DOI: 10.1038/nrd2075

[4] Sachan A, Singh S, Singh H, et al. An experimental study to evaluate the effect of *Mucuna pruriens* on learning and memory in mice. Journal of Innovation Sciences and Research. 2015;**4**(4):144-148

[5] Izzo AA, Hoon-Kim S, Radhakrishnan R, et al. A critical approach to evaluating clinical efficacy, adverse events and drug interactions of herbal remedies. Phytotherapy Research. 2016;**30**:691-700. DOI: 10.1002/ptr.5591

[6] Faillace MP, Zwiller J, Bernabeu RO. Effects of combined nicotine and fluoxetine treatment on adult hippocampal neurogenesis and conditioned place preference. Neuroscience. 2015;**300**:104-115. DOI: 10.1016/j.neuroscience.2015.05.017

[7] Zhang QJ, Li LB, Niu XL, et al. The pyramidal neurons in the medial prefrontal cortex show decreased response to 5-hydroxytryptamine-3 receptor stimulation in a rodent model of Parkinson's disease. Brain Research. 2011;**1384**:69-79. DOI: 10.1016/j.brainres.2011.01.086

[8] Kumar GP, Khanum F. Neuroprotective potential of phytochemicals. Pharmacognosy Reviews. 2012;**6**:81. DOI: 10.4103/0973-7847.99898

[9] Costa IM, Cavalcanti JRLP, Queiroz DB, et al. Supplementation with herbal extracts to promote behavioral and neuroprotective effects in experimental models of Parkinson's disease: A systematic review. Phytotherapy Research. 2017;**31**:959-970. DOI: 10.1002/ptr.5813

[10] Costa IM, Freire MAM, Cavalcanti JRLP, et al. Supplementation with *Curcuma longa* reverses neurotoxic and behavioral damage in models of Alzheimer's disease: A systematic review. Current Neuropharmacology. 2019;**17**(5):406-421. DOI: 10.2174/1570159X16666180117112610

[11] Hellewell SC, Ziebell JM, Lifshitz J, et al. Impact acceleration model of diffuse traumatic brain injury. Methods in Molecular Biology. 2016;**1462**:253-266. DOI: 10.1007/978-1-4939-3816-2_15

[12] Santiago LF, Rocha EG, Freire MA, et al. The organizational variability of the rodent somatosensory cortex. Reviews in the Neurosciences. 2007;**18**:283-294. DOI: 10.1515/REVNEURO.2007.18.3-4.283

[13] Rodríguez JJ, Verkhratsky A. Neuroglial roots of neurodegenerative diseases? Molecular Neurobiology. 2011;**43**(2):87-96. DOI: 10.1007/s12035-010-8157-x. Available from: https://www.ncbi.nlm.nih.gov/pubmed/21161612. [Accessed: 18 May 2018]

[14] Wruck CJ, Götz ME, Herdegen T, et al. Kavalactones protect neural cells against amyloid beta peptide-induced neurotoxicity via extracellular signal-regulated kinase 1/2-dependent nuclear

factor erythroid 2-related factor 2 activation. Molecular Pharmacology. 2008;**73**(6):1785-1795. DOI: 10.1124/mol.107.042499. Available from: https://www.ncbi.nlm.nih.gov/pubmed/18334601. [Accessed: 18 May 2018]

[15] Fragoulis A, Siegl S, Fendt M, et al. Oral administration of methysticin improves cognitive deficits in a mouse model of Alzheimer's disease. Redox Biology. 2017;**12**:843-853. DOI: 10.1016/j.redox.2017.04.024. Available from: https://www.ncbi.nlm.nih.gov/pmc/articles/PMC5406548/. [Accessed: 18 May 2018]

[16] Tanaka A, Hamada N, Fujita Y, et al. A novel kavalactone derivative protects against H_2O_2-induced PC12 cell death via Nrf2/ARE activation. Bioorganic and Medicinal Chemistry. 2010;**18**:3133-3139. DOI: 10.1016/j.bmc.2010.03.034. Available from: https://www.sciencedirect.com/science/article/pii/S0968089610002385?via%3Dihub. [Accessed: 18 May 2018]

[17] Garrett KM, Basmadjian G, Khan IA, et al. Extracts of kava (*Piper methysticum*) induce acute anxiolytic-like behavioral changes in mice. Psychopharmacology. 2003;**170**:33-41. DOI: 10.1007/s00213-003-1520-0. Available from: https://link.springer.com/article/10.1007/s00213-003-1520-0. [Accessed: 18 May 2018]

[18] Terazawa R, Akimoto N, Kato T, et al. A kavalactone derivative inhibits lipopolysaccharide-stimulated iNOS induction and NO production through activation of Nrf2 signaling in BV2 microglial cells. Pharmacological Research. 2013;**71**:34-43. DOI: 10.1016/j.phrs.2013.02.002 [Accessed: May 2018]

[19] Joshi G, Johnson JA. The Nrf2-ARE pathway: A valuable therapeutic target for the treatment of neurodegenerative diseases. Recent Patents on CNS Drug Discovery. 2012;7(3):218-229. Available from: https://www.ncbi.nlm.nih.gov/pmc/articles/PMC3625035/. [Accessed: 18 May 2018]

[20] Lobota A, Damulewicz M, Pyza E, et al. Role of Nrf2/HO-1 system in development, oxidative stress response and diseases: an evolutionarily conserved mechanism. Cellular and Molecular Life Sciences. 2016;**73**:3221-3247. DOI: 10.1007/s00018-016-2223-0. Available from: https://www.ncbi.nlm.nih.gov/pmc/articles/PMC4967105/. [Accessed: 18 May 2018]

[21] Lorenzi H, Matos FJ, Francisco JM. Plantas medicinais no Brasil: nativas e exóticas. 2nd ed. Nova Odessa: Plantarum; 2002

[22] Zhang L, Fang Y, Xu Y, et al. Curcumin improves amyloid β-peptide (1-42) induced spatial memory deficits through BDNF-ERK signaling pathway. PLoS One. 2015;**10**:e0131525. DOI: 10.1371/journal.pone.0131525

[23] Darvesh AS, Carroll RT, Bishayee A, et al. Curcumin and neurodegenerative diseases: A perspective. Expert Opinion on Investigational Drugs. 2012;**21**:1123-1140. DOI: 10.1517/13543784.2012.693479

[24] Strimpakos AS, Sharma RA. Curcumin: Preventive and therapeutic properties in laboratory studies and clinical trials. Antioxidants and Redox Signaling. 2008;**10**:511-546. DOI: 10.1089/ars.2007

[25] Ahmed T, Gilani AH. Therapeutic potential of turmeric in Alzheimer's disease: Curcumin or curcuminoids? 2014;**28**(4):517-525. DOI: 10.1002/ptr.5030

[26] Wright L, Frye JB, Gorti B, et al. Bioactivity of turmeric-derived curcuminoids and related metabolites in breast cancer. Current Pharmaceutical Design. 2013;**19**:6218-6225

[27] Garcia-Alloza M, Borrelli LA, Rozkalne A, et al. Curcumin labels amyloid pathology in vivo, disrupts existing plaques, and partially restores distorted neurites in an Alzheimer mouse model. Journal of Neurochemistry. 2007;**102**:1095-1104. DOI: 10.1111/j.1471-4159.2007.04613.x

[28] Lim GP, Chu T, Yang F, et al. The curry spice curcumin reduces oxidative damage and amyloid pathology in an Alzheimer transgenic mouse. The Journal of Neuroscience. 2001;**21**:8370-8377

[29] Li M, Li H, Fang F, et al. Astragaloside IV attenuates cognitive impairments induced by transient cerebral ischemia and reperfusion in mice via anti-inflammatory mechanisms. Neuroscience Letters. 2017;**639**:114-119

[30] Wagner H, Bauer R, Xiao PG, et al. Chinese Drug Monographs and Analysis: Radix Astragali (Huangqi). Verlag Wald Germany; 1997. pp. 1-17

[31] Zheng XY. Pharmacopoeia of the People's Republic of China. Vol. 1. Beijing: Chemical Industry Press; 2005

[32] Li ZP, Cao Q. Effects of astragaloside IV on myocardial calcium transport and cardiac function in ischemic rats. Acta Pharmacologica Sinica. 2002;**23**(10):898-904

[33] Yang J, Wang HX, Zhang YJ, et al. Astragaloside IV attenuates inflammatory cytokines by inhibiting TLR4/NF-κB signaling pathway in isoproterenol-induced myocardial hypertrophy. Journal of Ethnopharmacology. 2013;**150**:1062-1070

[34] Mancini M, Nicholson DW, Roy S, et al. The caspase-3 precursor has a cytosolic and mitochondrial distribution: Implications for apoptotic signaling. The Journal of Cell Biology. 1998;**140**:1485-1495. DOI: 10.1083/jcb.140.6.1485

[35] Mulugeta S, Maguire JA, Newitt JL, et al. Misfolded BRICHOS SP-C mutant proteins induce apoptosis via caspase-4- and cytochrome c-related mechanisms. American Journal of Physiology. Lung Cellular and Molecular Physiology. 2007;**293**:L720-L729. DOI: 10.1152/ajplung.00025.2007

[36] Chang CP, Liu YF, Lin HJ, et al. Beneficial effect of astragaloside on Alzheimer's disease condition using cultured primary cortical cells under beta-amyloid exposure. Molecular Neurobiology. 2016;**53**(10):7329-7340. DOI: 10.1007/s12035-015-9623-2

[37] Su C, Elfeki N, Ballerini P, et al. Guanosine improves motor behavior, reduces apoptosis, and stimulates neurogenesis in rats with parkinsonism. Journal of Neuroscience Research. 2009;**87**(3):617-625. DOI: 10.1002/jnr.21883

[38] Pérez-Hernández ZM, Villanueva-Porras D, Veja-Avila E, et al. A potential alternative against neurodegenerative diseases: Phytodrugs. Oxidative Medicine and Cellular Longevity. 2016;**2016**:8378613. DOI: 10.1155/2016/8378613

[39] Chan WS, Durairajan SS, Lu JH, et al. Neuroprotective effects of astragaloside IV in 6-hydroxydopamine-treated primary nigral cell culture. Neurochemistry International. 2009;**55**(6):414-442. DOI: 10.1016/j.neuint.2009.04.012

[40] Arulkumar S, Sabesan M. The behavioral performance tests of Mucuna pruriens gold nanoparticles in the 1-methyl4- phenyl-1,2,3,6-tetrahydropiridina treated mouse model of parkinsonism. Asian Pacific Journal of Tropical Disease. 2012;**2**:499-502. DOI: 10.1016/S2222-1808(12)60210-2

[41] Yu X, He GR, Sun L, et al. Assessment of the treatment effect of baicalein on a model Parkinsonian tremor and elucidation of the mechanism. Life Sciences. 2012;**91**(1-2): 5-13. DOI: 10.1016/j.lfs.2012.05.005

[42] Kim BW, Koppula S, Park SY, et al. Attenuation of neurinflamatory responses and behavioral déficits by *Ligusticum officinale* (Makino) kitag in stimulated microglia and MPTP-induced mouse model of Parkinson's disease. Journal of Ethnopharmacology. 2015;**164**:388-397. DOI: 10.1016/j.jep.2014.11.004

[43] Sankar RS, Manivasagam T, Surendran S. Ashwagandha leaf extract: A potential agent in treating oxidative damage and physiological abnormalities seen in a mouse model of Parkinson's disease. Neuroscience Letters. 2009;**454**(1):11-15. DOI: 10.1016/j.neulet.2009.02.044

[44] Jiang S, Bendjelloul F, Ballerini P, et al. Guanosine reduces apoptosis and inflammation associated with restoration of function in rats with acute spinal cord injury. Purinergic Signalling. 2007;**3**(4):411-442. Available from: https://link.springer.com/article/10.1007/s11302-007-9079-6. [Accessed: 31 July 2018]

[45] Calou I, Bandeira MA, Galvão WA, et al. Neuroprotective properties of a standardized extract from *Myracrodruon urundeuva* Fr. All. (Aroeira-do-Sertão), as evaluated by a Parkinson's disease model in rats. Parkinson's Disease. 2014;**2014**:1-11. DOI: 10.1155/2014/519615

[46] Guo S, Yan J, Yang T, et al. Protective effect of green tea polyphenols in the 6-OHDA rat model of Parkinson's disease through inhibition of ROS–NO pathway. Biological Psychiatry. 2007;**62**(12):1353-1362. DOI: 10.1016/j.biopsych.2007.04.020

[47] Choi HS, Park MS, Km SH, et al. Neuroprotective effects of herbal ethanol extracts from *Gynostemma pentaphyllum* in the 6-hydroxydopamine lesioned rat model of Parkinson's disease. Molecules. 2010;**15**(4):2814-2824. DOI: 10.3390/molecules15042814

[48] Zhu G, Wang X, Chen Y, et al. Puerarin protects dopaminergic neurons against 6-hydroxydopamine neurotoxicity via inhibiting apoptosis and upregulating glial cell line derived neurotrophic fator in a rat model of Parkinson's disease. Planta Medica. 2010;**76**(16):1820-1826. DOI: 10.1055/s-0030-1249976

[49] Zhang HN, An CN, Zhang HN, et al. Protocatechuic acid inhibits neurotoxicity induced by MPTP in vivo. Neuroscience Letters. 2010;**474**(2):99-103. DOI: 10.1016/j.neulet.2010.03.016

[50] Chen H, Jing FC, Li CH, et al. Echinacoside prevents the striatal extracellular levels of monoamine neurotransmitters from diminution in 6- hydroxydopamine lesion rats. Journal of Ethnopharmacology. 2007;**114**(3):285-289. DOI: 10.1016/j.jep.2007.07.035

[51] Zhao L, Pux XP. Neuroprotective effect of acteoside against MPTP-induced mouse model of Parkinson's disease. Chinese Pharmacological Bulletin. 2007;**23**(1):42-46

[52] Molz S, Dal-Cim T, Budni J, et al. Neuroprotective effect of guanosine against glutamate-induced cell death in rat hippocampal slices is mediated by the phosphatidylinositol-3 kinase/Akt/glycogen synthase kinase 3β pathway activation and inducible nitric oxide synthase inhibition. Journal of Neuroscience Research. 2011;**89**(9):1400-1408. DOI: 10.1002/jnr.22681. Available from: https://onlinelibrary.wiley.com/doi/full/10.1002/

jnr.22681?scrollTo=references. [Accessed: July 31, 2018]

[53] Singh YN. Kava: An overview. Journal of Ethnopharmacology. 1992;**37**(1):13-45. DOI: 10.1016/0378-8741(92)90003-a. Available from: https://www.sciencedirect.com/science/article/pii/037887419290003A. [Accessed: 18 May 2018]

[54] Chang R, Algird A, Bau C, et al. Neuroprotective effects of guanosine on stroke models in vitro and in vivo. Neuroscience Letters. 2008;**431**(2):101-105. DOI: 10.1016/j.neulet.2007.11.072. Available from: https://www.ncbi.nlm.nih.gov/pubmed/18191898. [Accessed: 31 July 2018]

[55] Backhauss C, Krieglstein J. Extract of kava (*Piper methysticum*) and its methysticin constituents protect brain tissue against ischemic damage in rodents. European Journal of Pharmacology. 1992;**215**(2-3):265-269. DOI: 10.1016/0014-2999(92)90037-5. Available from: https://www.ncbi.nlm.nih.gov/pubmed/1396990. [Accessed: 18 May 2018]

[56] Deng W, Aimone JB, Gage FH. New neurons and new memories: How does adult hippocampal neurogenesis affect learning and memory? Nature Reviews Neuroscience. 2010;**11**:339-350. Available from: https://www.ncbi.nlm.nih.gov/pubmed/20354534. [Accessed: 18 May 2018]

[57] Gerbatin RR, Cassol G, Dobrachinski F, et al. Guanosine protects against traumatic brain injury-induced functional impairments and neuronal loss by modulating excitotoxicity, mitochondrial dysfunction, and inflammation. Molecular Neurobiology. 2017;**54**(10):7585-7596. DOI: 10.1007/s12035-016-0238-z. Available from: https://www.ncbi.nlm.nih.gov/pubmed/27830534. [Accessed: 18 May 2018]

[58] Schmidt AP, Lara DR, Souza DO. Proposal of a guanine-based purinergic system in the mammalian central nervous system. Pharmacology and Therapeutics. 2007;**116**(3):401-416. DOI: 10.1016/j.pharmthera.2007.07.004. Available from: https://www.sciencedirect.com/science/article/pii/S0163725807001568. [Accessed: 31 July 2018]

[59] Bettio LEB, Freitas AE, Neis VB, et al. Guanosine prevents behavioral alterations in the forced swimming test and hippocampal oxidative damage induced by acute restraint stress. Pharmacology Biochemistry and Behavior. 2014;**127**:7-14. DOI: 10.1016/j.pbb.2014.10.002. Available from: https://www.sciencedirect.com/science/article/pii/S0091305714002767. [Accessed:31 July 2018]

[60] Bettio LEB, Neis VB, Pazini FL, et al. The antidepressant-like effect of chronic guanosine treatment is associated with increased hippocampal neuronal differentiation. European Journal of Neuroscience. 2016;**43**(8):1006-1015. DOI: 10.1111/ejn.13172. Available from: https://onlinelibrary.wiley.com/doi/abs/10.1111/ejn.13172. [Accessed: 31 July 2018]

[61] Duman RS, Nakagawa S, Malberg J. Regulation of adult neurogenesis by antidepressant treatment. Neuropsychopharmacology. 2001;**25**(6):836-844. DOI: 10.1016/S0893-133X(01)00358-X. Available from: https://www.ncbi.nlm.nih.gov/pubmed/11750177. [Accessed: 31 July 2018]

[62] Singh YN, Singh NN. Therapeutic potential of kava in the treatment of anxiety disorders. CNS Drugs. 2002;**16**(11):731-743. DOI: 10.2165/00023210-200216110-00002

[63] Bandelow B, Boerner JR, Kasper S, et al. The diagnosis and treatment of

generalized anxiety disorder. Deutsches Ärzteblatt International. 2013;**110**(17):300-309. DOI: 10.3238/arztebl.2013.0300. Available from: https://www.ncbi.nlm.nih.gov/pubmed/23671484. [Accessed: 18 May 2018]

[64] Saki K, Bahmani M, Rafieian-Kopaei M. The effect of most important medicinal plants on two importnt psychiatric disorders (anxiety and depression)—A review. Asian Pacific Journal of Tropical Medicine. 2014;**7**(1):S34-S42. DOI: 10.1016/S1995-7645(14)60201-7. Available from: https://www.sciencedirect.com/science/article/pii/S1995764514602017. [Accessed: 18 May 2018]

[65] Savage KM, Stough CK, Byrne GJ, et al. Kava for the treatment of generalised anxiety disorder (K-GAD): Study protocol for a randomised controlled trial. Trials. 2015;**16**(493):1-13. DOI: 10.1186/s13063-015-0986-5

[66] Pittler MH, Ernst E. Kava Extract Versus Placebo for Treating Anxiety (Review). New Jersey: John Wiley & Sons; 2010. Available from: https://www.cochranelibrary.com/cdsr/doi/10.1002/14651858.CD003383/epdf/abstract. [Accessed: 18 May 2018]

[67] Ooi SL, Henderson P, Pak SC. Kava for generalized anxiety disorder: A review of current evidence. Journal of Alternative and Complementary Medicine. 2018;**24**(8):770-780. DOI: 10.1089/acm.2018.0001

[68] Sahay A, Hen R. Adult hippocampal neurogenesis in depression. Nature Neuroscience. 2007;**10**(9):1110-1115. DOI: 10.1038/nn1969

[69] Wu D, Yu L, Nair MG, et al. Cyclooxygenase enzyme inhibitory compounds with antioxidant activities from *Piper methysticum* (kava kava) roots. Phytomedicine. 2002;**9**(1):41-47. DOI: 10.1078/0944-7113-00068

[70] Abuhamdah S, Abuhamdah R, Howes MJ, et al. Pharmacological and neuroprotective profile of an essential oil derived from leaves of *Aloysia citrodora* Palau. The Journal of Pharmacy and Pharmacology. 2015;**67**(9):1306-1315. DOI: 10.1111/jphp.12424

[71] Ahmadi L, Mirza M, Shahmir F. The volatile constituents of *Artemisia marschaliana* Sprengel and its secretory elements. Flavour and Fragrance Journal. 2002;**17**:141-143. DOI: 10.1002/ffj.1055

[72] Bezić N, Šamanić I, Dunkić V, et al. Essential oil composition and internal transcribed spacer (ITS) sequence variability of four south-Croatian Satureja species (Lamiaceae). Molecules. 2009;**14**:925-938. DOI: 10.3390/molecules14030925

[73] Ciccarelli D, Garbari F, Pagni AM. The flower of *Myrtus communis* (Myrtaceae): Secretory structures, unicellular papillae, and their ecological role. Flora. 2008;**203**(15):85-93. DOI: 10.1016/j.flora.2007.01.002

[74] Gershenzon J. Metabolic costs of terpenoid accumulation in higher plants. Journal of Chemical Ecology. 1994;**20**(6):1281-1328. DOI: 10.1007/BF02059810

[75] Liolios CC, Graikou K, Skaltsa E, et al. Dittany of Crete: A botanical and ethnopharmacological review. Journal of Ethnopharmacology. 2010;**131**:229-241. DOI: 10.1016/j.jep.2010.06.005

[76] Misharina TA, Polshkov AN. Antioxidant properties of essential oils: Autoxidation of essential oils from laurel and fennel and effects of mixing with essential oil from coriander. Prikladnaia Biokhimiia i Mikrobiologiia. 2005;**41**:693-702

[77] Santos JR, Gois AM, Mendonca DM, et al. Nutritional status, oxidative stress

and dementia: The role of selenium in Alzheimer's disease. Frontiers in Aging Neuroscience. 2014;**6**:206. DOI: 10.3389/fnagi.2014.00206

[78] Uttara B, Singh AV, Zamboni P, et al. Oxidative stress and neurodegenerative diseases: A review of upstream and downstream antioxidant therapeutic options. Current Neuropharmacology. 2009;**7**(1):65-74. DOI: 10.2174/157015909787602823

[79] Dunne TE. Alzheimer's Disease: Overview. 2nd ed. Oxford, UK: Academic Press; 2016. pp. 58-63

[80] Finkel T, Holbrook NJ. Oxidants, oxidative stress and the biology of ageing. Nature. 2000;**408**:239-247. DOI: 10.1038/35041687

[81] Freire MAM. Pathophysiology of neurodegeneration following traumatic brain injury. The West Indian Medical Journal. 2012;**61**:751-755

[82] Mattson MP. Contributions of mitochondrial alterations, resulting from bad genes and a hostile environment, to the pathogenesis of Alzheimer's disease. International Review of Neurobiology. 2002;**53**:387-409

[83] Ayaz M, Sadiq A, Junaid M, et al. Neuroprotective and anti-aging potentials of essential oils from aromatic and medicinal plants. Frontiers in Aging Neuroscience. 2017;**9**:168. DOI: 10.3389/fnagi.2017.00168

[84] Koulivand PH, Khaleghi Ghadiri M, Gorji A. Lavender and the nervous system. Evidence-based Complementary and Alternative Medicine. 2013;**2013**:681304. DOI: 10.1155/2013/681304

[85] Takahashi M, Satou T, Ohashi M, et al. Interspecies comparison of chemical composition and anxiolytic-like effects of lavender oils upon inhalation. Natural Product Communications. 2011;**6**(11):1769-1774

[86] Hancianu M, Cioanca O, Mihasan M, et al. Neuroprotective effects of inhaled lavender oil on scopolamine-induced dementia via anti-oxidative activities in rats. Phytomedicine. 2013;**20**(5):446-452. DOI: 10.1016/j.phymed.2012.12.005

[87] Hritcu L, Cioanca O, Hancianu M. Effects of lavender oil inhalation on improving scopolamine-induced spatial memory impairment in laboratory rats. Phytomedicine. 2012;**19**(6):529-534. DOI: 10.1016/j.phymed.2012.02.002

[88] Xu P, Wang K, Lu C, et al. The protective effect of lavender essential oil and its main component linalool against the cognitive deficits induced by D-Galactose and aluminum trichloride in mice. Evidence-based Complementary and Alternative Medicine. 2017;**2017**:7426538. DOI: 10.1155/2017/7426538

[89] Emerit J, Edeas M, Bricaire F. Neurodegenerative diseases and oxidative stress. Biomedicine and Pharmacotherapy. 2004;**58**:39-46. DOI: 10.1038/nrd1330

[90] Dasuri K, Zhang L, Keller JN. Oxidative stress, neurodegeneration, and the balance of protein degradation and protein synthesis. Free Radical Biology and Medicine. 2013;**62**:170-185. DOI: 10.1016/j.freeradbiomed.2012.09.016

[91] Halliwell B. Free radicals and antioxidants: Updating a personal view. Nutrition Reviews. 2012;**70**(5):257-265. DOI: 10.1111/j.1753-4887.2012.00476.x

[92] Gonzalez-Burgos E, Gomez-Serranillos MP. Terpene compounds in nature: A review of their potential antioxidant activity. Current Medicinal Chemistry. 2012;**19**(31):5319-5341. DOI: 10.2174/092986712803833335

[93] Guerra-Araiza C, Alvarez-Mejia AL, Sanchez-Torres S, et al. Effect of natural exogenous antioxidants on aging and on neurodegenerative diseases. Free Radical Research. 2013;**47**:451-462. DOI: 10.3109/10715762.2013.795649

[94] Porres-Martinez M, Gonzalez-Burgos E, Carretero ME, et al. Protective properties of *Salvia lavandulifolia* Vahl. essential oil against oxidative stress-induced neuronal injury. Food and Chemical Toxicology. 2015;**80**:154-162. DOI: 10.1016/j.fct.2015.03.002

[95] Gil A, Van Baren CM, Di Leo Lira PM, et al. Identification of the genotype from the content and composition of the essential oil of lemon verbena (*Aloysia citriodora* Palau). Journal of Agricultural and Food Chemistry. 2007;**55**(21):8664-8669. DOI: 10.1021/jf0708387

[96] Bush AI. The metallobiology of Alzheimer's disease. Trends in Neurosciences. 2003;**26**(4):207-214. DOI: 10.1016/S0166-2236(03)00067-5

[97] Small DL, Buchan AM. Mechanisms of cerebral ischemia: Intracellular cascades and therapeutic interventions. Journal of Cardiothoracic and Vascular Anesthesia. 1996;**10**:139-146. DOI: 10.1016/s1053-0770(96)80189-3

[98] Jivad N, Rabiei Z. Review on herbal medicine on brain ischemia and reperfusion. Asian Pacific Journal of Tropical Biomedicine. 2015;**5**(10):789-795. DOI: 10.1016/j.apjtb.2015.07.015

[99] Perazzo FF, Lima LM, Maistro EL, et al. Effect of *Artemisia annua* L. leaves essential oil and ethanol extract on behavioral assays. Revista Brasileira de Farmacognosia. 2008;**18**:686-689. DOI: 10.1590/S0102-695X2008000500008

[100] Peana AT, De Montis MG, Nieddu E, et al. Profile of spinal and supra-spinal antinociception of (−)-linalool. European Journal of Pharmacology. 2004;**485**:165-174. DOI: 10.1016/j.ejphar.2003.11.066

[101] Devi SL, Kannappan S, Anuradha CV. Evaluation of in vitro antioxidant activity of Indian bay leaf, *Cinnamomum tamala* (Buch. -ham.) T. Nees and Eberm using rat brain synaptosomes as model system. Indian Journal of Experimental Biology. 2007;**45**(9):778-784

[102] Batish DR, Singh HP, Setia N, et al. Chemical composition and inhibitory activity of essential oil from decaying leaves of *Eucalyptus citriodora*. Zeitschrift für Naturforschung. Section C. 2006;**61**:52-56. DOI: 10.1515/znc-2006-1-210

[103] Vakili A, Sharifat S, Akhavan MM, et al. Effect of lavender oil (*Lavandula angustifolia*) on cerebral edema and its possible mechanisms in an experimental model of stroke. Brain Research. 2014;**1548**:56-62. DOI: 10.1016/j.brainres.2013.12.019

Chapter 5

Glycodendrimers as Potential Multitalented Therapeutics in Alzheimer's Disease

Oxana Klementieva

Abstract

Finding successful therapies for the treatment of Alzheimer's disease (AD) is one of the most challenging tasks existing for human health. Several drugs have been found and validated in preclinical studies with some success, but not with the desired breakthroughs in the following clinical development phases. AD causes multiple brain dysfunctions that can be described as a brain organ failure, resulting in significant cognitive decline. Aggregation of amyloid proteins and neuronal loss are the hallmarks of AD. Thus, one of the strategies to treat AD is to find a multifunctional drug that may combine both anti-aggregation and neuroprotective properties. Such a candidate could be chemically modified dendrimers. Dendrimers are branched, nonlinear molecules with multiple reactive groups located on their surface. Chemical modification of reactive surface groups defines the property of the dendrimers. In this chapter, I will discuss poly(propylene imine) dendrimers with the surface functionalized with histidine and maltose as an example of a multifunctional therapeutic drug candidate able to protect the memory of AD transgenic model mice.

Keywords: dendrimer, histidine, aggregation, synapse, memory, Alzheimer's disease

1. Introduction

Alzheimer's disease (AD) is a complex neurological disease, which already in its earliest clinical phase is characterized by remarkable memory impairment. Multiple pieces of evidence suggest that in AD, memory impairment begins with dysfunction of synapses, a unique characteristic of nerve cells. Early neurochemical analyses of AD brain tissue revealed that the deficits in numerous neurotransmitters (including corticotropin-releasing factor, somatostatin, GABA, and serotonin) and the early symptoms correlate with dysfunction of cholinergic and glutamatergic synapses [1]. In addition to the deficits of the transmitters, many other biochemical and morphological indicators suggest that in early AD, synapses are under attack as reviewed in [2]. It has been shown that in biopsied AD cortex, there is a significant decrease in the numerical density of synapses in the brain and the number of synapses per cortical neuron [3]. The amyloid cascade hypothesis, one of the widely accepted theories, suggests that progressive accumulation and aggregation of amyloid-β proteins (Aβ) could be the main cause of AD, which triggers AD neuropathology. Aβ proteins are the proteolytic products of amyloid precursor protein (APP), a type-I transmembrane protein which is highly expressed in neurons, known to regulate synaptic function and neurite outgrowth [4]. There are two main alternative enzymatic pathways to process APP [5]:

1. Non-amyloidogenic pathway, where APP is subjected to consecutive cleavage by α-and γ-secretases that cut APP within the Aβ fragment

2. Amyloidogenic APP pathway, where APP is subjected to cleavage by β-and γ-secretases generating Aβ, a mix of short peptides ranging from 38 to 43 amino acids in length able to form polymorphous aggregates, so-called oligomers, and fibrils [6]

APP processing is regulated by neuronal activity, and neuronal activity may favor β-secretase-mediated amyloidogenic cleavage of APP during which Aβ proteins are generated [7]. It was accepted that after APP cleavage, Aβ peptides are first secreted, and then, extracellularly, soluble Aβ peptides aggregate into amyloid plaques. This extracellular Aβ, which is the main constituent of amyloid plaques, is thought to be toxic to the neurons. More recently, the intraneuronal Aβ has been demonstrated and reported to be involved in neuronal damage [8, 9]. It has been demonstrated that Aβ attacks synapses, small membranous protrusions that permit one neuron to pass a signal (electrical or chemical) to another neuron.

It has been shown that synaptic activity may affect Aβ secretion [5], and it has been hypothesized that synaptic activity may stimulate the generation of Aβ although why this occurs and whether Aβ might have a normal function in neuronal synapse have not been understood well [10]. Strikingly, it has been shown that Aβ selectively binds to synapses when added to cultured neurons [11]. Further, the level of Aβ is shown to be increased in synaptosomes in early AD [12]. Immunoelectron microscopy and high-resolution immunofluorescence microscopy studies show that this early subcellular Aβ accumulation leads to progressive damage of neurites and synapses [13]. Thus, synapses could be sites of early accumulation of pathogenic Aβ. It is believed that soluble Aβ oligomers rather than monomeric or fibrillar Aβ are the main neurotoxic species. However, a structure of neurotoxic Aβ oligomers and the nature of their effects on synapses are not identified [14].

Despite advances, the efforts to target neurotoxic Aβ oligomers in the brain are confounded by high polymorphism of amyloid structures [15]. Oligomer specific antibodies may interact mainly with a specific type of Aβ conformers against which these antibodies were produced [16]. Therefore, to target polymorphic Aβ oligomers, a cocktail from several antibodies might be required. Another way to modulate Aβ aggregation could be via establishing H-bond interactions [17] to favor the formation of less toxic Aβ species [18].

To fight a brain disease such as AD pathology, both synapse protection and anti-amyloid modulation would be desired properties of a possible therapeutic drug. However, to protect synapses and to modulate Aβ aggregation, amyloid aggregation modulator and neuroprotective therapeutics have to be delivered to the synapse. One way to deliver both therapeutic molecules is to use a compound which may carry both molecules simultaneously. Such multifunctional compound could be a dendrimer.

Dendrimers are three-dimensionally branched, globular macromolecules built by a series of iterative steps from a small core molecule which defines the type of the dendrimer [19]. They were first synthesized and described in 1978 [20], and since then dendrimers are in focus, due to their outstanding complexation properties. The most important features of dendrimers are controlled molecular structure, nanoscopic size, and high tunable availability of multiple functional groups at the dendrimer surface. Dendrimers are composed of three elements: a core branched

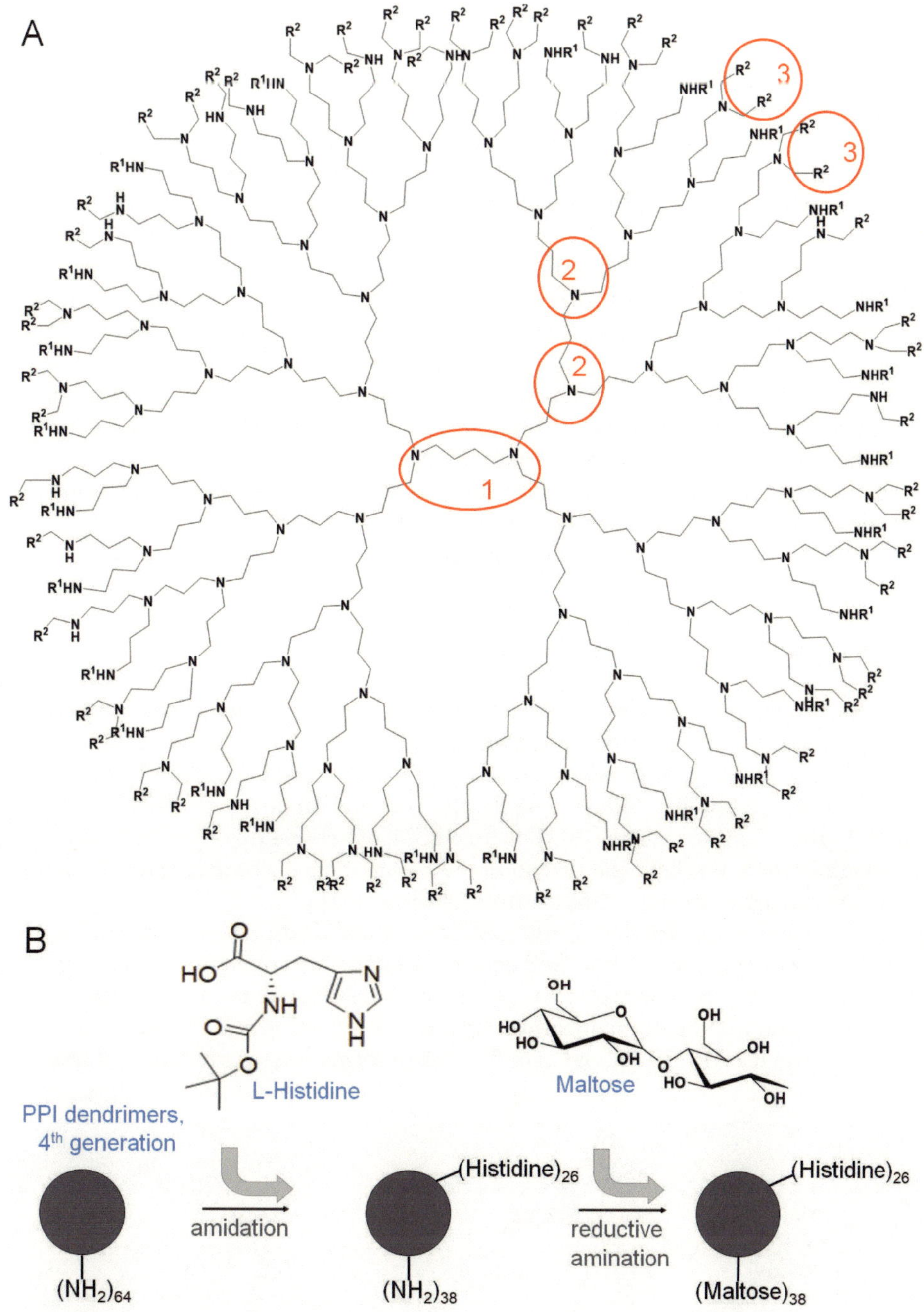

Figure 1.
Structure and chemical modification of dendrimers. (A) Molecular structure of poly(propylene imine) dendrimers of the fourth generation. Circle 1 shows the core; circle 2 indicates branching points of the dendrimers; circle 3 shows the terminal groups, R^1 and R^2. Fifth-generation PPI dendrimer (Eindhoven, the Netherlands) was renamed as fourth-generation (G4) PPI dendrimers following the uniform nomenclature [21]. (B) Example of surface modification of the PPI dendrimer. A reaction pathway shows the synthesis of G4 histidine-maltose PPI dendrimers first with histidine (R^1) and then with maltose (R^2). Conjugation with histidine and maltose neutralizes the positive charge of the primary amino groups [22].

dendron and terminal groups which could be used for dendrimer functionalization. The number of surface functional groups of the dendrimer depends on the degree of dendrimer branching (**Figure 1**). For example, PPI or PAMAM dendrimers of the second generation have 16 functional groups on their surface, the third generation has 32, and the fourth dendrimer generation has 64 functional groups. Strikingly, the number of terminal groups increases exponentially, while the size increases linearly. The terminal groups on the dendrimer surface can be used for surface modification and dendrimer functionalization. Such modifications could change dendrimers' surface charge and, for example, reduce toxicity associated with a cationic surface charge as reviewed by Appelhans et al. [23]. Dendrimers are most commonly synthesized using divergent or convergent different synthetic pathways [24]. Importantly, the high tunability of dendrimers' surface allows endless possibilities for dendrimers' biomedical applications, for example, for pharmaceutical applications, the terminal groups can be functionalized with different active conjugates such as specifically targeting antibodies, drugs, metal ions or imaging agents, and more [25]. Moreover, several research groups demonstrated that some types of dendrimers are able to cross the BBB [22, 26–28], showing their applicability for the research and possibly treatment of brain diseases.

In the present chapter, I summarize the experimental evidence showing that functionalized poly(propylene imine) dendrimers may provide multitargeting properties for dendrimers increasing their potential for the treatment of AD.

2. Amyloid aggregation and dendrimers

According to the amyloid cascade hypothesis, Aβ peptides are important players triggering the AD development. Multiple in vitro studies have demonstrated that the Aβ peptides can form fibrils and other aggregates called oligomers. The formation of insoluble Aβ fibril follows a nucleation-dependent polymerization mechanism (**Figure 2**) as described [29]. The formation of soluble Aβ oligomers in vivo is largely unknown; it is believed that soluble Aβ oligomers may precede fibril formation [30] and are more toxic than mature Aβ fibrils [31].

In the search for drugs that would inhibit neuronal death in Alzheimer's disease, one of the ways one can use is to find compounds that interfere with Aβ, cleaning the brain tissues from neurotoxic Aβ oligomers. It has been demonstrated that PPI dendrimers modified with maltose are capable of interfering with the amyloid formation in vitro [18, 28, 32, 33]. Amyloid fibril formation is usually monitored

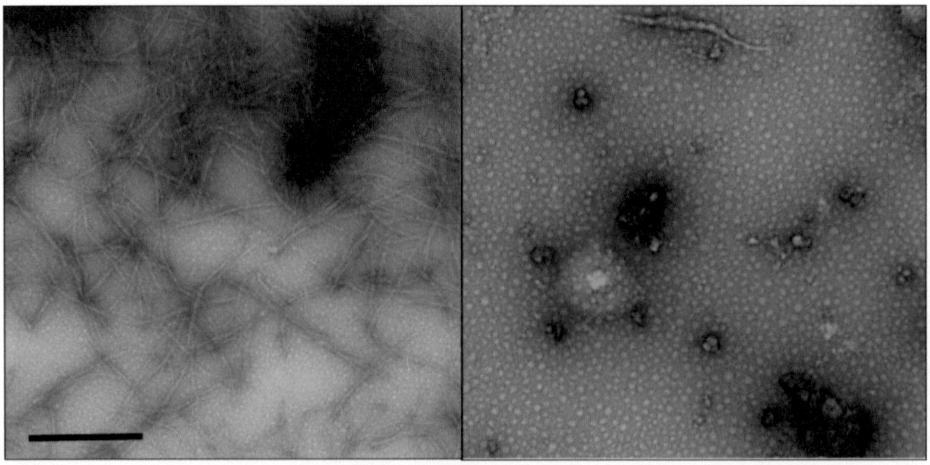

Figure 2.
Example of amyloid fibrils and amyloid oligomers. (A) Electron micrographs of the Aβ(1–40) fibrils (B) Aβ(1–40) oligomers prepared as described [9]. Scale bar is 200 nm.

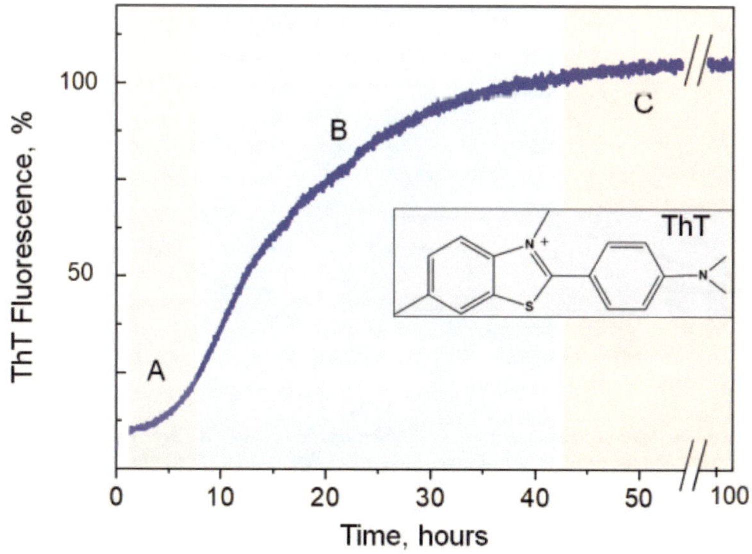

Figure 3.
Characteristic aggregation curve for amyloid fibril formation. Sigmoid-shaped curve 5 μM recombinant Aβ(1–42) kinetics as detected by ThT fluorescence over time and displayed as % of total ThT binding. Area (A) corresponds to the lag phase (nucleation), area (B) corresponds to the growing phase, and area (C) corresponds to final ThT fluorescence plateau. Inset: molecular structure of ThT.

using the fluorescence dye thioflavin T (ThT). The dye becomes fluorescent when interacting with the ordered β-sheet structures characteristic for amyloid fibrils. With the fibril growth, the ThT fluorescence increases until its value reaches a plateau. **Figure 3** demonstrates the sigmoid-shaped line corresponding to the ThT kinetics corresponding to the fibril growth of Aβ(1–40), where the lag (nucleation) phase is followed by the elongation phase and plateau; when all ThT molecules have intercalated into β-sheets of the amyloid fibrils, the aggregation kinetics of amyloids is reviewed [34].

PPI dendrimers modified with maltose may, in the case of Aβ(1–40) or Aβ(1–42), interfere with amyloid fibril formation in a concentration-dependent manner, indicating that maltose PPI dendrimers bind amyloid proteins [18]. **Figure 4** demonstrates the ThT fluorescent kinetics of Aβ(1–40) and Aβ(1–42) in the presence of maltose PPI dendrimers. As expected, Aβ alone forms the typical amyloid fibrils [30]. However, when the maltose PPI dendrimers are present, the morphology of amyloid fibrils is altered, demonstrating binding of the dendrimers to Aβ [18, 28, 35, 36]. The electron micrograph shows the morphology of amyloid fibril in the presence of maltose PPI dendrimers. Fibril clumps were generated by incubating maltose PPI dendrimers with Aβ(1–40). As it has been suggested that dendrimers interact with Aβ thus, fibrils seem to be varnished by maltose dendrimers and clumped together, and importantly, no Aβ oligomers were observed in the presence of maltose PPI dendrimers [18]. Thus it is reasonable to think that maltose dendrimers interacting with Aβ may form hybrid fibrils, shifting the balance between oligomeric and fibrillar forms of Aβ toward less toxic hybrid products.

Dendrimers' intrinsic toxicity is an important issue in relation to their potential biological applications [37]. It was observed that unmodified PPI dendrimers have high intrinsic toxicity for cells [38, 39]. It was hypothesized that this toxicity could be related to the dendrimer capacity of establishing strong interactions of electrostatic nature [40]. It has been demonstrated that dendrimers with a surface decorated by polysaccharides, such as maltose or maltotriose, confer less toxicity [41, 42]. The charge of the dendrimer covered by polysaccharides is close to neutral;

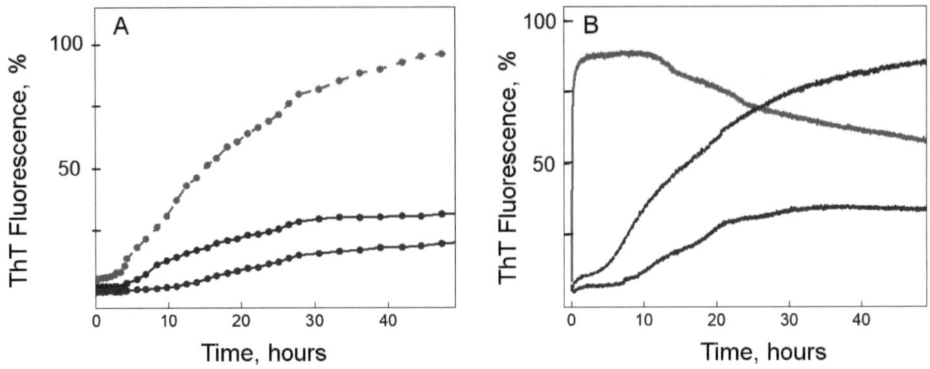

Figure 4.
Effect of G4 histidine-maltose PPI dendrimers on the fibrillization of Aβ. (A) Aggregation of 20 μM Aβ(1–40) in the absence (red) and the presence of histidine-maltose PPI dendrimers. (Magenta) 20 μM Aβ(1–40) in the presence of dendrimers at dendrimer/peptide ratio = 0.1, (blue) 20 μM Aβ(1–40) in the presence of dendrimers at dendrimer/peptide ratio = 1. (B) Aggregation of 25 μm Aβ(1–42) in the absence (red) and in the presence of histidine-maltose PPI dendrimers. (Magenta) 25 μM Aβ(1–42) in the presence of dendrimers at dendrimer/peptide ratio = 0.1, (blue) 25 μM Aβ(1–42) in the presence of dendrimers at dendrimer/peptide ratio = 1. The temperature was 37°C, the pH was set to 7.4, and the concentration of ThT was 6 μM (adapted with permission from [22]).

thus the interaction of dendrimer with other biomolecules is driven by hydrogen bonds, which is less strong; therefore, dendrimers covered by polysaccharides are less toxic [38, 39, 41].

In collaborations between the research groups of Dietmar Appelhans (Leibniz Institute of Polymer Research, Dresden, Germany), Josep Cladera (Autonomous University of Barcelona, Spain), and Isidro Ferrer in Barcelona (University of Barcelona, Spain), it has been shown that distinct PPI dendrimers with electroneutral maltose shell, with cationic maltose or maltotriose shell, were tested against amyloid toxicity in vivo and in vitro. The evaluation of the toxicity of Aβ in the presence of PPI maltose dendrimers showed that the dendrimers could significantly reduce the Aβ toxicity compared to Aβ alone [28].

Interestingly, only the electroneutral maltose dendrimers were able to reduce the toxicity of Alzheimer's disease brain extracts in cultured SH-SY5Y neuroblastoma cells [28]. Moreover, maltose PPI dendrimers with electroneutral or cationic surface penetrated the cytoplasm of cultured cells. Additionally, they penetrated inside the brain when administered to AD transgenic mice intranasally [28]. These PPI maltose dendrimers were able to modify amyloid plaque load in the brains of AD transgenic animals, showing anti-amyloid potential for in vivo applications. However, the studied maltose PPI dendrimers could not reverse memory impairment in APP/PS1 mice following chronic administration. Strikingly, cationic maltose dendrimers were neurotoxic in vivo and caused cognitive decline in non-transgenic mice [28]. Taken together, these results suggest that maltose PPI dendrimers require further optimization of biocompatibility.

3. Modified PPI dendrimers as potential multifunctional therapeutics for Alzheimer's disease

As it has been mentioned at the beginning of the chapter, Alzheimer's disease is a fatal neurodegenerative disorder. AD is characterized by a decade-long presymptomatic phase, and it is during the presymptomatic phase, before synaptic damage and neuronal loss, that therapies are most likely to be effective [43]. Thus, a preventive treatment which could protect synapses and reduce the neurotoxicity of Aβ oligomers is one such strategy. Such successful drug candidates for AD treatment have to possess both anti-amyloidogenic and neuroprotective properties. Therefore, a modification of maltose dendrimers with a molecule with neuroprotective characteristics was the next logical step in search of the new drug candidate for the treatment of AD.

To further improve the pharmacological properties of maltose PPI dendrimers, it was decided to modify PPI dendrimers of the fourth generation with maltose and histidine. Maltose was used due to anti-amyloidogenic properties; histidine was added due to several reasons: it is selectively transported through the BBB [44]. Histidine has chelating properties for Cu^{2+} ions [45]. Thus these properties were considered to be important since Cu ion dyshomeostasis may play a detrimental role in AD progression [46], and importantly, histidine has been shown to have some neuroprotective capacity [47]. After the modification, G4 PPI dendrimers modified with maltose and histidine were supposed to possess both anti-amyloid and neuroprotective properties simultaneously.

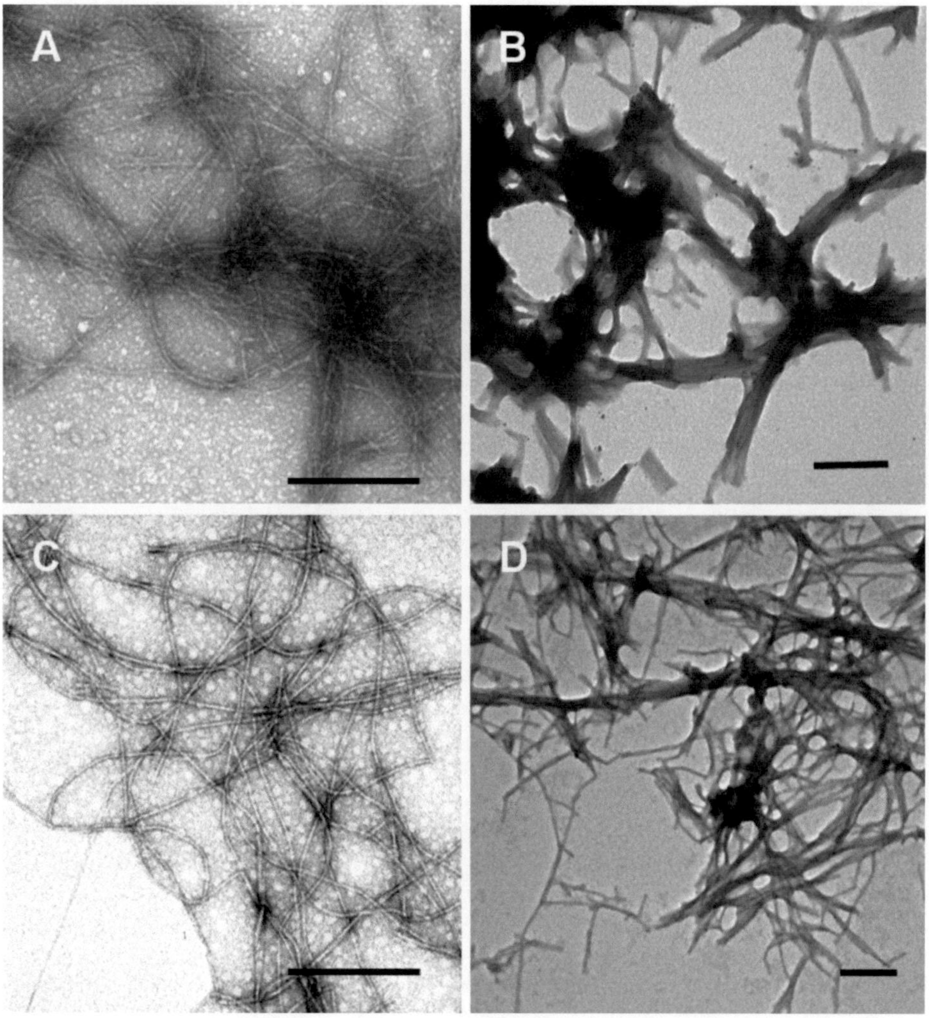

Figure 5.
Effect of G4 histidine-maltose PPI dendrimers on Aβ morphology. (A) Electron microscopy micrographs of 25 μM Aβ(1–40) incubated at pH 7.4 for 24 h. (B) 25 μM Aβ(1–40) incubated at pH 7.4 in the presence of G4 histidine-maltose PPI dendrimers at the ratio 1 to 1. (C) Aβ(1–42) incubated at pH 7.4 for 24 h. (D) Aβ(1–42) incubated in the presence of G4 histidine-maltose PPI dendrimers (clumped fibrils). Scale bar is 200 nm.

In vitro evaluations demonstrated that histidine-maltose PPI dendrimers could interact with Aβ. As maltose PPI dendrimers, G4 histidine-maltose PPI dendrimers did not prevent fibril formation but clump Aβ fibrils (**Figure 5**). Importantly, small oligomeric aggregates were not present in the studied suspensions in the presence of the dendrimers. Interestingly, the intensity of ThT was significantly decreased following the aggregation of Aβ probably due to the competition of the dendrimers with ThT for binding to Aβ(1–40) or due to change of structure, resulting in lower ThT fluorescence quantum yield [48, 49]. To test if G4 histidine-maltose PPI dendrimers could reduce the neurotoxicity of Aβ, primary neurons derived from wild-type mouse were treated with 1 μM Aβ(1–42) in the presence of the dendrimers at the ratio 1 to 1. As it was demonstrated by cell viability assay, histidine-maltose PPI dendrimers significantly reduced the neurotoxicity of soluble Aβ oligomers [22]. **Figure 6** shows the neuronal viability in the presence of the dendrimers and Aβ(1–42) oligomers as assessed by a lactate dehydrogenase (LDH) activity assay. 1 μM G4 histidine-maltose PPI dendrimers were added to primary neurons and incubated 24 h before the assay; as it was documented, the dendrimers alone were not toxic to the neurons. 1 μM recombinant Aβ(1–42) monomers, oligomers, and fibrils were added to primary neurons and incubated 1 h at 37°C in the presence and the absence of dendrimers. The results demonstrate that G4 histidine-maltose PPI dendrimers significantly reduced the toxicity of Aβ(1–42) for primary neurons.

In vivo evaluations demonstrated that chronic treatment with histidine-maltose PPI dendrimers of APP/PS1 mice prevented AD-related memory impairment [22]. **Figure 7** shows the results of the memory test after the treatment. APP/PS1 mice harbor two human genes: APP with the KM670/671NL, the Swedish mutation, and PSEN1 with the L166P mutation [50]. In APP/PS1 mice, human Aβ increases with age, but Aβ42 is preferentially generated over Aβ40, and the expression of the human APP transgene is approximately 3-fold higher than the endogenous murine APP [51]. For the treatment, APP/PS1 and wild-type mice were randomly divided into four groups, two groups (transgenic and wild type) were treated intranasally with histidine-maltose PPI dendrimers, and two groups (transgenic and wild type) were given intranasally phosphate saline. Administration lasted 3 months until animals reached the age of 6 months, the age when the first cognitive decline is detected [52]. Memory evaluation tests were performed at the end of treatment using two object recognition tests in a Vmaze[R] as described [52].

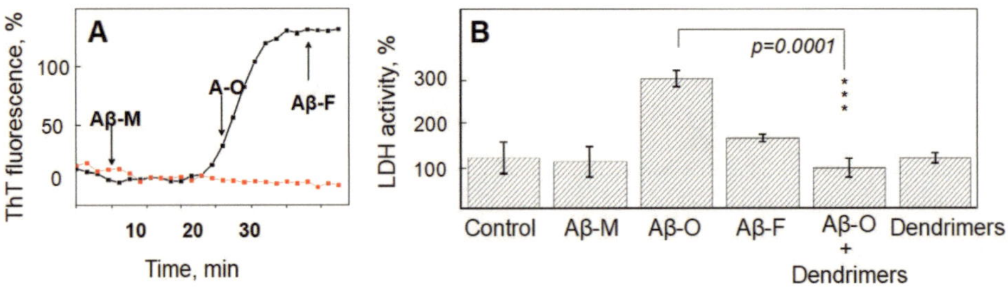

Figure 6.
G4 histidine-maltose PPI dendrimers reduce the toxicity of Aβ oligomers for cultured primary neurons. (A) ThT fluorescence variation was used to monitor aggregation of 10 μM Aβ(1–42) in PBS at 37°C (black line); red line corresponds to ThT alone. The arrows indicate the time when aliquots of Aβ(1–42) were taken for neuronal viability assay. Aβ-M, a monomeric form of Aβ(1–42); Aβ-O, an oligomeric form of Aβ(1–42); Aβ-F, mature fibrils of Aβ(1–42); (B) 1 μM of G4 histidine-maltose PPI dendrimers were added to primary neurons and incubated 24 h before a cell viability assay. Cell viability was assessed by a lactate dehydrogenase activity assay. For the assay, 1 μM Aβ(1–42) of monomers, oligomers, and fibrils were added to wild-type primary neurons and incubated 1 h at 37°C. statistics: one-way ANOVA followed by Tukey's post hoc test; data are expressed as mean ± SD. Primary neurons were derived from the brains of wild-type mouse embryos and cultured for 19 days. The experiment was performed in triplicate, one embryo per replica (adapted with permission from [22]).

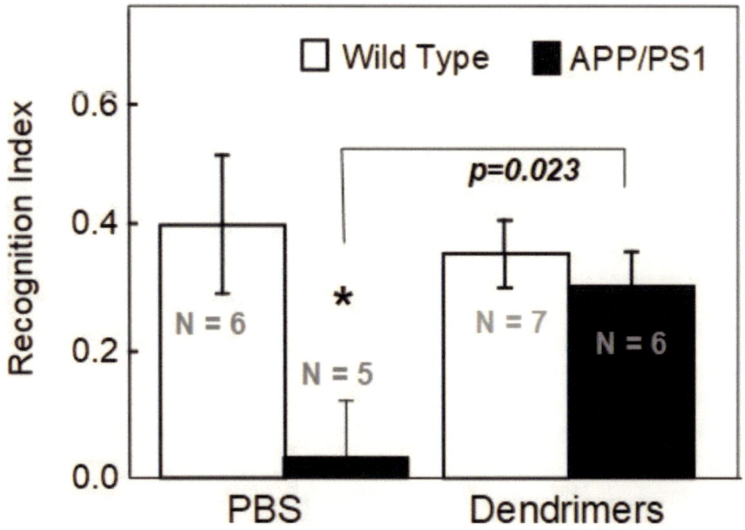

Figure 7.
G4 histidine-maltose PPI dendrimers can protect memory in vivo. Memory performance in the V-maze shows significant improvement after preventive treatment with histidine-maltose PPI dendrimers. Treatment procedure: at the age of 3 months, animals were randomly divided into four groups; two groups control and APP/PS1 mice were given intranasally 5 µL of PBS, and two groups received intranasally 5 µg/day of G4 histidine-maltose PPI dendrimers (dendrimers). Treatment lasted 3 months until animals reached the age of 6 months when APP/PS1 mice display cognitive impairment [52]. Statistics: two-way ANOVA with genotype and treatment as between factors followed by Tukey's post hoc test; data are expressed as mean ± SEM (adapted with permission from [22]).

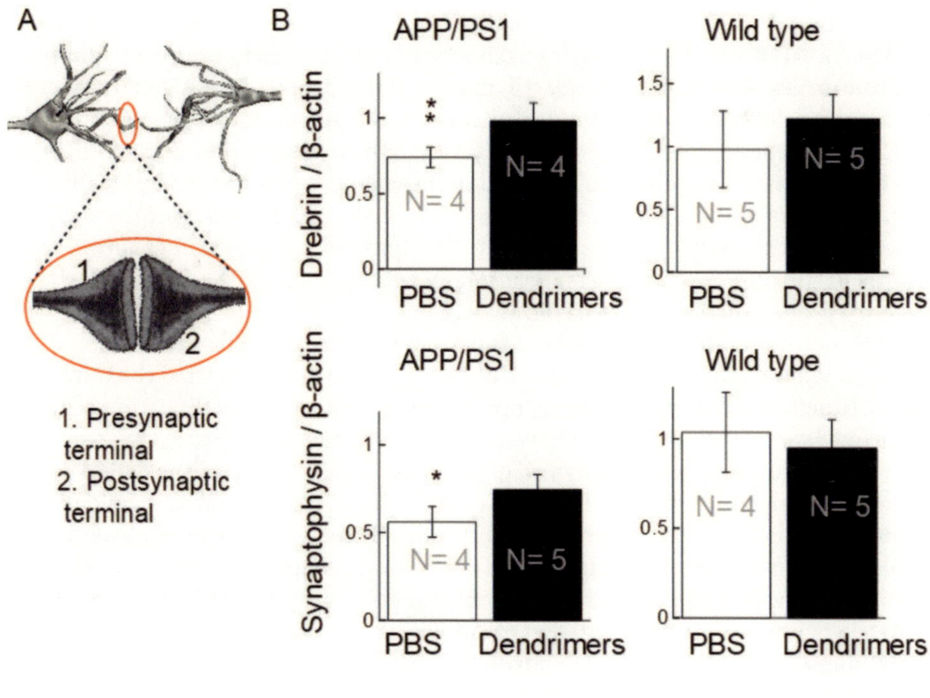

Figure 8.
G4 histidine-maltose PPI dendrimers protect synapses in vivo. (A) Synapse is a junction between two neurons, which consist of pre- and postsynaptic terminals characterized by specific pre- and postsynaptic proteins. Synaptophysin was used to assess presynapse, while drebrin was used to evaluate postsynapse. Brain tissue homogenates of control mice and mice treated with G4 histidine-maltose PPI dendrimers (dendrimers) were analyzed using Western blotting; β-actin was used for protein normalization. Statistics: Student's t-test (N is the number of animals per group, Western blotting was done in triplicate). Data are expressed as mean ± SD.

To understand a possible mechanism behind the memory rescue, the levels of pre- and postsynaptic markers in the brain of treated APP/PS1 mice were evaluated by Western blotting. Pre- and postsynaptic markers, such as drebrin and synaptophysin, play a crucial role in the synaptic plasticity and are downregulated in AD [53, 54]. Loss of synaptophysin correlates with cognitive impairments in AD patients and AD transgenic models [54, 55]; Psd95 knockout animals have impaired basal synaptic transmission and learning deficit [56]; transgenic animals lacking synaptophysin have reduced novel object recognition [57]. Importantly, it has been shown that loss of synaptophysin immunoreactivity precedes amyloid plaque formation [58, 59]. Preventive treatment of AD transgenic mice with G4 histidine-maltose PPI dendrimers prevented a decrease in synaptic proteins compared to PBS-treated mice [22].

In contrast, G4 histidine-maltose PPI dendrimers did not change the level of these synaptic proteins in WT mice, indicating that, most likely, the level of their mRNA expression was not affected [22]. Thus it is reasonable to think that the increased levels of pre- and postsynaptic proteins are more likely an effect of reduced synaptic loss in the treated AD transgenic animals (**Figure 8**). Thus a possible mechanism of memory protection in APP/PS1 could be the synapses were shielded by the dendrimers from toxic Aβ oligomers or the toxicity of Aβ oligomers were inactivated in the presence of the dendrimers.

4. Conclusions and perspectives

Dendrimers, which represent a type of 3D polymers, have been in the spotlight for three decades in biomedical and pharmaceutical research, and their chemistry and synthesis are continuously progressing by efforts from many research groups and companies. Although there are still many unclear problems in AD, in this chapter, functionalization of dendrimers dedicated to the prevention of memory decline in AD pathogenesis has been discussed. Based on the reviewed literature, PPI dendrimers have been shown to be useful in the way of the surface functionalization, which tuned their biochemical properties. Strikingly, the effect of the surface functionalization with histidine and maltose magnified exponentially neuroprotective properties of PPI dendrimers, resulting in an unprecedented outcome, such as memory protection in AD transgenic animals.

In this chapter, I have analyzed the functionalization of PPI dendrimers, which tuned the intrinsic properties of PPI dendrimers and converted them into a multifunctional drug candidate against Alzheimer's disease. Modification of the dendrimer surface with maltose allowed dendrimers successfully to interfere with Aβ(1–42) by forming nontoxic hybrid glycofibrils. Modification of the dendrimer surface with histidine improved the ability of the dendrimers to cross the blood–brain barrier and resulted in synaptic protection. By reducing the level of soluble amyloid oligomers, on the one hand, and conferring synapse protection, on the other hand, the dendrimers were given multifunctionality against main features of AD, synaptic loss, and aggregation of Aβ. These observations, coming out of the studies on the interaction of dendrimers with amyloid peptides [18, 22, 28, 32, 42], carried out in vitro and in vivo, point toward a possible use of dendrimers (in particular functionalization of PPI dendrimers with histidine and maltose) as a multifunctional drug candidate against Alzheimer's disease.

However, to find a successful drug against AD, other modifications of histidine-maltose PPI dendrimers might be required. For example, the ability to cross the blood-brain barrier, cell wall penetration, distribution in the specific tissue, and biodegradation could be tuned for a particular dendrimer application.

Acknowledgements

I acknowledge Dr. Dietmar Appelhans (Leibniz Institute of Polymer Research Dresden, Dresden, Germany) for the generation of histidine-maltose PPI dendrimers, collaboration, and valuable discussions.

The work is supported by MultiPark (Lund University), Vinnova, Swedish Research Council grants.

Thanks

I thank Dr. Stefan Broselid for fruitful discussions and editorial help.

Author details

Oxana Klementieva
Department of Experimental Medical Science, Faculty of Medicine, Lund University, Lund, Sweden

*Address all correspondence to: oxana.klementieva@med.lu.se

References

[1] Selkoe DJ. Alzheimer's disease is a synaptic failure. Science. 2002;**298**(5594):789-791

[2] Small DH, Mok SS, Bornstein JC. Alzheimer's disease and Aβ toxicity: From top to bottom. Nature Reviews. Neuroscience. 2001;**2**(8):595-598

[3] Davies CA, Mann DM, Sumpter PQ, Yates PO. A quantitative morphometric analysis of the neuronal and synaptic content of the frontal and temporal cortex in patients with Alzheimer's disease. Journal of the Neurological Sciences. 1987;**78**(2):151-164

[4] Martinsson I, Capetillo-Zarate E, Faideau M, Willén K, Esteras N, Frykman S, et al. APP depletion alters selective pre- and post-synaptic proteins. Molecular and Cellular Neurosciences. 2019;**95**:86-95

[5] Kamenetz F, Tomita T, Hsieh H, Seabrook G, Borchelt D, Iwatsubo T, et al. APP processing and synaptic function. Neuron. 2003;**37**(6):925-937

[6] Xue C, Tran J, Wang H, Park G, Hsu F, Guo Z. Aβ42 fibril formation from predominantly oligomeric samples suggests a link between oligomer heterogeneity and fibril polymorphism. Royal Society Open Science. 2019;**6**(7):190179

[7] Li X, Uemura K, Hashimoto T, Nasser-Ghodsi N, Arimon M, Lill CM, et al. Neuronal activity and secreted amyloid β lead to altered amyloid β precursor protein and presenilin 1 interactions. Neurobiology of Disease. 2013;**50**:127-134

[8] Takahashi RH, Nagao T, Gouras GK. Plaque formation and the intraneuronal accumulation of β-amyloid in Alzheimer's disease: Intraneuronal accumulation of β-amyloid. Pathology International. 2017;**67**(4):185-193

[9] Klementieva O, Willén K, Martinsson I, Israelsson B, Engdahl A, Cladera J, et al. Pre-plaque conformational changes in Alzheimer's disease-linked Aβ and APP. Nature Communications. 2017;**8**:14726

[10] Spires-Jones TL, Hyman BT. The intersection of amyloid Beta and tau at synapses in Alzheimer's disease. Neuron. 2014;**82**(4):756-771

[11] Lacor PN. Synaptic targeting by Alzheimer's-related amyloid oligomers. The Journal of Neuroscience. 2004;**24**(45):10191-10200

[12] Bilousova T, Miller CA, Poon WW, Vinters HV, Corrada M, Kawas C, et al. Synaptic amyloid-β oligomers precede p-tau and differentiate high pathology control cases. The American Journal of Pathology. 2016;**186**(1):185-198

[13] Takahashi RH. Oligomerization of Alzheimer's-amyloid within processes and synapses of cultured neurons and brain. The Journal of Neuroscience. 2004;**24**(14):3592-3599

[14] Bayer TA. Intracellular accumulation of amyloid-beta—A predictor for synaptic dysfunction and neuron loss in Alzheimer's disease. Frontiers in Aging Neuroscience. 2010. Available from: http://journal.frontiersin.org/article/10.3389/fnagi.2010.00008/abstract.[Accessed: 01 August 2019]

[15] Close W, Neumann M, Schmidt A, Hora M, Annamalai K, Schmidt M, et al. Physical basis of amyloid fibril polymorphism. Nature Communications. 2018;**9**(1):699

[16] Baghallab I, Reyes-Ruiz JM, Abulnaja K, Huwait E, Glabe C. Epitomic characterization of the specificity of the anti-amyloid Aβ monoclonal antibodies 6E10 and 4G8. Journal of Alzheimer's Disease. 2018;**66**(3):1235-1244

[17] Dhanavade MJ, Sonawane KD. Insights into the molecular interactions between aminopeptidase and amyloid beta peptide using molecular modeling techniques. Amino Acids. 2014;**46**(8):1853-1866

[18] Klementieva O, Benseny-Cases N, Gella A, Appelhans D, Voit B, Cladera J. Dense shell glycodendrimers as potential nontoxic anti-amyloidogenic agents in Alzheimer's disease. Amyloid–dendrimer aggregates morphology and cell toxicity. Biomacromolecules. 2011;**12**(11):3903-3909

[19] Svenson S, Tomalia DA. Dendrimers in biomedical applications—Reflections on the field. Advanced Drug Delivery Reviews. 2012;**64**:102-115

[20] Buhleier E, Wehner W, Vögtle F. "Cascade"- and "nonskid-chain-like" syntheses of molecular cavity topologies. Synthesis. 1978;**1978**(02):155-158

[21] Mark JE. Polymer Data Handbook. 2nd ed. Oxford, New York: Oxford University Press; 2009. p. 1250

[22] Aso E, Martinsson I, Appelhans D, Effenberg C, Benseny-Cases N, Cladera J, et al. Poly(propylene imine) dendrimers with histidine-maltose shell as novel type of nanoparticles for synapse and memory protection. Nanomedicine: Nanotechnology, Biology and Medicine. 2019;**17**:198-209

[23] Appelhans D, Klajnert-Maculewicz B, Janaszewska A, Lazniewska J, Voit B. Dendritic glycopolymers based on dendritic polyamine scaffolds: View on their synthetic approaches, characteristics and potential for biomedical applications. Chemical Society Reviews. 2015;**44**(12):3968-3996

[24] Mlynarczyk DT, Kocki T, Goslinski T. Dendrimer structure diversity and tailorability as a way to fight infectious diseases. In: Seehra MS, editor. Nanostructured Materials—Fabrication to Applications. London, United Kingdom: IntechOpen Limited; 2017

[25] Najlah M, D'Emanuele A. Synthesis of dendrimers and drug-dendrimer conjugates for drug delivery. Current Opinion in Drug Discovery and Development. 2007;**10**(6):756-767

[26] Wu G. Targeted delivery of methotrexate to epidermal growth factor receptor-positive brain tumors by means of cetuximab (IMC-C225) dendrimer bioconjugates. Molecular Cancer Therapeutics. 2006;**5**(1):52-59

[27] Huang R-Q, Qu Y-H, Ke W-L, Zhu J-H, Pei Y-Y, Jiang C. Efficient gene delivery targeted to the brain using a transferrin-conjugated polyethyleneglycol-modified polyamidoamine dendrimer. The FASEB Journal. 2007;**21**(4):1117-1125

[28] Klementieva O, Aso E, Filippini D, Benseny-Cases N, Carmona M, Juvés S, et al. Effect of poly(propylene imine) glycodendrimers on β-amyloid aggregation in vitro and in APP/PS1 transgenic mice, as a model of brain amyloid deposition and Alzheimer's disease. Biomacromolecules. 2013;**14**(10):3570-3580

[29] Arosio P, Cukalevski R, Frohm B, Knowles TPJ, Linse S. Quantification of the concentration of Aβ42 propagons during the lag phase by an amyloid chain reaction assay. Journal of the American Chemical Society. 2014;**136**(1):219-225

[30] Benseny-Cases N, Cócera M, Cladera J. Conversion of non-fibrillar β-sheet oligomers into amyloid fibrils in Alzheimer's disease amyloid peptide aggregation. Biochemical and Biophysical Research Communications. 2007;**361**(4):916-921

[31] Taneja V, Verma M, Vats A. Toxic species in amyloid disorders: Oligomers or mature fibrils. Annals of Indian Academy of Neurology. 2015;**18**(2):138

[32] McCarthy JM, Franke M, Resenberger UK, Waldron S, Simpson JC, Tatzelt J, et al. Anti-prion drug mPPIg5 Inhibits PrPC conversion to PrPSc. PLoS One. 2013;**8**(1):e55282

[33] McCarthy JM, Rasines Moreno B, Filippini D, Komber H, Maly M, Cernescu M, et al. Influence of surface groups on poly(propylene imine) dendrimers antiprion activity. Biomacromolecules. 2013;**14**(1):27-37

[34] Arosio P, Knowles TPJ, Linse S. On the lag phase in amyloid fibril formation. Physical Chemistry Chemical Physics. 2015;**17**(12):7606-7618

[35] Klajnert B, Peng L, Ceña V. Dendrimers in Biomedical Applications. Cambridge: European Cooperation in the Field of Scientific and Technical Research (Organization), Royal Society of Chemistry (Great Britain), RSC Publishing; 2013. 204 p

[36] Ottaviani FM, Cangiotti M, Fiorani L, Fattori A, Wasiak T, Appelhans D, et al. Kinetics of amyloid and prion fibril formation in the absence and presence of dense Shell sugar-decorated dendrimers. Current Medicinal Chemistry. 2012;**19**(34):5907-5921

[37] Jain K, Kesharwani P, Gupta U, Jain NK. A review of glycosylated carriers for drug delivery. Biomaterials. 2012;**33**(16):4166-4186

[38] Ziemba B, Janaszewska A, Ciepluch K, Krotewicz M, Fogel WA, Appelhans D, et al. In vivo toxicity of poly(propyleneimine) dendrimers. Journal of Biomedical Materials Research. Part A. 2011;**99A**(2):261-268

[39] Ciepluch K, Ziemba B, Janaszewska A, Appelhans D, Klajnert B, Bryszewska M, et al. Modulation of biogenic amines content by poly(propylene imine) dendrimers in rats. Journal of Physiology and Biochemistry. 2012;**68**(3):447-454

[40] Palmerston Mendes L, Pan J, Torchilin V. Dendrimers as nanocarriers for nucleic acid and drug delivery in cancer therapy. Molecules. 2017;**22**(9):1401

[41] Klajnert B, Appelhans D, Komber H, Morgner N, Schwarz S, Richter S, et al. The influence of densely organized maltose shells on the biological properties of poly(propylene imine) dendrimers: New effects dependent on hydrogen bonding. Chemistry: A European Journal. 2008;**14**(23):7030-7041

[42] Fischer M, Appelhans D, Schwarz S, Klajnert B, Bryszewska M, Voit B, et al. Influence of surface functionality of poly(propylene imine) dendrimers on protease resistance and propagation of the scrapie prion protein. Biomacromolecules. 2010;**11**(5):1314-1325

[43] Sperling R, Mormino E, Johnson K. The evolution of preclinical Alzheimer's disease: Implications for prevention trials. Neuron. 2014;**84**(3):608-622

[44] Yamakami J, Sakurai E, Sakurada T, Maeda K, Hikichi N. Stereoselective blood-brain barrier transport of histidine in rats. Brain Research. 1998;**812**(1-2):105-112

[45] Oshima T, Oshima C, Baba Y. Selective extraction of histidine derivatives by metal affinity with a copper(II)-chelating ligand complex in an aqueous two-phase system. Journal of Chromatography B. 2015;**990**:73-79

[46] Wang H, Wang M, Wang B, Li M, Chen H, Yu X, et al. The distribution profile and oxidation states of biometals in APP transgenic mouse brain: Dyshomeostasis with age and as a function of the development of Alzheimer's disease. Metallomics. 2012;**4**(3):289

[47] Tang S-C, Arumugam TV, Cutler RG, Jo D-G, Magnus T, Chan SL, et al. Neuroprotective actions of a

histidine analogue in models of ischemic stroke: Histidine analogue in models of ischemic stroke. Journal of Neurochemistry. 2007;**101**(3):729-736

[48] Jimenez JL, Nettleton EJ, Bouchard M, Robinson CV, Dobson CM, Saibil HR. The protofilament structure of insulin amyloid fibrils. Proceedings of the National Academy of Sciences. 2002;**99**(14):9196-9201

[49] Sulatskaya AI, Kuznetsova IM, Turoverov KK. Interaction of thioflavin T with amyloid fibrils: Fluorescence quantum yield of bound dye. The Journal of Physical Chemistry. B. 2012;**116**(8):2538-2544

[50] APPPS1. ALZFORUM [Internet]. Available from: https://www.alzforum.org/research-models/appps1 [Accessed: 01 August 2019]

[51] Radde R, Bolmont T, Kaeser SA, Coomaraswamy J, Lindau D, Stoltze L, et al. Aβ42-driven cerebral amyloidosis in transgenic mice reveals early and robust pathology. EMBO Reports. 2006;**7**(9):940-946

[52] Aso E, Lomoio S, López-González I, Joda L, Carmona M, Fernández-Yagüe N, et al. Amyloid generation and dysfunctional immunoproteasome activation with disease progression in animal model of familial Alzheimer's disease: Amyloid generation and UPS in FAD mice. Brain Pathology. 2012;**22**(5):636-653

[53] Shim KS, Lubec G. Drebrin, a dendritic spine protein, is manifold decreased in brains of patients with Alzheimer's disease and down syndrome. Neuroscience Letters. 2002;**324**(3):209-212

[54] Poirel O, Mella S, Videau C, Ramet L, Davoli MA, Herzog E, et al. Moderate decline in select synaptic markers in the prefrontal cortex (BA9) of patients with Alzheimer's disease at various cognitive stages. Scientific Reports. 2018;**8**(938):1-14

[55] Terry RD, Masliah E, Salmon DP, Butters N, DeTeresa R, Hill R, et al. Physical basis of cognitive alterations in Alzheimer's disease: Synapse loss is the major correlate of cognitive impairment. Annals of Neurology. 1991;**30**(4):572-580

[56] Nagura H, Ishikawa Y, Kobayashi K, Takao K, Tanaka T, Nishikawa K, et al. Impaired synaptic clustering of postsynaptic density proteins and altered signal transmission in hippocampal neurons, and disrupted learning behavior in PDZ1 and PDZ2 ligand binding-deficient PSD-95 knockin mice. Molecular Brain. 2012;**5**(1):43

[57] Schmitt U, Tanimoto N, Seeliger M, Schaeffel F, Leube RE. Detection of behavioral alterations and learning deficits in mice lacking synaptophysin. Neuroscience. 2009;**162**(2):234-243

[58] Mucke L, Masliah E, Yu GQ, Mallory M, Rockenstein EM, Tatsuno G, et al. High-level neuronal expression of a beta 1-42 in wild-type human amyloid protein precursor transgenic mice: Synaptotoxicity without plaque formation. Journal of Neuroscience: The Official Journal of the Society for Neuroscience. 2000;**20**(11):4050-4058

[59] Tampellini D, Capetillo-Zarate E, Dumont M, Huang Z, Yu F, Lin MT, et al. Effects of synaptic modulation on -amyloid, synaptophysin, and memory performance in Alzheimer's disease transgenic mice. The Journal of Neuroscience. 2010;**30**(43):14299-14304

Chapter 6

Alzheimer's Disease Neuroprotection: Associated Receptors

Alice Barros Câmara

Abstract

Research with humans and animals has been developed over the past few years to identify receptors involved in Alzheimer's disease, aiming at a better understanding of the mechanisms and pathophysiological aspects associated with the disease. Such receptors, whether or not directly associated with current AD therapy, are relevant since their blockage or activation might result in improving or worsening the clinical scenario of the disease. In other words, such receptors might be involved in the AD prognosis. This chapter discusses some relevant points about the receptors involved with AD.

Keywords: neuroprotection, Alzheimer disease, receptors, beta-amyloid peptides, central nervous system, agonists, antagonists

1. Introduction

Alzheimer's disease (AD) is the most recurring chronic and incurable neurodegenerative disorder. The main neuropathological findings on AD are beta-amyloid protein plaque (APP) deposition, an accumulation of hyperphosphorylated neurofibrillary tangles, inflammation, neurotransmitter signaling dysregulation, brain atrophy, and neuronal changes. AD affects the central nervous system (CNS) and results in an impaired emotional state, loss of synapses, neuronal death, and progressive cognitive decline. Some risk factors such as advanced age, genetic factors, and head trauma (among others) are involved in AD progression. Alzheimer's disease is responsible for marked morbidity and mortality due to the difficulty in treatment and irreversible damage. However, there is condition stabilization in some cases, and the individual can postpone their life expectancy for years [1].

2. Alzheimer's disease-associated receptors

2.1 Nicotinic acetylcholine receptor

Nicotinic acetylcholine receptors (nAChR) are involved with neuroprotective effects in AD. Furthermore, nAChR agonists and antagonists have been shown to have positive effects on memory. Cotinine and methyl cyclonite are examples of nAChR ligands associated with brain protection when in vitro and in vivo tests have been performed. In addition, nAChR and the muscarinic acetylcholine receptor family (mAChR) are acetylcholine targets in the brain. The nAChR family is affected in AD because beta-amyloid peptides (Aβ) can interact with these receptors [1]. Acetylcholine (Ach) plays a crucial role in CNS. Choline acetyltransferase enzyme is responsible for ACh synthesis from acetyl-CoA and choline in the cytoplasm. The acetylcholine vesicular transporter absorbs the neurotransmitter in synaptic vesicles. After depolarization, ACh undergoes exocytosis in reaching the synaptic cleft, where it can bind with its receptors. The ACh in the synaptic cleft is readily hydrolyzed by the acetylcholinesterase enzyme, forming acetate and choline, which is recycled at the presynaptic nerve terminal by the high-affinity choline transporter. Cholinergic neurons located in the basal forebrain, including the neurons which form Meynert's basal nucleus, are severely affected in AD. The loss of cholinergic neurons contributes to memory and attention deficits. Therefore, drugs acting on the cholinergic system represent a promising option for treating AD patients [2]. The conventional therapeutic prescription for AD consists of three acetylcholinesterase inhibitors and one NMDA receptor antagonist. Researchers around the world are developing new nAChR agonists to develop drugs with lower risks and adverse effects [3].

2.2 Estrogen receptor

Another important target in AD is the estrogen receptor (ER), which may represent a promising therapeutic approach since its activation through agonists prolongs survival, improves spatial recognition memory, and decreases the amyloid pathology progression in animal models of AD. On the other hand, estrogen receptor genetic polymorphisms have been associated with cognitive impairment, accelerated brain aging, and increased risk of AD, predominantly in women. A methylation promoter in estrogen receptor α is also related to impaired cognitive function and quality of life in AD patients by inhibiting ERα mRNA expression and transcription [4]. Estrogen can increase neural plasticity, cognitive functions, and the brain's regenerative potential. The beneficial effects of estrogen on neural plasticity occur at three levels: cellular, morphological, and synaptic function. Studies have shown that estradiol can increase neurogenesis in several brain regions, such as the hippocampal gyrus. These estrogen-induced hippocampal neurons contribute to learning and memory. Estradiol can also rapidly increase the number of dendritic spines in the hippocampus, amygdala, and hypothalamus and thus improve the performance in a hippocampal-dependent memory task. Moreover, estradiol is an effective enhancer of synaptic transmission in the hippocampal system. Estradiol plays an important role in promoting neurogenesis and neuronal plasticity to maintain healthy cognitive function and protect against women's cognitive decline during aging [5]. Therefore, estrogen with selective effects on ERα or G protein-coupled estrogen receptors (GPER1 or GqMER) can be used to influence the inflammation process resolution, with positive effects on AD progression [6].

2.3 Ryanodine receptor

Ryanodine receptors (RyR) are an ion channel family responsible for calcium release from intracellular reserves during muscle contraction. Calcium homeostasis is known to be related to cognition; thus, RyR may be associated with AD, especially RyR 3, which is found in various nervous system areas. In addition, RyR 1 and RyR 2 are also found in the brain, although they are not predominantly present in the nervous system. Ryanodine receptors can be regulated by several proteins and ions, as well as redox modifications. Antioxidants importantly prevent cognitive decline, long-term depolarization, and memory loss by inhibiting RyR sensitization [7]. Calcium-dependent signaling pathways are related to AD pathogenesis. A pharmacological approach (using a RyR stabilizing drug) or gene therapy of calcium leakage (mediated by RyR2) improved synaptic plasticity, and behavioral and cognitive functions and reduced Aβ loading. Genetically, altered mice (congenital leaking of RyR2) exhibited premature and severe defects in synaptic plasticity, and behavioral and cognitive function. These data provide an underlying mechanism for RyR2 channels, which can be considered as possible therapeutic targets in AD [8]. Additionally, calcium accumulation may result in the calpain and CaMKK2 activation, contributing to Aβ production and tau phosphorylation. Ryanodine receptor dysfunction can also lead to abnormal activation and accumulation of PKR kinase in AD brains. PKR kinase is linked to calcium accumulation and PKR autophosphorylation can be triggered by Aβ peptides in neuronal cultures in a calcium-dependent manner. In turn, PKR activation may lead to Aβ production by regulating BACE1 levels and abnormal tau protein phosphorylation by GSK3 activation. Dantrolene, a RyR inhibitor, may be an AD treatment [9].

2.4 Gamma-Aminobutyric Acid receptor

Gamma-Aminobutyric Acid receptor (GABAR) inhibition is also related to a better prognosis in AD. Gamma-Aminobutyric Acid receptor regulates learning, memory, and cognition, inhibits Adenylyl Cyclase and the cAMP cascade, as well as controls GABA and glutamate release. CGP35348 is a GABA receptor antagonist, and the CGP35348 hippocampal concentration is a crucial point for improving memory by reducing APP toxicity. Several neurological and psychiatric disorders occur with neuronal hyperexcitability in specific regions of the brain or spinal cord, partly due to some loss and/or dysfunction of GABAergic inhibitory interneurons [10]. Strategies which improve inhibitory neurotransmission in the affected brain regions may decrease deficits associated with these disorders. This perception has prompted an interest in testing the efficacy of GABAergic interneuron grafting in the brain or spinal cord regions which exhibit hyperexcitability, GABAergic interneurons scarcity, or impaired inhibitory neurotransmission, using preclinical models of neurological and psychiatric disorders [10]. Defective GABAergic neuronal functions can lead to cortical network hyperactivity and aberrant neuronal oscillations and thereby generate a detrimental change in memory processes [11]. In this context, GABAergic cell therapy may decrease neurological deficits in AD preclinical models [10]. Alzheimer patients have low GABA levels in the brain and spinal cerebrospinal fluid (SCF), and these changes are more severe in ApoE4 allele carriers. ApoE4 is associated with increased brain activity at rest and memory tasks, possibly reflecting impaired GABAergic inhibitory control. In addition, GABA levels in human SCF change with aging, constituting the strongest AD risk factor. Therefore, ApoE4 may at least partially contribute to the AD pathogenesis, causing age-dependent impairment in GABAergic interneurons [12].

2.5 Receptor for advanced glycation end products

The relationship between the receptor for advanced glycation end products (RAGE) and AD has also recently been established; RAGE is widely expressed and regulated in the AD brain. Furthermore, RAGE is involved with the transport of beta-amyloid protein through the blood-brain barrier (BBB) to the brain parenchyma. Interactions between RAGE and APP result in inflammatory responses and oxidative stress, as well as reduce cerebral blood flow. The receptor also inhibits the elimination of APP and RAGE ligands such as AGE, HMGB1, and S100β, which are involved in the neurodegenerative disease progression. Additionally, RAGE/AGE interactions induce the apoptosis cascade and neuronal inflammation [7]. In addition, RAGE has been considered as a therapeutic approach in AD; in fact, a RAGE antagonist demonstrated a protective effect in an animal model. Chronic oral dosing of PF-04494700 antagonist in transgenic AD mice reduced Aβ levels, improved performance in spatial memory testing, and normalized the electrophysiological recordings of hippocampal slices. According to the results of the Phase II clinical study [13], the RAGE inhibitor has an excellent safety profile and is well-tolerated for over 10 weeks in patients with oral AD. These inhibitors block the binding of Aβ peptides to the RAGE V domain as well as inhibit the cell stress induced by Aβ in cells expressing RAGE in vitro, as well as in the brains of mice [14].

Moreover, a RAGE inhibitor (FPS-ZM1) has no animal toxic activity and easily crosses the BBB. In aged mice with AD, FPS-ZM1 can inhibit the RAGE-mediated influx of Aβ40 and Aβ42 in the brain. FPS-ZM1 binds exclusively to RAGE in the brain, inhibiting Aβ production and suppressing microglia activation and neuroinflammatory response. Blocking RAGE actions in the SCF and brain normalizes cognitive performance and cerebral blood flow. FPS-ZM1 is a potent RAGE blocker, thereby controlling the progression of Aβ-mediated brain disorder [14]. Furthermore, metabolic syndrome is a risk factor for cognitive decline in AD, and RAGE has been associated with metabolic syndrome, as this receptor directly contributes to an inflammatory process and oxidative stress. Thus, the RAGE inhibition is able to reduce cellular toxicity, and therefore, RAGE inhibitors have therapeutic potential in retarding AD progression [15].

2.6 Vitamin D receptor

Vitamin D (VD) acts through the vitamin D receptor (VDR), expressed in various tissues, including the nervous system. Vitamin D receptor is related to memory and cognitive functions. Research has reported a higher prevalence of VD deficiency in AD patients and individuals with VD deficiency had twice the risk of developing AD compared with individuals with sufficient VD concentrations. Several potential mechanisms which link low VD levels to the risk of dementia have been identified. First, VDR is expressed throughout the brain, including areas involved in memory, such as the hippocampus. The enzyme which synthesizes the active form of VD, 1α-hydroxylase, is also produced in various brain areas. Second, the VD active form (1,25dihydroxyvitamin D3 or 1,25-D3) regulates neurotrophin expression, such as neurotrophin 3, Glial cell-derived neurotrophic factor (GDNF) and neural growth factor (NGF). NGF has been implicated in maintaining and regulating the normal function of the septohippocampal pathway, which is involved in learning and memory. In addition, NGF levels are substantially reduced in AD patients and NGF negatively modulates APP protein gene expression, while increased APP expression is observed after NGF suppression. Furthermore, VD analogs increase APP binding to the NGF promoter, inducing NGF expression. Therefore, 1,25-D3 contributes to the development, survival, and function of neural cells [16].

Third, VD can stimulate macrophages, which increases amyloid plaque clearance. Fourth, the antioxidant effect of VD may be related to the modulation of antioxidant gene expression. Oxidative stress is known to contribute to the pathophysiology of neurodegenerative diseases, which leads to impaired cognitive and behavioral function. Genetic analyses of the human genome have pointed to several genes playing a role in susceptibility to AD, such as genes which are involved in inflammation and oxidative stress [7]. Fifth, VD also plays a role in vascular protection. Sixth, VD regulates neurotransmitter metabolism in the CNS, such as acetylcholine, dopamine, serotonin, and aminobutyric gamma acid. Finally, VD also reduces Aβ-induced cytotoxicity and apoptosis in primary cortical neurons. A recent study found that Aβ induction of nitric oxide synthase, part of the AD inflammatory process, depends on the VDR pathway disruption. VD supplementation improves age-related cognitive decline, learning, and memory in older rats. A cross-sectional study found that VD deficiency was associated with increased white matter volume and reduced gray matter volume. In summary, low VD concentrations may increase the risk of dementia and AD through vascular and neurodegenerative mechanisms [16].

2.7 Retinoid X receptor

Vitamin D receptor interacts with the retinoid receptor X (RXR) to perform VD actions. Retinoid receptor X activation can stimulate the normal physiological processes by which APP is eliminated from the brain. Thus, RXR agonists may be useful in treating AD. Two-week treatment with an RXR agonist (bexarotene) in an AD animal model resulted in clearance of intraneuronal amyloid deposits. Additionally, treatment with bexarotene improved remote memory stabilization in fear-conditioned mice and improved olfactory habituation. In addition, bexarotene pretreatment improved neuronal survival in response to glutamate-induced excitotoxicity. The bexarotene effects were accompanied by reduced amyloid plaque levels, decreased astrogliosis and suppression of inflammatory gene expression. Therefore, treatment with RXR agonists can decrease neuron loss, reverse cognitive deficits, and improve neural circuit function in aggressive AD models [17]. Retinoid receptor X agonists can increase the expression of ApoE, ABCA1, and ABCG1 by activating RXR heterodimers. On the other hand, these beneficial effects are blocked by the RXR antagonist, which can accentuate cellular oxidative stress [18].

Interestingly, RXR decreased expression was identified in the AD mouse model and in cells treated with Aβ peptides [19]. However, the action mechanism of RXR ligands remains unknown, particularly in the context of human ApoE [20]. Retinoids have effects on various physiological and pathological processes in the brain. For example, retinoic acid (RA) signaling is widely detected in the adult CNS, including the amygdala, cortex, hypothalamus, hippocampus, and other brain areas. Retinoids are mainly involved in neural patterns, axon differentiation, and cell growth. Retinoids also play a key role in preserving the differentiated state of adult neurons. Impaired RA signaling may result in neurodegeneration and AD progression. Recent studies have shown severe deficiencies in mouse learning and memory during RA deprivation, indicating its importance in preserving memory. Defective cholinergic neurotransmission is related to cognitive deficits in AD. Retinoic acid is also known to increase choline acetyltransferase expression and the activity in neuronal cell lines. In addition, retinoids have been shown to inhibit the expression of proinflammatory chemokines and cytokines in microglia and astrocytes, which are activated in AD [21].

2.8 N-methyl-d-aspartate receptors

N-methyl-d-aspartate receptors (NMDAR) participate in CNS development and are involved in synaptic plasticity, which is essential for learning and memory. Cognitive symptoms associated with learning and memory deficits have been associated with glutaminergic neurotransmission disorders. Excitatory glutaminergic neurotransmission via NMDAR is critical for synaptic plasticity and neuron survival. However, excessive neuron stimulation by the glutamate neurotransmitter causes cytotoxicity and results in neuronal damage and death, underlying a potential mechanism of neurodegeneration in AD. Therefore, blocking NMDAR receptor-mediated glutaminergic neurotransmission can decrease cytotoxicity, thereby preventing further damage to neurons and cellular oxidative damage [22]. Therefore, NMDAR antagonists have emerged as potential compounds for AD patients since the receptor itself has many subunits and its variants have several brain functions. For example, conantokine acts as an NMDA receptor antagonist and plays an important role in understanding the importance of NMDA receptor inhibition in the AD treatment. Moreover, NMDAR activation might be blocked by an AD drug, memantine, an NMDAR antagonist which selectively blocks the function of extra synaptic NMDARs, but does not affect normal neurotransmission. However, memantine (and other current medications used to treat AD) only relieve the symptoms and do not alter the disease progression [23].

2.9 Cholesterol receptors

Regarding cholesterol receptors, some specific genotypes have been related to a higher or lower risk of dementia and AD. Even genotypes associated with AD neuropathology attenuation could be associated with late-onset of dementia. Liver nuclear X receptors (LXRs) are the main regulators of cholesterol homeostasis and CNS inflammation. The brain, which contains about 25% of total body cholesterol, requires a complex and balanced cholesterol metabolism to maintain neuronal function. Deregulation of cholesterol metabolism has been implicated in several neurodegenerative diseases, including AD. Due to their anti-inflammatory activities, LXRs play a crucial role in CNS function. Although LXR agonists have therapeutic potential in neurological diseases, the use of LXR in these pathologies remains problematic. The recent discovery of cholesterol derivatives which function as LXR agonists has shown new roles for LXRs in midbrain neurogenesis. Elucidating the repertoire of endogenous ligands for LXR will improve the understanding of how this receptor regulates CNS lipid metabolism [24].

Nuclear X receptor signaling affects AD development through various pathways. Studies indicate that LXR genetic loss in transgenic mice results in increased amyloid plaques. Studies also suggest that LXRs activation in mice improves the expression of cholesterol efflux-linked genes (ApoE and ABCA-1), induces APP processing, and reduces Aß synthesis, with significant improvement in memory. Furthermore, LXR agonists have also been shown to inhibit neuroinflammation by modulating microglial phagocytosis and repressing COX2, MCP1, and INOS expression in glial cells [25]. The T allele of NR1H2 (rs2695121) presents the most significant risk for AD among all LXR-β gene polymorphisms. Taken together, these findings suggest that brain-penetrable LXR agonists or LXR modulators may be useful therapeutic agents for AD treatment and prevention [26].

Additionally, chromosome 12p has been recognized as an AD-associated region. This chromosome includes genes for LDL receptor 1 (LRP1) and oxidized low-density lipoprotein receptor 1 (OLR1). OLR1 is a class E scavenger receptor and is a transmembrane glycoprotein. In vitro factors such as oxidized LDL, oxidative stress, and inflammatory cytokines, as well as in vivo factors such as diabetes mellitus, hyperlipidemia, and hypertension, may induce OLR1 expression. Increased oxidized LDL levels induce endothelial cell activation and dysfunction, apoptosis, and impaired vessel relaxation, thus contributing to atherosclerosis development and progression through OLR1. Epidemiological and clinical literature has reported an association between atherosclerosis, vascular risk factors, and AD. Therefore, ORL1 variations may lead to low efficiency in the oxidized LDL removal and therefore increased Aβ levels, which may result in neuronal death. Indeed, a single nucleotide polymorphism in OLR1 located in the 3′ untranslated region of the gene may influence regulatory microRNA binding and OLR1 homeostasis. Several studies have reported an association between this variant and AD [27].

2.10 Toll-like receptors

Toll-like receptors (TLRs) are innate immune system receptors which are activated by pathogens (PAMP) or damage-associated molecular patterns (DAMPs). Toll-like receptors are associated with neuronal injury in chronic inflammatory conditions but also with functional recovery after nerve injury. Amyloid aggregates seem to be a type of DAMP and may interact and activate standard recognition receptors. Two TLR actions (ligand binding and immune signaling) may have beneficial effects on AD pathology. Moreover, microglial activation represents an important AD hallmark. Analysis of genetic polymorphisms suggested relationships between TLR polymorphisms and AD risk, further supporting the hypothesis that TLRs are involved in AD [28]. In fact, TLR2 is elevated in the hippocampus and cortex of AD patients and mice. In this context, it was observed that a TLR2-binding peptide (WT TIDM) inhibited Aβ-induced microglial activation, reduced Aβ load, attenuated neuronal apoptosis, and improved memory and learning in mice. However, WT TIDM peptide was not effective in TLR2 knockout mice [29].

Importantly, TLR5 binds to APP with high-affinity, forming complexes which block APP toxicity. In turn, APP fibrils modulate the human TLR5 activation via flagellin, but APP cannot activate TLR5 signaling by themselves. Thus, TLR5-related biological data suggest this receptor as a potential agent in AD therapy [30]. A new TLR9 signaling pathway has recently been associated with the immune-inflammatory response, reducing Aβ levels in AD mice. Therefore, TLR9 may represent a functional candidate gene for AD [31]. Moreover, TLR4 has also been described in the brain and seems to regulate some physiological processes such as neurogenesis. In this sense, TLR4 plays an important role during neurodegenerative disorders. PRDX6 has been shown to inhibit neural stem cell neurogenesis by down-regulating the TLR4 signaling pathway [32]. An early TLR3-mediated signal improves Aβ neuronal autophagy, although it increases neuronal apoptosis in the late stage of AD. Similarly, TLR7, TLR8, and TLR9 may improve early Aβ microglial uptake, but over time, they contribute to neuroinflammation. Therefore, TLRs, in particular TLR2 and TLR4, represent suitable targets for therapeutic intervention in AD and carefully targeting them may increase Aβ autophagy and phagocytosis, as well as reduce inflammatory responses. Several modulators with selective TLR agonist or antagonist activity have been developed, and many of them could produce a therapeutic benefit in AD patients [33].

2.11 Chemokine receptors

Another molecule involved in AD is the chemokine receptor CX3C1 (CX3CR1), which performs IL-1β-dependent cognitive functions. It is known that CX3CR1 maintains microglial homeostasis and is essential for microglia function in synaptic support since it is highly expressed in microglia. In vivo, CX3CR1-GFP knock-in mice (in which GFP replaced a CX3CR1 allele) were used to study the role of microglia in AD and other brain diseases. Under physiological conditions, decreased CX3CR1 function affects cognitive functions in an IL-1β-dependent manner, as well as exacerbates LPS-induced inflammation, suggesting that CX3CR1 is essential for nerve synapses. In this context, CX3CL1/CX3CR1 axis dysregulation in AD may have neuroprotective and neurotoxic effects depending on the model used. It is also possible that CX3CR1 is involved in the death of neurons with intracellular TAU deposits and the subsequent TAU release [34]. Still, regarding chemokine receptors, CCL2 receptor (CCR2) was also associated with AD since CCR2 promotes the recruitment of bone marrow monocytes into the APP deposition sites in the parenchyma, where APP phagocytosis occurs. In mice, CCR2 deficiency accelerated early AD progression, impairing mononuclear phagocyte accumulation. CCR2−/− mice exhibited high APP levels and low CD11b+ cell recruitment in the brain. Importantly, these mice had increased mortality in a dose-dependent manner of the CCR2 gene. Subsequent studies showed that APP reduction is due to the monocyte accumulation in the perivascular spaces and possibly its infiltration into the brain parenchyma. These findings were corroborated by the fact that CCR2 deficiency worsened memory and increased soluble APP levels in mice [34].

2.12 Glucocorticoid receptors

The main AD risk factor is aging, but there is growing evidence that chronic stress or stress-related disorders may increase the chance of developing AD. Thus, depressive disorder may be a risk factor for AD [35]. Stress promotes AD progression on neurons and glial cells, supporting an important pro-inflammatory role of glucocorticoid (GC) in the CNS [36]. Glucocorticoids act via two receptors: mineralocorticoid and glucocorticoid receptors (GR) and can participate in APP generation and APP activity in the brain. There is a cross-talk between APP and GRs in hippocampal excitatory synapses, which may contribute to abnormal brain activity during the AD pathogenesis. Both AD patients and AD mice have dysregulated hypothalamic-pituitary-adrenal (HPA) axis, marked by hypercortisolemia early in the AD pathology. Thus, in early AD, while APP levels slowly increase in the brain, GR activity is probably abnormally high [37]. Moreover, GRs hyperactivation induces brain changes similar to AD changes. In the brain, GCs are regulators of dendritic spine renewal and microglia activity, two strongly altered phenomena in AD. Although well established that GCs initiate the brain neuroinflammatory response, it is not known whether GRs modulate dendritic spine plasticity and microglial activity in AD [36].

Several strategies aiming GR has been tested to counteract HPA axis dysregulation and GC overproduction. Given the GR ubiquitous expression, antagonists have many side effects, limiting the GR therapeutic potential. However, a new class of selective molecules has been developed, acting as GR modulators. They selectively reduce GR-dependent pathogenic processes while retaining the beneficial aspects of GR signaling. Indeed, these "selective GR modulators" induce receptor conformations that allow the activation of only a subset of downstream signaling pathways, explaining their ability to combine agonistic and antagonistic properties. Therefore, targeting GR with selective modulators, alone or in association with current strategies, is attractive to develop new strategies aiming disorders associated with HPA axis dysregulation [35]. Dexamethasone, a GR agonist, was able to reduce the dendritic spine density, induced the microglia proliferation, and activated the microglia in the mouse hippocampus. Besides, in vitro microglial cells were activated by dexamethasone. In contrast, treatment with mifepristone, a GRs antagonist, strongly increased dendritic column density, decreased microglia density, and improved mice behavioral performance [36].

2.13 G-protein-coupled receptor 40

There are a large number of polyunsaturated fatty acids in the nervous system, such as docosahexaenoic acid (DHA), an omega 3 carboxylic acid. The DHA binds to G-protein-coupled receptor 40 (GPR40) and exerts protective effects on the nervous system. For example, GPR40 can increase synaptic plasticity, neuronal activity, and inhibits neuronal apoptosis. In this context, GPR40 was considered a possible target in dementia [38]. The receptor is expressed in several brain areas, including the hippocampus, which is involved in learning and spatial memory. However, few studies are investigating the functional role of GPR40 in the brain [39]. One study evaluated the GPR40 functional role in the AD mouse model. Groups treated with GPR40 significantly improved cognitive performance and GPR40 agonist-treated groups improved learning and memory skills in various tests. Besides, GPR40 activation caused CREB phosphorylation and increased neurotrophic factors levels, including brain-derived neurotrophic factor (BDNF), nerve growth factor (NGF), neurotrophin-3 (NT-3), and neurotrophin-4 (NT-4) in hippocampal neurons. These results suggest that GPR40 can be a therapeutic candidate for neurogenesis and neuroprotection in AD treatment and prevention [39] since GPR40 agonists can promote adult neurogenesis, inhibit neuronal apoptosis, and play a vital role in protecting nerves and decreasing brain damage [38].

2.14 Triggered receptor expressed on myeloid cells 2

The triggered receptor expressed in myeloid cells 2 (TREM2) is a soluble protein carried by macrophages through ventricles and choroid plexus, entering the brain parenchyma through radial glial cells. TREM2 is important for innate immunity, but it is also essential for neuroplasticity and myelination. During later stages of life, the TREM2 absence can accelerate aging processes, neuronal cell loss and reduce microglial activity, leading to neuroinflammation. Inflammation plays an important role in neurodegenerative diseases and TREM2 can be important to immunomodulation and neuroprotection [40]. As a member of the immunoglobulin superfamily, TREM2 can suppress inflammatory responses, mediates phagocytic pathways, is involved with neuronal survival and neurogenesis, as well as contributes to CNS neuroimmune homeostasis. Changes in TREM2 are involved in AD-related neuropathology, including Aβ deposition, tau hyperphosphorylation, neuroinflammation, and neuronal and synaptic losses in AD animal models. However, the precise underlying mechanisms about TREM2 have not yet been fully characterized [41]. Besides, TREM2 might be related to microglial activation, promoting the association of microglial cells with APP plaques. Therefore, microglia can decrease APP plaque growth, limiting APP toxicity. On the other hand, this phagocytotic capacity is impaired by TREM2 deficiency. Moreover, different mutations in TREM2 are associated with AD [42, 43]. Interestingly, recent findings also suggested that the association between TREM2 variants and the AD risk varies according to different ethnicities and populations [41].

2.15 5-Hydroxytryptamine 6 receptor

The serotoninergic neurotransmitter system has been implicated in AD pathogenesis. The 5-hydroxytryptamine 6 receptor (5HTR6) is expressed in brain areas involved with cognitive processes and has been investigated as a possible therapeutic target in AD symptomatology. Besides, 5HTR6 may be added to currently approved "Food and Drug Administration" therapies: cholinesterase inhibitors and NMDA receptor antagonists since 5HTR6 controls the pyramidal neurons' migration during corticogenesis. In addition, 5HTR6 is a TOR signaling activator and seems to regulate GABAergic, glutamatergic, and cholinergic activity. Therefore, 5HTR6 is involved in cognition, anxiety, memory, affective state, among others [44]. Several kinds of research have been conducted with selective 5HTR6 antagonists. These antagonists act by modulating the glutamate and GABA levels, consequently increasing dopamine, ACh, and norepinephrine concentrations in the brain, all compromised in AD. Besides, 5HTR6 agonists have also been shown to have pro-cognitive effects. Partial or inverse agonists may produce promising cognitive effects [44, 45]. Moreover, 5HTR6 gene variants can be a genetic risk factor for late-onset AD and 5HTR6 polymorphisms are possibly involved with AD susceptibility, such as the C267T polymorphism [44]. However, there are relatively few genetic studies investigating the association between AD and gene variants involved in the serotonergic system.

2.16 Cannabinoid receptors

Evidence regarding the involvement of the endocannabinoid system (ECS) in the AD pathogenesis raised questions about the development of new therapeutic approaches for AD based on endocannabinoid regulation. The endocannabinoid system is composed of receptors, endogenous ligands, and enzymes, which are involved in AD pathogenesis [46]. Endocannabinoid system-directed drugs can exert beneficial effects on mood, as well as modulate neuroinflammation, synaptic plasticity, neurotoxicity, apoptosis, cell proliferation, cell differentiation, and oxidative stress [47, 48]. Moreover, cannabis tetrahydrocannabinol (THC) induces neurogenesis, removes Aβ peptides, and decreases neurofibrillary tangles. The hippocampus and microglia, key actors in dementia pathophysiology, express 1 and 2 cannabinoid receptors, respectively [49]. Type 2 cannabinoid receptor (CNR2) is overexpressed in activated microglia in different areas of the nervous system. Activated CNR2 has the potential to disrupt the AD process and treat the symptoms, reducing neurodegeneration, neuroinflammation, and improving spatial memory [50]. The role of the type 1 cannabinoid receptor (CNR1) is unclear. However, CNR1 can up-regulate anti-apoptotic proteins in rats [49].

2.17 Peroxisome proliferator-activated γ receptor

Peroxisome proliferator-activated γ receptor (PPARγ) regulates the transcription of several genes involved in inflammation, immune response, insulin sensitivity, and lipid metabolism. The pathways governed by PPARγ overlap the biological pathways implicated in AD pathogenesis according to various pieces of evidence. Besides, PPARγ regulates the expression of seven AD-associated genes, including ApoE, ABCA1, and ABCG1. Increasing ApoE lipid levels facilitate soluble Aβ degradation. Studies using AD animal models have suggested that PPARγ exerts direct and indirect effects on APP protein metabolism [51]. Peroxisome proliferator-activated γ receptor is up-regulated in AD due to existing neuroinflammation and PPARγ agonists can be used in AD and shows anti-inflammatory effects, as well as improve learning and memory. Thus, PPARγ might be a significant new therapeutic target in AD treatment [52]. In addition, emerging evidence suggests that PPARγ effectively regulates microglia activation under physiological and pathological conditions, facilitating Aβ microglial phagocytosis [53]. In addition, PPARγ polymorphisms have been studied in AD; however, the results are controversial and inconclusive [54].

2.18 NOD-like receptor pyrin domain-containing-3

The NOD-like receptor pyrin domain-containing-3 (NLRP3) is the best known member of the NLR family. Importantly, APP can activate the NLRP3 inflammasome and increase NLRP3, caspase1, and IL1-β genes expression [55]. In microglia, NLRP3 activation is essential for interleukin-1β (IL1-β) maturation and subsequent inflammatory events. Besides, NLRP3 is possibly involved in AD pathogenesis through oxidative stress [56]. One study showed that NLRP3 knock-out mice were largely protected from spatial memory loss and other AD-associated sequelae, showing reduced caspase-1 and IL1-β activation, as well as increased Aβ clearance. Microglial activation by Aβ can initiate innate immune responses in CNS via NLRP3, even before the Aβ deposition. These results show an important role of the NLRP3 axis in the AD pathogenesis and suggest that NLRP3 inflammasome inhibition might be a new therapeutic intervention for the disease [57]. Non-steroidal anti-inflammatory drugs can inhibit NLRP3 inflammasome via reversible blockade of volume-regulated anionic channels in the plasma membrane, inhibiting cognitive impairment in AD mice models [58]. The loss of NLRP3 inflammasome function also reduced tau hyperphosphorylation and aggregation (involved in AD pathogenesis) by regulating tau kinases and phosphatases. Tau, in turn, activated the NLRP3 inflammasome. The intracerebral injection containing Aβ induced tau pathology in an NLRP3-dependent manner. Therefore, these data suggest an important role of NLRP3, microglia, and inflammasome activation in AD tauopathies [59]. Finally, virgin coconut oil improved hippocampal health, memory, and learning in AD mice models by inhibiting NLRP3 and reducing oxidative stress [55].

3. Conclusion

Nuclear receptors family and G-protein-coupled receptors are probably the receptors families most involved with AD (**Table 1**). Additionally, the cerebral cortex is the main area where most of the receptors involved in AD express themselves. The cerebral cortex's physical area, its complexity, and its involvement with several relevant functions in AD probably justify this fact. Despite the small size of the hippocampus, this region is significantly affected in AD. While the cerebral cortex is mainly involved in decision making, subjective thinking, consequences of action assessment, perception, and attention, the hippocampus is mainly related to memory. As a key component of cortico-hippocampal networks, the perirenal cortex plays an important role in memory processes, especially familiarity-based recognition memory. Therefore, disrupted functional connectivity of this cortical region as a result of early neurodegeneration may contribute to altered brain rhythms and cognitive failures observed in the early clinical phase of AD patients [11].

Although few receptors involved with AD are expressed in the hypothalamus and amygdala (when compared to the expression in the cortex, hippocampus, pons, medulla, and basal ganglia), it is known that AD is closely associated with changes in mood and motivation. However, these associations depend on the AD stage. Most of the receptors involved with AD are expressed in more than one nervous system area, showing the involvement of several brain regions in AD. Additionally, microglia is one of the main cell types in which AD-associated receptors express themselves, highlighting the relevance of microglia in AD, especially in the removal of toxic peptides. Additionally, AD-associated receptors are involved with several metabolic pathways, which may be directly or indirectly related to the disease. The APP elimination or the blockage of pathways related to the APP synthesis is the main function performed by the receptors involved with AD (**Table 1**, **Figure 1**). Besides, many receptors are directly involved with cognitive, memory, and/or learning functions and many receptors are associated with more than one AD-related function (**Table 1**, **Figure 1**). Finally, AD-associated receptors are also related to nervous system plasticity, including neuronal and microglial survival, nervous system development (positive plasticity), and neuronal death (negative plasticity).

Receptor/family	Main expression area in human CNS	Main roles in AD
Acetylcholine receptors (AChR) Nicotinic Receptors	Cerebral cortex and cerebellum	Interacts with APP protein and exert positive effects on memory and attention [1, 2].
Estrogen receptors (ER) Nuclear receptor family	Basal ganglia and hippocampus	Increases neural plasticity and neurogenesis, affecting cognitive functions and the brain regenerative potential. May play beneficial effects in reducing the brain inflammatory process [4–6].
Ryanodine receptor 3 (RyR3) Calcium channels	Basal ganglia	Plays negative effects related to synaptic transmission and synaptic plasticity. Associated with memory loss and age-related cognition decline [7–9].
Gamma-Aminobutyric Acid receptor (GABAR) Ionotropic receptor	Cerebral cortex	Regulates learning, memory, cognitive function, controls the glutamate release, and reduces APP toxicity [10–12].
Receptor for advanced glycation end products (RAGE) Immunoglobulins superfamily	Cerebellum	Contributes to neuronal death and inflammation and is involved with the APP transport, oxidative stress, and cerebral blood flow [14, 15].
Vitamina D receptor (VDR) Nuclear receptor family	Cerebral cortex and hippocampus	Interacts with SMAD3, regulating APP transcription through TGFβ signaling. Suppress APP gene promoter activity [16].
Retinoid X receptor (RXR) Nuclear receptor family	Cerebral cortex	Stimulates physiological mechanisms of APP elimination, decreasing APP-induced deficits [17, 18, 21].
N-methyl-D-aspartate receptors (NMDAR) Ionotropic receptor	Cerebral cortex and hypothalamus	Participates in CNS development and is involved in synaptic plasticity, essential for learning and memory [22, 23].
Liver X receptor β (LXR) Nuclear receptor family	Cerebral cortex	Regulates the cholesterol homeostasis and inflammation in CNS. May play roles in neurogenesis, APP processing, and microglial phagocytosis modulation [24–26].
Low-density lipoprotein receptor (LDLR) Lipoprotein receptor family	Pons and medulla	Mediates the increase in ApoE expression induced by APP protein [27].
Oxidized low-density lipoprotein receptor 1 (OLR1) Lipoprotein receptor family	Midbrain	Mediates the uptake and internalization of low-density oxidized lipoprotein (oxLDL), which may be involved in AD [27].
Toll-like receptor 4 (TLR4) Toll-like receptor family	Hippocampus	Induces CREB signaling, which regulates neuron survival, neuronal gene expression, and neurogenesis in the adult subventricular zone [28, 32, 33].
Toll-like receptor 5 (TLR5) Toll-like receptor family	Thalamus	Binds to APP oligomers and fibrils, forming complexes that block APP toxicity [28, 30, 31].
C-C chemokine receptor type 2 (CCR2) Chemokine receptor family	Pons and medulla	Promotes monocyte recruitment to APP deposition sites, where these cells can phagocyte APP proteins [34].
Chemokine receptor CX3C 1 (CX3CR1) Chemokine receptor family	Midbrain, pons, and medulla	Maintains microglial function in synaptic support and performs IL-1β dependent cognitive functions [34].

Receptor/family	Main expression area in human CNS	Main roles in AD
Glucocorticoid receptor (GCRs) Glucocorticoid receptor family	Cerebellum	Participates in the generation and activity of APP protein in the brain [36, 37].
G-protein-coupled receptor 40 (GPR40) G-protein-coupled receptor family	Spinal cord	Promotes neurogenesis, inhibits neuronal apoptosis, and plays a role in protecting nerves and decreasing brain damage [38, 39].
Triggered receptor expressed on myeloid cells 2 (TREM-2) Immunoglobulins superfamily	Midbrain	Participates in microglial survival, inflammatory response, phagocytosis, dendritic cell maturation and others [40–43].
5-hydroxytryptamine 6 receptor (5 HTR6) G-protein-coupled receptor family	Basal ganglia	Controls the pyramidal neurons migration during corticogenesis, activates TOR signaling, and regulates the GABAergic, glutamatergic, and cholinergic activity. Involved in cognition, anxiety, memory, mood, among others [44, 45].
Cannabinoid receptor (CNR) G-protein-coupled receptor family	Cerebral cortex	Disrupt the AD process, reduce symptoms, neurodegeneration, neuroinflammation, and improve spatial memory [47–50].
Peroxisome proliferator-activated γ receptor (PPARγ) Nuclear receptor family	Amygdala	Participates in pathways involved with lipid metabolism and immune response implicated in AD etiology. PPARγ acts as a transcriptional regulator of several genes involved in AD pathogenesis [51–53].
NOD-like receptor pyrin domain-containing-3 (NLRP3) NOD-like receptor family	Pons and medulla	The NLRP3 activation leads to IL-1β and IL-18 production that play a role in the inflammatory response and oxidative stress in AD pathogenesis. [56–59].
Sigma-1 receptor (σ1R) Chaperone protein	Cerebral cortex	Inhibits enzymes involved in AD, such as acetylcholinesterase, 5-lipoxygenase, and monoamine oxidase. Protects neurons against oxidative stress, contributing to neuronal tissues repair [64].
Calcium sensing receptor (CaSR) G-protein-coupled receptor family	Cerebral cortex and hippocampus	Role in hippocampal neurons degeneration. APP is able to increase intracellular calcium by opening calcium-permeable cationic channels in hippocampal neurons [65].

Table 1.
Alzheimer's disease associated receptors.

This suggests that these receptors participate in several long-term changes in the nervous system (long-term plasticity) [60].

Finally, most of the receptors involved in AD (67%) are associated with beneficial effects on the disease. These receptors include nuclear receptors, such as VDR, membrane receptors, such as TLR5, and cytoplasmic receptors, such as GABAR. Most of the AD-associated receptors are found in the membrane of nerve cells (61%). Among the neuroprotective receptors, we can highlight the vitamin D receptor, responsible for vitamin D actions. Vitamin D is increasingly recognized as a substance involved in neuronal survival, taking part in psychiatric and

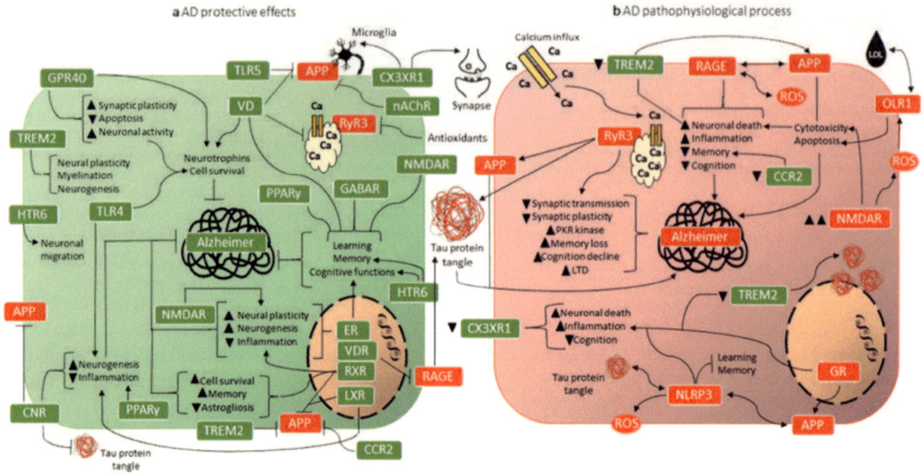

Figure 1.
Proteins associated with AD. Proteins related to AD are shown according to their protective (a) or pathological (b) effects in AD. The receptors located in the green boxes are associated with neuroprotective effects on AD. Receptors located in red boxes are associated with AD pathophysiology. Proteins are shown according to their location in the cell (nucleus, membrane, intracellular or extracellular). Arrows/triangles represent activation, induction or increase. Inverted bars/triangles represent inhibition, deficit or decrease. Protein associated to AD protection are related to proteins involved in AD pathophysiological process. Two triangles represent overactivation. Elements in the figure are not showed in real scale. ROS, reactive oxygen.

neurodegenerative diseases such as AD. The participation of vitamin D in neuronal survival may be related to its role in inhibiting the cellular oxidative stress and APP synthesis. Therefore, supplementation with vitamin D can help in the current AD treatment [61]. A beneficial role in inflammation, played by some receptors acting on inflammatory pathways, such as TLRs, has also been shown to be beneficial in the AD treatment [62]. More and more new treatments are being researched for AD, but unfortunately, the improvements have not been significant. What has been sought are combinations of treatments, which can result in some side effects in the elderly patient. Besides, current treatments are only symptomatic, that is, they do not modify the AD stage. These are cholinesterase inhibitors, used in all AD stages as they result in some beneficial effects on cognition and behavior. However, therapies affecting the AD stage are still under development. Therefore, efficient research must be conducted in this direction, instead of alleviating only the symptoms. Immunotherapy, for example, can be a viable option soon [63].

Author details

Alice Barros Câmara
Federal University of Rio Grande do Norte, Natal, Brazil

*Address all correspondence to: alicecamara@hotmail.com

References

[1] Lombardo S, Maskos U. Role of the nicotinic acetylcholine receptor in Alzheimer's disease pathology and treatment. Neuropharmacology. 2015;**96**:255-262

[2] Ferreira-Vieira TH, Guimaraes MI, Silva RF, Ribeiro MF. Alzheimer's disease: Targeting the cholinergic system. Current Neuropharmacology. 2016;**14**(1):101-115

[3] Verma S, Kumar A, Tripathi T, Kumar A. Muscarinic and nicotinic acetylcholine receptor agonists: Current scenario in Alzheimer's disease therapy. Journal of Pharmacy and Pharmacology. 2018;**70**(8):985-993

[4] Li KX, Sun Q, Wei LL, Du GH, Huang X, Wang JK. ERα gene promoter methylation in cognitive function and quality of life of patients with Alzheimer disease. Journal of Geriatric Psychiatry and Neurology. 2019;**32**(4):221-228

[5] Cui J, Shen Y, Li R. Estrogen synthesis and signaling pathways during aging: From periphery to brain. Trends in Molecular Medicine. 2013;**19**(3):197-209

[6] Coman L, Păunescu H, Catană R, Coman LI, Voiculescu Ş, Coman OA. Alzheimer's DiseAse–estrogens AnD selective estrogen receptor moDulAtors, frienDs or foes? Acta Endocrinologica (Bucharest). 2017;**13**(1):77

[7] Câmara AB, de Souza ID, Dalmolin RJS. Sunlight incidence, vitamin D deficiency, and Alzheimer's disease. Journal of Medicinal Food. 2018;**21**(9):841-848

[8] Lacampagne A, Liu X, Reiken S, Bussiere R, Meli AC, Lauritzen I, et al. Post-translational remodeling of ryanodine receptor induces calcium leak leading to Alzheimer's disease-like pathologies and cognitive deficits. Acta Neuropathologica. 2017;**134**(5):749-767

[9] Hugon J, Paquet C. Could ryanodine receptor dysfunction be linked to PKR brain accumulations in Alzheimer's disease? Medical Hypotheses. 2018;**113**:45-45

[10] Shetty AK, Bates A. Potential of GABA-ergic cell therapy for schizophrenia, neuropathic pain, and Alzheimer's and Parkinson's diseases. Brain Research. 2016;**1638**:74-87

[11] Sanchez-Mejias E, Nuñez-Diaz C, Sanchez-Varo R, Gomez-Arboledas A, Garcia-Leon JA, Fernandez-Valenzuela JJ, et al. Distinct disease-sensitive GABAergic neurons in the perirhinal cortex of Alzheimer's mice and patients. Brain Pathology. 2019;**30**(2):345-363

[12] Huang Y, Mucke L. Alzheimer mechanisms and therapeutic strategies. Cell. 2012;**148**(6):1204-1222

[13] Yan SS, Chen D, Yan S, Guo L, Chen JX. RAGE is a key cellular target for Aβ-induced perturbation in Alzheimer's disease. Frontiers in Bioscience (Scholar Edition). 2012;**4**:240

[14] Galasko D, Bell J, Mancuso JY, Kupiec JW, Sabbagh MN, van Dyck C, et al. Clinical trial of an inhibitor of RAGE-Aβ interactions in Alzheimer disease. Neurology. 2014;**82**(17):1536-1542

[15] Etchegoyen M, Nobile MH, Baez F, Posesorski B, González J, Lago N, et al. Metabolic syndrome and neuroprotection. Frontiers in Neuroscience. 2018;**12**:196

[16] Littlejohns TJ, Henley WE, Lang IA, Annweiler C, Beauchet O, Chaves PH, et al. Vitamin D and the

risk of dementia and Alzheimer disease. Neurology. 2014;**83**(10):920-928

[17] Mariani MM, Malm T, Lamb R, Jay TR, Neilson L, Casali B, et al. Neuronally-directed effects of RXR activation in a mouse model of Alzheimer's disease. Scientific Reports. 2017;**7**:42270

[18] Wang W, Nakashima KI, Hirai T, Inoue M. Neuroprotective effect of naturally occurring RXR agonists isolated from Sophora tonkinensis Gagnep. On amyloid-β-induced cytotoxicity in PC12 cells. Journal of Natural Medicines. 2019;**73**(1):154-162

[19] Dheer Y, Chitranshi N, Gupta V, Abbasi M, Mirzaei M, You Y, et al. Bexarotene modulates retinoid-X-receptor expression and is protective against neurotoxic endoplasmic reticulum stress response and apoptotic pathway activation. Molecular Neurobiology. 2018;**55**(12):9043-9056

[20] Koster KP, Smith CC, Valencia-Olvera AC, Thatcher GR, Tai LM, MJ LD. Rexinoids as therapeutics for Alzheimer's disease: Role of APOE. Current Topics in Medicinal Chemistry. 2017;**17**(6):708-720

[21] Chakrabarti M, McDonald AJ, Will Reed J, Moss MA, Das BC, Ray SK. Molecular signaling mechanisms of natural and synthetic retinoids for inhibition of pathogenesis in Alzheimer's disease. Journal of Alzheimer's Disease. 2016;**50**(2):335-352

[22] Wang R, Reddy PH. Role of glutamate and NMDA receptors in Alzheimer's disease. Journal of Alzheimer's Disease. 2017;**57**(4):1041-1048

[23] Pinheiro L, Faustino C. Therapeutic strategies targeting amyloid-β in Alzheimer's disease. Current Alzheimer Research. 2019;**16**(5):418-452

[24] Courtney R, Landreth GE. LXR regulation of brain cholesterol: From development to disease. Trends in Endocrinology and Metabolism. 2016;**27**(6):404-414

[25] Sodhi RK, Singh N. Liver X receptors: Emerging therapeutic targets for Alzheimer's disease. Pharmacological Research. 2013;**72**:45-51

[26] Cao G, Bales KR, DeMattos RB, Paul SM. Liver X receptor-mediated gene regulation and cholesterol homeostasis in brain: Relevance to Alzheimer's disease therapeutics. Current Alzheimer Research. 2007;**4**(2):179-184

[27] Kong Y, Wu JB, Wang X, Zhao JF, Song H, Yuan LD. Polymorphism of the OLR1 3'UTR potential microRNA binding site and risk of Alzheimer's disease: A meta-analysis. Genetics and Molecular Research. 2014;**13**(4):10162-10172

[28] Su F, Bai F, Zhou H, Zhang Z. Reprint of: Microglial toll-like receptors and Alzheimer's disease. Brain, Behavior, and Immunity. 2016;**55**:166-178

[29] Rangasamy SB, Jana M, Roy A, Corbett GT, Kundu M, Chandra S, et al. Selective disruption of TLR2-MyD88 interaction inhibits inflammation and attenuates Alzheimer's pathology. The Journal of Clinical Investigation. 2018;**128**(10):4297-4312

[30] Chakrabarty P, Li A, Ladd TB, Strickland MR, Koller EJ, Burgess JD, et al. TLR5 decoy receptor as a novel anti-amyloid therapeutic for Alzheimer's disease. Journal of Experimental Medicine. 2018;**215**(9):2247-2264

[31] Wang YL, Tan MS, Yu JT, Zhang W, Hu N, Wang HF, et al. Toll-like receptor 9 promoter polymorphism is associated with decreased risk of

Alzheimer's disease in Han Chinese. Journal of Neuroinflammation. 2013;**10**(1):886

[32] Trotta T, Porro C, Calvello R, Panaro MA. Biological role of toll-like receptor-4 in the brain. Journal of Neuroimmunology. 2014;**268**(1-2):1-12

[33] Gambuzza ME, Sofo V, Salmeri FM, Soraci L, Marino S, Bramanti P. Toll-like receptors in Alzheimer's disease: a therapeutic perspective. CNS & Neurological Disorders-Drug Targets (Formerly Current Drug Targets-CNS & Neurological Disorders). 2014;**13**(9):1542-1558

[34] Guedes JR, Lao T, Cardoso AL, El Khoury J. Roles of microglial and monocyte chemokines and their receptors in regulating Alzheimer's disease-associated amyloid-β and tau pathologies. Frontiers in Neurology. 2018;**9**:549

[35] Canet G, Chevallier N, Zussy C, Desrumaux C, Givalois L. Central role of glucocorticoid receptors in Alzheimer's disease and depression. Frontiers in Neuroscience. 2018;**12**:739

[36] Pedrazzoli M, Losurdo M, Paolone G, Medelin M, Jaupaj L, Cisterna B, et al. Glucocorticoid receptors modulate dendritic spine plasticity and microglia activity in an animal model of Alzheimer's disease. Neurobiology of Disease. 2019;**132**:104568

[37] Kootar S, Frandemiche ML, Dhib G, Mouska X, Lorivel T, Poupon-Silvestre G, et al. Identification of an acute functional cross-talk between amyloid-β and glucocorticoid receptors at hippocampal excitatory synapses. Neurobiology of Disease. 2018;**118**:117-128

[38] Chen JJ, Gong YH, He L. Role of GPR40 in pathogenesis and treatment of Alzheimer's disease and type 2 diabetic dementia. Journal of Drug Targeting. 2019;**27**(4):347-354

[39] Khan MZ, Zhuang X, He L. GPR40 receptor activation leads to CREB phosphorylation and improves cognitive performance in an Alzheimer's disease mouse model. Neurobiology of Learning and Memory. 2016;**131**:46-55

[40] Raha AA, Henderson JW, Stott SR, Vuono R, Foscarin S, Friedland RP, et al. Neuroprotective effect of TREM-2 in aging and Alzheimer's disease model. Journal of Alzheimer's Disease. 2017;**55**(1):199-217

[41] Gao L, Jiang T, Yao X, Yu L, Yang X, Li Y. TREM2 and the progression of Alzheimer's disease. Current Neurovascular Research. 2017; **14**(2):177-183

[42] Deming Y, Li Z, Benitez BA, Cruchaga C. Triggering receptor expressed on myeloid cells 2 (TREM2): A potential therapeutic target for Alzheimer disease? Expert Opinion on Therapeutic Targets. 2018;**22**(7):587-598

[43] Shi Y, Holtzman DM. Interplay between innate immunity and Alzheimer disease: APOE and TREM2 in the spotlight. Nature Reviews Immunology. 2018;**18**(12):759-772

[44] Kan R, Wang B, Zhang C, Yang Z, Ji S, Lu Z, et al. Association of the HTR6 polymorphism C267T with late-onset Alzheimer's disease in Chinese. Neuroscience Letters. 2004;**372**(1-2):27-29

[45] Khoury R, Grysman N, Gold J, Patel K, Grossberg GT. The role of 5 HT6-receptor antagonists in Alzheimer's disease: An update. Expert Opinion on Investigational Drugs. 2018;**27**(6):523-533

[46] Takkinen JS, López-Picón FR, Kirjavainen AK, Pihlaja R, Snellman A, Ishizu T, et al. [18F] FMPEP-d2 PET imaging shows age-and genotype-dependent impairments in the

availability of cannabinoid receptor 1 in a mouse model of Alzheimer's disease. Neurobiology of Aging. 2018;**69**:199-208

[47] Liu CS, Chau SA, Ruthirakuhan M, Lanctôt KL, Herrmann N. Cannabinoids for the treatment of agitation and aggression in Alzheimer's disease. CNS Drugs. 2015;**29**(8):615-623

[48] Crunfli F, Vrechi TA, Costa AP, Torrão AS. Cannabinoid receptor type 1 agonist ACEA improves cognitive deficit on STZ-induced neurotoxicity through apoptosis pathway and NO modulation. Neurotoxicity Research. 2019;**35**(3):516-529

[49] Bahji A, Meyyappan AC, Hawken ER. Cannabinoids for the neuropsychiatric symptoms of dementia: A systematic review and meta-analysis. The Canadian Journal of Psychiatry. 2019:0706743719892717. DOI: 10.1177/0706743719892717

[50] Çakır M, Tekin S, Doğanyiğit Z, Erden Y, Soytürk M, Çiğremiş Y, et al. Cannabinoid type 2 receptor agonist JWH-133, attenuates Okadaic acid induced spatial memory impairment and neurodegeneration in rats. Life Sciences. 2019;**217**:25-33

[51] Barrera J, Subramanian S, Chiba-Falek O. Probing the role of PPARγ in the regulation of late-onset Alzheimer's disease-associated genes. PLoS One. 2018;**13**(5):e0196943, 1-12. DOI: 10.1371/journal.pone.0196943

[52] Vallée A, Lecarpentier Y, Guillevin R, Vallée JN. Effects of cannabidiol interactions with Wnt/β-catenin pathway and PPARγ on oxidative stress and neuroinflammation in Alzheimer's disease. Acta Biochimica et Biophysica Sinica. 2017;**49**(10):853-866

[53] Zhang M, Qian C, Zheng ZG, Qian F, Wang Y, Thu PM, et al. Jujuboside a promotes Aβ clearance and ameliorates cognitive deficiency in Alzheimer's disease through activating Axl/HSP90/PPARγ pathway. Theranostics. 2018;**8**(15):4262

[54] Lee YH, Song GG. PPARγ Pro12Ala and His447His polymorphisms and susceptibility to Alzheimer's disease: A meta-analysis. Genetics and Molecular Research. 2015;**14**(2):7248-7257

[55] Mirzaei F, Khazaei M, Komaki A, Amiri I, Jalili C. Virgin coconut oil (VCO) by normalizing NLRP3 inflammasome showed potential neuroprotective effects in amyloid-β induced toxicity and high-fat diet fed rat. Food and Chemical Toxicology. 2018;**118**:68-83

[56] Bai H, Zhang QF, Duan JJ, Yu DJ, Liu LJ. Downregulation of signal transduction and STAT3 expression exacerbates oxidative stress mediated by NLRP3 inflammasome. Neural Regeneration Research. 2018;**13**(12):2147

[57] Heneka MT, Kummer MP, Stutz A, Delekate A, Schwartz S, Vieira-Saecker A, et al. NLRP3 is activated in Alzheimer's disease and contributes to pathology in APP/PS1 mice. Nature. 2013;**493**(7434):674-678

[58] Daniels MJ, Rivers-Auty J, Schilling T, Spencer NG, Watremez W, Fasolino V, et al. Fenamate NSAIDs inhibit the NLRP3 inflammasome and protect against Alzheimer's disease in rodent models. Nature Communications. 2016;**7**(1):1-10

[59] Ising C, Venegas C, Zhang S, Scheiblich H, Schmidt SV, Vieira-Saecker A, et al. NLRP3 inflammasome activation drives tau pathology. Nature. 2019;**575**(7784):669-673

[60] Câmara AB. Receptores neurais e a doença de Alzheimer: uma revisão sistemática da literatura

sobre as famílias de receptores mais associadas a doença, suas funções e áreas de expressão. Jornal Brasileiro de Psiquiatria. 2019;**68**(3):161-176

[61] Câmara AB, Brandão IA. The relationship between vitamin D deficiency and oxidative stress can be independent of age and gender. International Journal for Vitamin and Nutrition Research. 2019. DOI: 10.1024/0300-9831/a000614

[62] Süß P, Schlachetzki JCM. Microglia in Alzheimer's disease. Current Alzheimer Research. 2020;**17**(1):29-43

[63] Chu LW. Alzheimer's disease: Early diagnosis and treatment. Hong Kong Medical Journal. 2012;**18**(3):228-237

[64] Ryskamp D, Wu L, Wu J, Kim D, Rammes G, Geva M, et al. Pridopidine stabilizes mushroom spines in mouse models of Alzheimer's disease by acting on the sigma-1 receptor. Neurobiology of Disease. 2019;**124**:489-504

[65] Chiarini A, Armato U, Whitfield JF, Pra ID. Targeting human astrocytes' calcium-sensing receptors for treatment of Alzheimer's disease. Current Pharmaceutical Design. 2017;**23**(33):4990-5000

Section 2

Neuroprotection in Cerebral Ischemia and Other Neurological Diseases

Chapter 7

In Vivo Studies of Protein Misfolding and Neurodegeneration Induced by Metabolic Syndrome Relative to Chronic Cerebral Hypoperfusion: A Critical Review

María I. Herrera, Juan P. Luaces, Lucas D. Udovin, Nicolás Toro-Urrego, Matilde Otero-Losada and Francisco Capani

Abstract

Metabolic syndrome (MetS) leads to microvascular dysfunction and chronic cerebral hypoperfusion (CCH) in an insidious way. Clinical evidence and several rodent models have contributed to determining the neurodegenerative effect of a sustained decrease in cerebral blood flow (CBF). Protein misfolding and aggregation derived from CCH might account for the establishment of vascular cognitive impairment and dementia (VCID) and Alzheimer's disease (AD). However, the complex and multifactorial etiology of cerebrovascular disease demands the combination of experimental models in scientific research. In this sense, the present work aims at summarizing the differential available rodent paradigms for studying the establishment of cognitive decline resulting from protein misfolding induced by MetS in association with CCH. Revising experimental findings in the field will help further basic research on the pathophysiology of cerebrovascular disease and the future testing of protein-remodeling factors as neuroprotective agents for the prevention of cognitive impairment.

Keywords: metabolic syndrome (MetS), chronic cerebral hypoperfusion (CCH), protein misfolding, experimental models, cognitive impairment

1. Introduction

Metabolic syndrome (MetS) is the resulting condition of specific concurrent maladies, whose common pathogenic component is insulin resistance. Difficult to diagnose in clinical practice, there is consensus on its presence provided a cluster of risk factors be present, including abdominal obesity, hyperglycemia, hypertriglyceridemia, and hypertension [1–3]. Several murine models have contributed to the knowledge of this vascular risk factors' constellation, which has been studied for over 80 years [4]. The experimental evidence shows that MetS silently, though relentlessly, leads to microvascular dysfunction and chronic cerebral hypoperfusion (CCH) [5]. Clinical findings, including the multivariate association between functional microvascular variables and laboratory-anthropometrical measurements [6], have reinforced the linkage of MetS with CCH [7], which leads to cognitive decline in late middle-aged adults [8]. As much as CCH might explain the considerable overlap between features of vascular cognitive impairment and dementia (VCID) and Alzheimer's disease (AD), it might also underly as a common pathophysiological mechanism [9]. Experimental models of CCH have also contributed to exploring the interplay between hypoperfusion and amyloid β (Aβ) deposition, as it relates to AD [9]. Scientific evidence has underscored the importance of treating dementia comorbid disease conditions, including hypometabolism and diminished cerebral blood flow (CBF) [10]. An alternative target in neuroprotection is the regulation of the proteostasis network since protein aggregates link MetS-induced CCH and sporadic AD late-onset [11]. Therefore, the present work aims at revising different murine models of MetS and CCH, summarizing those experimental findings of relevance in the establishment of cerebrovascular disease. Plus, this overview intends to shed light on the usefulness of experimental models for the study of protein misfolding as a mechanism of neurodegeneration in CCH. Thirdly, this review attempts to discuss the requirement of combining MetS and CCH experimental models in order to resemble multifactorial conditions like VCID and AD and to test protein-remodeling factors as potential neuroprotective mechanisms for cognitive decline in the aging brain [12].

2. Experimental models of MetS and CCH: relevant findings to vascular dementia

Although MetS is a multifactorial and complex condition, several rat strains have been developed to assemble a profile of anomalies described in human subjects that exhibit cerebrovascular disease. Obese Zucker rats constitute the most representative rat strain to study this syndrome since animals present changes similar to those seen in patients [1]. This widely extended model of insulin resistance and obesity was discovered in 1961 by Lois Zucker. The mutation in the leptin receptor fa leads to noticeable obesity from the third week of life [13]. Leptin is synthesized by adipose tissue. This hormone acts in the brain on leptin receptors [14]. Elevated levels of leptin represent the molecular base of the characteristic phenotype of Zucker rats, which includes hyperphagia, deposition of energy in adipose tissue, dyslipidemia, mild glucose intolerance, hyperinsulinemia, and vascular changes [1, 15]. In contraposition to obese Zucker rats, the Wistar Ottawa Karlsburg W (WOKW) rat model is not induced by a single-gene mutation, resembling the context in which this pathology is developed in human subjects. However, these animals exhibit signs of MetS between 8 and 10 weeks of age, much later than Zucker rats [1].

Several murine models of MetS derive from the spontaneously hypertensive rat (SHR), which represents the of-choice experimental model of essential (or primary) hypertension. While the SHR rats show hypertriglyceridemia and abdominal obesity, corpulent SHR rats are preferable for reproducing MetS [1]. Different strains have been developed, including obese SHR or Koletsky rats, SHR/NIH-corpulent (SHR/N-cp) rats and its subline, the SHR/NDmc-corpulent rats, and stroke-prone-SHR fatty rats. The first strain, originally developed by Koletsky in 1970, shows premature vascular pathology mimicking human atherosclerosis [16]. The SHR/N corpulent model was established to reproduce obesity and non-insulin-dependent diabetes mellitus (NIDDM) [17]. Spontaneously hypertensive rats (SHR), an animal model of essential (or primary) hypertension, and SHR/NDmc-corpulent rats are also obese, presenting hyperphagia and metabolic alterations, while stroke-prone-SHR fatty rats are characterized by severe hypertension, which induces atherosclerosis and stroke. The spontaneously hypertensive/NIH-corpulent (SHR/N-cp) rat is a genetic model doomed to developing both non-insulin-dependent diabetes mellitus and hypertension.

Low-capacity runner (LCR) rats have been lately described, when cardiovascular risk factors were observed to emerge after artificial selection of low aerobic capacity [18]. These animals are selectively bred according to their performance in a running task. The LCR group is represented by rats capable of running short distances due to their low intrinsic aerobic capacity and bred with each other. After 11 generations, elevated blood pressure, insulin resistance, hyperinsulinemia, and endothelial dysfunction were registered in this strain [1]. Finally, from a translational perspective, both high-fat diet (HFD) and sweet carbonated beverage drinking represent two interesting rodent models of MetS evoking unhealthy dietary habits, increasing cardiovascular risk [19]. The former experimental paradigm reproduces impaired glucose tolerance (IGT) and type 2 diabetes. Rodents fed a HFD containing near 58% of total energy supply from fat develop obesity over the first week of life due to higher energy intake in combination with lower metabolic efficiency [20]. In the latter, 6-month ad libitum coke beverage drinking as the only liquid source results in hyperglycemia, hypertriglyceridemia, hypercholesterolemia, overweight, systolic hypertension, cardiac, renal alterations, and oxidative stress [2, 3, 21–24]. **Table 1** offers a translational overview of the abovementioned experimental models of MetS.

Disruption of CBF has been studied using focal or global ischemia. Focal ischemia models are used for resembling stroke pathophysiology and consist in the occlusion of a specific vessel, which reduces CBF by 70% due to restrictions in the vessel's territory. This condition is generally induced by transient or permanent middle cerebral artery occlusion. Multiple infarcts can be reproduced via intra-arterial injection of emboli (heterogeneous localization) or by inducing spontaneous strokes (SHRSP). Higher reductions of CBF are developed in global ischemia models, which include transient common carotid artery occlusion (TCAO), three- and four-vessel occlusion, and cardiac arrest [9].

Since focal and global ischemia leads to severe reductions in CBF, alternative models have been developed to reproduce CCH, i.e., the subtle yet sustained decrease in CBF relevant to VCID. Early pathological events provoking VCID were studied through the ligation or occlusion of unilateral or bilateral common carotid arteries (two-vessel occlusion) [25]. Bilateral common carotid artery occlusion (BCCAO) was refined to resemble modest reductions in CBF. Bilateral common carotid artery stenosis (BCCAS) was developed to reduce flow to 50% of baseline [26]. However, flow largely recovered 1 month later, which was overcome by establishing a gradual stenosis model. Aneroid devices were used to absorb extracellular fluid and provoke the constriction of arteries, resulting in a slower and progressive onset of hypoperfusion. This experimental condition is known as gradual common carotid artery stenosis [27]. Consequently, murine models of CCH include a wide spectrum of disease severity, ranging from traditional occlusion mechanisms to gradual stenosis methods. Despite these variants, experimental models of CCH induce sustained and moderate blood flow reductions by 30–50%, in contraposition to ischemic models that reduce CBF in 70% acutely [9].

Although stenosis represents a better theoretical approach from a clinical perspective, it involves difficult techniques, rendering BCCAO the most commonly used model [28]. An alternative experimental model of CCH comprises the

Name of the model	Experimental induction of MetS	Characteristic phenotype	Translational advantages
Obese Zucker rats	Mutation in leptin receptor fa causes obesity in rats from the 3rd week of life.	Hyperphagia, energy deposition in adipose tissue, dyslipidemia, mild glucose intolerance, hyperinsulinemia, and vascular changes.	Reproduces phenotypic changes resembling those in patients with MetS.
Wistar Ottawa Karlsburg W (WOKW) rats	Derived from a Wistar rat outbred strain, WOKW rats first exhibit signs of MetS at 8–10 weeks of age.	Obesity, moderate hypertension, dyslipidemia, hyperinsulinemia, and glucose intolerance.	Resembles MetS in a polygenetic context, as in humans.
Spontaneously hypertensive rats (SHR)	Rats bred with high blood pressure develop hypertension around 5–6 weeks of age.	Hypertension, hypertriglyceridemia, and abdominal obesity. The phenotype varies according to the respective corpulent strain: a. Obese SHR or Koletsky rats b. SHR/NIH-corpulent (SHR/N-cp) rats c. SHR/NDmc-corpulent rats d. Stroke-prone-SHR fatty rats	The of-choice experimental model of essential (or primary) hypertension. Corpulent SHR rats are preferable for reproducing MetS. Some strains resemble human-like atherosclerosis (a,d) or non-insulin-dependent (type II) diabetes mellitus (NIDDM) (b,c), respectively.
Low-capacity runner (LCR) rats	Rats capable of running short distances due to their low intrinsic aerobic capacity are selectively bred with each other along various generations.	Elevated blood pressure, insulin resistance, hyperinsulinemia, and endothelial dysfunction.	Represents metabolic dysfunction associated with low aerobic capacity.
High-fat diet (HFD)	Rodents fed a diet containing near 58% of total energy supply from fat become obese over the 1st. week of life due to higher energy intake.	Obesity and low metabolic efficiency.	Evokes impaired glucose tolerance (IGT) and type-2 diabetes due to unhealthy dietary habits.
Sweet carbonated beverage drinking	6-month ad libitum coke beverage drinking as the only liquid source causes metabolic dysfunction in rats.	Hyperglycemia, hypertriglyceridemia, hypercholesterolemia, overweight, systolic hypertension, cardiorenal alterations, and oxidative stress.	It mimics MetS derived from unhealthy dietary habits.

Table 1.
Experimental models of MetS: summary of phenotypic features from a translational perspective.

asymmetric common carotid artery surgery. Differential procedures are used for each common carotid artery (CCA), allowing interesting comparisons between both hemispheres. Gradual occlusion of the right artery lasts 1 month, while the

Name of the model	Experimental induction of CCH	Characteristic phenotype	Translational advantages
Bilateral common carotid artery occlusion (BCCAO)	Both common carotid arteries are ligated.	Cerebral blood flow (CBF) CBF rapidly decreases.	Represents a widely used model of CCH, characterized by its feasibility.
Bilateral common carotid artery stenosis (BCCAS)	Microcoils are placed on both CCAs.	CBF decreases and gradually recovers.	Mimics the clinical scenario of modest reductions in CBF.
Gradual common carotid artery stenosis (GCCAS)	Aneroid devices are used to absorb extracellular fluid and provoke the constriction of arteries.	CBF gradually decreases without recovery.	Reproduces a progressive onset of hypoperfusion, slower than induced by BCCAS.
Asymmetric common carotid artery surgery (ACCAS)	An aneroid constrictor is placed on the right common carotid artery (CCA), inducing a gradual occlusion for 1 month. The left CCA undergoes 50% stenosis by placing a micro-coil.	CBF decreases to different extents between the right and left CCAs.	Resembles differential reductions in CBF between both hemispheres.

Table 2.
Experimental models of CCH: Summary of phenotypic features from a translational perspective.

left artery undergoes 50% stenosis by placing a micro-coil. Further investigation is necessary to assess CBF reductions at longer time points, discarding the complete occlusion of carotid arteries in the long term [9]. **Table 2** summarizes the main features of the described models of CCH. For more details regarding experimental paradigms of CCH, including primate models, see [29].

Recent evidence using the abovementioned experimental models of CCH has shown that disruption of CBF leads to vascular cognitive impairment (VCI). Because of BCCAS induction in mice, selective recognition alterations were encountered in the novel object recognition (NOR) test, together with damage to the perirhinal cortex [30]. When CBF was gradually reduced, progressive motor impairment and working memory decline were found in the rotarod and Y-maze tests, respectively. Loss of oligodendrocytes in the white matter might underlie these behavioral deficits, suggesting that the GCCAS model could closely replicate the clinical pathogenesis of hypoperfusive vascular dementia in humans [31]. After implanting an aneroid constrictor on the left CCA and provoking stenosis on the right CCA, mice exhibited sustained motor, learning, and memory dysfunction, inferred from the balance beam maze, a fear conditioning task, and the NOR test. Histopathological analysis showed neurodegeneration in the cerebral cortex, dorsal striatum, and hippocampus. These findings support the usefulness of the ACCAS experimental model for reproducing the effect of microvascular occlusions on cognitive impairment [32].

3. Experimental findings supporting protein misfolding as a neurodegenerative mechanism in CCH

The causative role of CCH in cognitive impairment and AD has been reported in several studies using the BCCAO model, an experimental paradigm of easy application [28]. Differential mechanisms have been proposed as a potential link between CCH and neurodegeneration, including synaptic dysfunction, oxidative stress, neuronal loss, white matter lesion, neuroinflammation, and protein misfolding [28].

The latter appears as a novel target for neuroprotection, according to cumulative evidence [11]. **Figure 1** illustrates how CCH alters proteostasis network, leading to protein misfolding and neurodegeneration.

Degeneration of hippocampal neurons was attributed to proteostasis network destruction and protein aggregation induced by BCCAO [33]. This murine model has also led to a sustained increase in autophagy related-proteins Beclin-1, light chain 3B (LC3-B), and P62, suggesting a defensive reaction against protein misfolding. In this study, although CBF returned to baseline, cognitive failure was irreversible and attributed to Aβ aggregation in the hippocampus [34]. This brain region is characterized by its vulnerability to CCH [35] and its association with memory and learning dysfunction in AD [36]. Hippocampal degeneration has also been related to BCCAO-induced macroautophagy and endoplasmic reticulum (ER) stress, as it was inferred from the expression of light chain 3 II (LC3-II), Beclin 1, CCAAT/enhancer-binding protein, and C/EBP homologous protein [37].

Besides BCCAO, oxygen-glucose deprivation (OGD) provokes autophagy upregulation and apoptosis [35]. Recent evidence extended these findings, reporting CCH-induced high levels of LC3-II and Beclin-1 along with ultrastructural markers of apoptosis in CA1 neurons, including nuclear pycnosis, autophagosomes, and autolysosomes. ER fragmentation and spatial working memory impairment appeared as subcellular and functional correlates [38]. In addition to autophagy [34, 35, 38] and macroautophagy [37], ubiquitin-proteasome system (UPS) appears as another proteostatic pathway altered as a consequence of experimental CCH, which leads to CA1 degeneration. Long-term decrease peptidase activity and accumulation of ubiquitinated protein aggregates were observed after ligating the left vein and draining the transverse sinus and the bilateral external carotid arteries [39]. Previous studies from this laboratory had suggested the removal of misfolded proteins was impaired by UPS downregulation [40], and cognitive decline might be associated with long-term potentiation inhibition [41].

Along with aggregation of extracellular Aβ, intracellular phosphorylated tau protein deposition constitutes a hallmark of AD [42]. Tau hyperphosphorylation was observed as a result of unilateral common carotid artery occlusion (UCCAO),

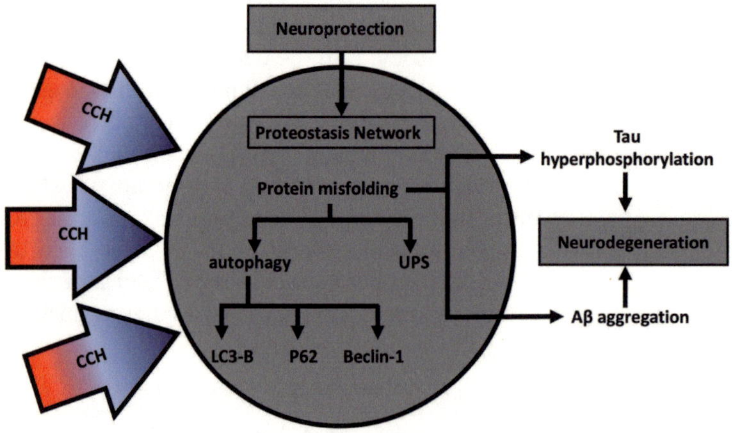

Figure 1.
Protein misfolding as a neurodegenerative mechanism and novel neuroprotective target in CCH. Chronic cerebral hypoperfusion impairs proteostasis network, inducing protein misfolding. Under cell stress, proteostasis network surveillance systems degrade proteins through different mechanisms. Depending on the nature of misfolded proteins, different systems are activated such as ubiquitin-proteasome system or macroautophagy. Protein aggregates, are recognized by molecular chaperones, ubiquitinated and delivered to the autophagosome via Beclin-1 complex. Neuroprotective agents, which target proteostasis network, emerge as promising treatments for cognitive impairment following CCH.

together with decreased post-translational tau O-GlcNAcylation by β-N-acetylglucosamine, dysregulation of synaptic proteins, and memory deficits [43]. According to previous findings, brain glucose metabolic dysfunction might down-regulate tau O-GlcNAcylation mediated by tau hyperphosphorylation [44–46]. Recent studies have confirmed and extended this finding, suggesting CCH might exacerbate tau hyperphosphorylation in AD-rodents, either after UCCAO in mice [47] or BCCAO in rats [48]. Similarly, previous evidence prompted CCH might precipitate AD neuropathology since BCAS seemed to accelerate Aβ aggregation, the same process found in amyloid protein precursor (APP)-transgenic (APP-Tg) mice [49]. In fact, aberrant processing of APP has been reported after BCCAO [50].

4. Combining experimental models

Since MetS is associated with an increased risk of cerebral ischemia, recent investigations developed murine models of MetS combined with experimental paradigms of ischemia-reperfusion injury to study the impact of ischemia associated with MetS. Wistar rats fed a high-fat diet for 20 weeks were more susceptible to BCCAO-reperfusion than normal diet (ND)-fed animals, showing worsening in microvascular dysfunction and oxidative stress. These results show that MetS increases the vulnerability of the ischemic brain to damage, whereby BCCAO exacerbates cerebrovascular disease previously induced by HFD [51]. Similarly, BCCAO, followed by reperfusion, aggravated microvascular alterations in obese Zucker rats compared with lean Wistar controls. Lesions in the cortex and striatum were largely more pronounced in obese Zucker rats, suggesting MetS could increase the risk of adverse outcomes following a brain hypoperfusion-reperfusion event [52].

Novel findings support the hypothesis that the brain under obesity's conditions is more vulnerable to ischemic injury. A brief episode of transient ischemia (TI) was provoked in obese gerbils, commonly known as desert rats. After 12 weeks of HFD, the rodents underwent a 2-min experimental TI. Hyperglycemia, cholesterolemia, and triglyceridemia observed in gerbils fed with a HFD were associated with a massive loss of pyramidal neurons in the hippocampal CA1 region 5 days after TI, indicating that a short-lived episode of TI could evoke neuronal damage along with pre-existing MetS. Increased levels of dihydroethidium, 4-hydroxynonenal, tumor necrosis factor-α, and interleukin-1β indicated brain injury was mediated by oxidative stress and neuroinflammation. On the contrary, ND gerbils did not exhibit neuronal death as a consequence of acute TI. In addition, these control animals could develop cerebral ischemic tolerance against a subsequent severer episode of TI [53]. Previous studies from the same laboratory have deepened the role of mammalian target of rapamycin (mTOR) in the pathogenesis of metabolic and neurological diseases and demonstrated that obesity and its related metabolic dysfunction might exacerbate the impact of TI in certain brain areas, including cerebral cortex, striatum, and hippocampus (CA1-3 regions) [54–56].

Conversely, cerebral ischemia itself might lead to glucose deregulation, a pathognomonic feature of MetS. Experimental evidence combining rodent models of ischemia and MetS shows that ischemic hippocampal neuronal death hampers glucose homeostasis, decreasing insulin secretion, which is later exacerbated by a HFD. In this study, gerbils were subjected to an 8-min BCCAO or a sham operation followed by either 11 or 40% fat diet for 7, 14, or 28 days. Although the initial occlusion provoked a 70% decrease in CA1 neurons, only HFD and longer ischemic periods resulted in larger hippocampal cell death. Similarly, glucose intolerance measured through the oral glucose tolerance test (OGTT) was overrated in gerbils fed a HFD as the ischemic periods became longer. During the OGTT, insulin levels were significantly lower in gerbils subjected to BCCAO than in sham-operated controls. In addition, insulin secretion decrease was elevated the most after 28 days of HFD in ischemic gerbils [57]. These interesting findings using a combination of rodent models suggest that ischemic damage is a risk factor for glucose homeostasis, which might be worsened by the experimental induction of MetS in a HFD paradigm.

5. Future directions

Scientific findings combining rodent models have shown that chronic MetS is associated with poor stroke outcomes following experimental cerebrovascular events [58] since HFD or the way of inducing MetS modulates ischemic mechanisms of brain damage [59]. Also, experimental CBF restriction seems to hamper glucose homeostasis, posing a risk factor for developing MetS. When artery occlusion models are followed by the experimental induction of metabolic dysfunction features, the resulting MetS might exacerbate previously ischemia-induced glucose deregulation [57]. Therefore, combining experimental models offers an interesting scientific paradigm for elucidating the complexity of pathophysiological mechanisms underlying chronic cerebrovascular disease. In terms of Zhao and Gong [28], differential clinical scenarios may coexist in chronic pathologies where risk factors rarely exist alone or may even exert a causative role in some patients while acting as a consequence in others. In this regard, experimental studies using the combined application of murine models could help to close the gap between rodent models and human disease [9].

However, this complex translational perspective is still necessary for studying the interaction between MetS and CCH inducing neurodegeneration. Although brain microvascular dysfunction has been confirmed in several murine models of MetS, including HFD [60, 61], Zucker [62], and SHR rats [63], whether MetS causes cognitive impairment due to a decrease in CBF has not been fully addressed yet [64]. In addition, since protein misfolding is a hallmark of neurodegenerative diseases [65], dissecting the exact role of MetS in association with CCH in protein aggregation represents a relevant challenge in the field. Detailed studies on the time-dependent proteostatic changes after experimental MetS and CCH will shed light on the roles and mechanisms of these clinical conditions in the establishment of VCID and AD. Furthermore, these studies will contribute to testing protein-remodeling factors [12] as putative neuroprotective agents for the prevention of cerebrovascular disease and cognitive decline.

Author details

María I. Herrera[1,2†*], Juan P. Luaces[2†], Lucas D. Udovin[2], Nicolás Toro-Urrego[2], Matilde Otero-Losada[2†] and Francisco Capani[2,3,4†]

1 Centro de Investigaciones en Psicología y Psicopedagogía, Facultad de Psicología y Psicopedagogía, Universidad Católica Argentina, Buenos Aires, Argentina

2 Instituto de Investigaciones Cardiológicas, Universidad de Buenos Aires, Consejo Nacional de Investigaciones Científicas y Técnicas, ININCA, UBA-CONICET, Buenos Aires, Argentina

3 Facultad de Medicina, Universidad Católica Argentina, Buenos Aires, Argentina

4 Universidad Autónoma de Chile, Santiago de Chile, Chile

*Address all correspondence to: ines_herrera@uca.edu.ar

† Share authorship.

References

[1] de Artiñano AA, Castro MM. Experimental rat models to study the metabolic syndrome. British Journal of Nutrition. 2009;**102**(9):1246-1253. DOI: 10.1017/S0007114509990729

[2] Otero-Losada M, González J, Müller A, Ottaviano G, Cao G, Azzato F, et al. Exercise ameliorates endocrine pancreas damage induced by chronic cola drinking in rats. PLoS One. 2016;**11**(5):e0155630. DOI: 10.1371/journal.pone.0155630

[3] Otero-Losada M, Gómez Llambí H, Ottaviano G, Cao G, Müller A, Azzato F, et al. Cardiorenal involvement in metabolic syndrome induced by cola drinking in rats: Proinflammatory cytokines and impaired antioxidative protection. Mediators of Inflammation. 2016;**2016**:5613056. DOI: 10.1155/2016/5613056

[4] Burton-Freeman B. Dietary fiber and energy regulation. The Journal of Nutrition. 2000;**130**(2):272S-275S. DOI: 10.1093/jn/130.2.272S

[5] Aoqui C, Chmielewski S, Scherer E, Eißler R, Sollinger D, Heid I, et al. Microvascular dysfunction in the course of metabolic syndrome induced by high-fat diet. Cardiovascular Diabetology. 2014;**13**(1):31. DOI: 10.1186/1475-2840-13-31

[6] Panazzolo DG, Sicuro FL, Clapauch R, Maranhão PA, Bouskela E, Kraemer-Aguiar LG. Obesity, metabolic syndrome, impaired fasting glucose, and microvascular dysfunction: A principal component analysis approach. BMC Cardiovascular Disorders. 2012;**12**(1):102. DOI: 10.1186/1471-2261-12-102

[7] Czernichow S, Thomas D, Bruckert E. n-6 fatty acids and cardiovascular health: A review of the evidence for dietary intake recommendations. British Journal of Nutrition. 2010;**104**(6):788-796. DOI: 10.1017/S0007114510002096

[8] Birdsill AC, Carlsson CM, Willette AA, Okonkwo OC, Johnson SC, Xu G, et al. Low cerebral blood flow is associated with lower memory function in metabolic syndrome. Obesity. 2013;**21**(7):1313-1320. DOI: 10.1002/oby.20170

[9] Duncombe J, Kitamura A, Hase Y, Ihara M, Kalaria RN, Horsburgh K. Chronic cerebral hypoperfusion: A key mechanism leading to vascular cognitive impairment and dementia. Closing the translational gap between rodent models and human vascular cognitive impairment and dementia. Clinical Science. 2017;**131**(19):2451-2468. DOI: 10.1042/CS20160727

[10] Daulatzai MA. Cerebral hypoperfusion and glucose hypometabolism: Key pathophysiological modulators promote neurodegeneration, cognitive impairment, and Alzheimer's disease. Journal of Neuroscience Research. 2017;**95**(4):943-972. DOI: 10.1002/jnr.23777

[11] Herrera MI, Udovin LD, Toro-Urrego N, Kusnier CF, Luaces JP, Otero-Losada M, et al. Neuroprotection targeting protein misfolding on chronic cerebral hypoperfusion in the context of metabolic syndrome. Frontiers in Neuroscience. 2018;**12**(339):1-9. DOI: 10.3389/fnins.2018.00339

[12] Jackrel ME, Shorter J. Protein-remodeling factors as potential therapeutics for neurodegenerative disease. Frontiers in Neuroscience. 2017;**11**:99. DOI: 10.3389/fnins.2017.00099

[13] Phillips MS, Liu Q, Hammond HA, Dugan V, Hey PJ, Caskey CT, et al.

Leptin receptor missense mutation in the fatty Zucker rat. Nature Genetics. 1996;**13**(1):18. DOI: 10.1038/ng0596-18

[14] Ahima RS, Flier JS. Leptin. Annual Review of Physiology. 2000;**62**(1):413-437. DOI: 10.1146/annurev.physiol.62.1.413

[15] Picó C, Sánchez J, Oliver P, Palou A. Leptin production by the stomach is up-regulated in obese (fa/fa) Zucker rats. Obesity Research. 2002;**10**(9):932-938. DOI: 10.1038/oby.2002.127

[16] Kastin AJ, Pan W, Maness LM, Koletsky RJ, Ernsberger P. Decreased transport of leptin across the blood–brain barrier in rats lacking the short form of the leptin receptor. Peptides. 1999;**20**(12):1449-1453. DOI: 10.1016/s0196-9781(99)00156-4

[17] Michaelis OE, Carswell N, Velasquez MT, Hansen CT. The role of obesity, hypertension and diet in diabetes and its complications in the spontaneous hypertensive/NIH-corpulent rat. Nutrition (Burbank, Los Angeles County, Calif.). 1989;**5**(1):56-59

[18] Wisløff U, Najjar SM, Ellingsen Ø, Haram PM, Swoap S, Al-Share Q, et al. Cardiovascular risk factors emerge after artificial selection for low aerobic capacity. Science. 2005;**307**(5708):418-420. DOI: 10.1126/science.1108177

[19] Abdel-Megeid FY, Abdelkarem HM, El-Fetouh AM. Unhealthy nutritional habits in university students are a risk factor for cardiovascular diseases. Saudi Medical Journal. 2011;**32**(6):621-627

[20] Winzell MS, Ahrén B. The high-fat diet–fed mouse: A model for studying mechanisms and treatment of impaired glucose tolerance and type 2 diabetes. Diabetes. 2004;**53**(suppl 3):S215-S219. DOI: 10.2337/diabetes.53.suppl_3.S215

[21] Otero-Losada M, Grana DR, Müller A, Ottaviano G, Ambrosio G, Milei J. Lipid profile and plasma antioxidant status in sweet carbonated beverage-induced metabolic syndrome in rat. International Journal of Cardiology. 2011;**146**(1):106-109. DOI: 10.1016/j.ijcard.2010.09.066

[22] Otero-Losada M, Mc Loughlin S, Rodríguez-Granillo G, Müller A, Ottaviano G, Moriondo M, et al. Metabolic disturbances and worsening of atherosclerotic lesions in ApoE$^{-/-}$ mice after cola beverages drinking. Cardiovascular Diabetology. 2013;**12**(1):57. DOI: 10.1186/1475-2840-12-57

[23] Otero-Losada M, Cao G, Mc Loughlin S, Rodríguez-Granillo G, Ottaviano G, Milei J. Rate of atherosclerosis progression in ApoE$^{-/-}$ mice long after discontinuation of cola beverage drinking. PLoS One. 2014;**9**(3):e89838. DOI: 10.1371/journal.pone.0089838

[24] Otero-Losada M, Cao G, González J, Muller A, Ottaviano G, Lillig C, et al. Functional and morphological changes in endocrine pancreas following cola drink consumption in rats. PLoS One. 2015;**10**(3):e0118700. DOI: 10.1371/journal.pone.0118700

[25] Farkas E, Luiten PG, Bari F. Permanent, bilateral common carotid artery occlusion in the rat: A model for chronic cerebral hypoperfusion-related neurodegenerative diseases. Brain Research Reviews. 2007;**54**(1):162-180. DOI: 10.1016/j.brainresrev.2007.01.003

[26] Shibata M, Ohtani R, Ihara M, Tomimoto H. White matter lesions and glial activation in a novel mouse model of chronic cerebral hypoperfusion. Stroke. 2004;**35**(11):2598-2603. DOI: 10.1161/01.STR.0000143725.19053.60

[27] Kitamura A, Fujita Y, Oishi N, Kalaria RN, Washida K, Maki T, et al. Selective white matter abnormalities in a novel rat model of vascular dementia.

Neurobiology of Aging. 2012;**33**(5):1012.e25-1012.e35. DOI: 10.1016/j.neurobiolaging.2011.10.033

[28] Zhao Y, Gong CX. From chronic cerebral hypoperfusion to Alzheimer-like brain pathology and neurodegeneration. Cellular and Molecular Neurobiology. 2015;**35**(1):101-110. DOI: 10.1007/s10571-014-0127-9

[29] Washida K, Hattori Y, Ihara M. Animal models of chronic cerebral hypoperfusion: From mouse to primate. International Journal of Molecular Sciences. 2019;**20**(24):6176. DOI: 10.3390/ijms20246176

[30] Patel A, Moalem A, Cheng H, Babadjouni RM, Patel K, Hodis DM, et al. Chronic cerebral hypoperfusion induced by bilateral carotid artery stenosis causes selective recognition impairment in adult mice. Neurological Research. 2017;**39**(10):910-917. DOI: 10.1080/01616412.2017.1355423

[31] Hattori Y, Enmi JI, Iguchi S, Saito S, Yamamoto Y, Tsuji M, et al. Gradual carotid artery stenosis in mice closely replicates hypoperfusive vascular dementia in humans. Journal of the American Heart Association. 2016;**5**(2):e002757. DOI: 10.1161/JAHA.115.002757

[32] Mehla J, Lacoursiere S, Stuart E, McDonald RJ, Mohajerani MH. Gradual cerebral hypoperfusion impairs fear conditioning and object recognition learning and memory in mice: Potential roles of neurodegeneration and cholinergic dysfunction. Journal of Alzheimer's Disease. 2018;**61**(1):283-293. DOI: 10.3233/JAD-170635

[33] Jian H, Yi-Fang W, Qi L, Xiao-Song H, Gui-Yun Z. Cerebral blood flow and metabolic changes in hippocampal regions of a modified rat model with chronic cerebral hypoperfusion. Acta Neurologica Belgica. 2013;**113**(3):313-317. DOI: 10.1007/s13760-012-0154-6

[34] Zou W, Song Y, Li Y, Du Y, Zhang X, Fu J. The role of autophagy in the correlation between neuron damage and cognitive impairment in rat chronic cerebral hypoperfusion. Molecular Neurobiology. 2017;**55**(1):776-791. DOI: 10.1007/s12035-016-0351-z

[35] Liu L, Li CJ, Lu Y, Zong XG, Luo C, Sun J, et al. Baclofen mediates neuroprotection on hippocampal CA1 pyramidal cells through the regulation of autophagy under chronic cerebral hypoperfusion. Scientific Reports. 2015;**5**:14474. DOI: 10.1038/srep14474

[36] Ashraf MG, Greig HN, Khan TA, Hassan I, Tabrez S, Shakil S, et al. Protein misfolding and aggregation in Alzheimer's disease and type 2 diabetes mellitus. CNS & Neurological Disorders Drug Targets. 2014;**13**(7):1280-1293. DOI: 10.2174/1871527313666140917095514

[37] Jia Y, Jin W, Xiao Y, Dong Y, Wang T, Fan M, et al. Lipoxin A4 methyl ester alleviates vascular cognition impairment by regulating the expression of proteins related to autophagy and ER stress in the rat hippocampus. Cellular and Molecular Biology Letters. 2015;**20**(3):475-487. DOI: d10.1515/cmble-2015-0027

[38] Wang D, Lin Q, Su S, Liu K, Wu Y, Hai J. URB597 improves cognitive impairment induced by chronic cerebral hypoperfusion by inhibiting mTOR-dependent autophagy. Neuroscience. 2017;**344**:293-304. DOI: 10.1016/j.neuroscience.2016.12.034

[39] Hai J, Lin Q, Wu YF, Huang XS, Zhang GY, Wang F. Effects of N-stearoyl-L-tyrosine on the hippocampal ubiquitin-proteasome system in rats with chronic cerebral hypoperfusion. Neurological

Research. 2013;**35**(7):734-743. DOI: 10.1179/1743132812Y.0000000154

[40] Hai J, Lin Q, Su SH, Zhang L, Wan JF, Lu Y. Chronic cerebral hypoperfusion in rats causes proteasome dysfunction and aggregation of ubiquitinated proteins. Brain Research. 2011;**1374**:73-81. DOI: 10.1016/j.brainres.2010.12.030

[41] Hai J, Wan JF, Lin Q, Wang F, Zhang L, Li H, et al. Cognitive dysfunction induced by chronic cerebral hypoperfusion in a rat model associated with arteriovenous malformations. Brain Research. 2009;**1301**:80-88. DOI: 10.1016/j.brainres.2009.09.001

[42] Ozcan L, Tabas I. Role of endoplasmic reticulum stress in metabolic disease and other disorders. Annual Review of Medicine. 2012;**63**:317-328. DOI: 10.1146/annurev-med-043010-144749

[43] Zhao Y, Gu JH, Dai CL, Liu Q, Iqbal K, Liu F, et al. Chronic cerebral hypoperfusion causes decrease of O-GlcNAcylation, hyperphosphorylation of tau and behavioral deficits in mice. Frontiers in Aging Neuroscience. 2014;**6**:10. DOI: 10.3389/fnagi.2014.00010

[44] Liu F, Iqbal K, Grundke-Iqbal I, Hart GW, Gong CX. O-GlcNAcylation regulates phosphorylation of tau: A mechanism involved in Alzheimer's disease. Proceedings of the National Academy of Sciences. 2004;**101**(29):10804-10809. DOI: 10.1073/pnas.0400348101

[45] Liu F, Shi J, Tanimukai H, Gu J, Gu J, Grundke-Iqbal I, et al. Reduced O-GlcNAcylation links lower brain glucose metabolism and tau pathology in Alzheimer's disease. Brain. 2009;**132**(7):1820-1832. DOI: 10.1093/brain/awp099

[46] Liu Y, Liu F, Grundke-Iqbal I, Iqbal K, Gong CX. Brain glucose transporters, O-GlcNAcylation and phosphorylation of tau in diabetes and Alzheimer's disease. Journal of Neurochemistry. 2009;**111**(1):242-249. DOI: 10.1111/j.1471-4159.2009.06320.x

[47] Qiu L, Ng G, Tan EK, Liao P, Kandiah N, Zeng L. Chronic cerebral hypoperfusion enhances tau hyperphosphorylation and reduces autophagy in Alzheimer's disease mice. Scientific Reports. 2016;**6**:23964. DOI: 10.1038/srep23964

[48] Li JF, Wang Z, Sun QJ, Du YF. Expression of tau protein in rats with cognitive dysfunction induced by cerebral hypoperfusion. International Journal of Clinical and Experimental Medicine. 2015;**8**(10):19682-19688

[49] Kitaguchi H, Tomimoto H, Ihara M, Shibata M, Uemura K, Kalaria RN, et al. Chronic cerebral hypoperfusion accelerates amyloid β deposition in APPSwInd transgenic mice. Brain Research. 2009;**1294**:202-210. DOI: 10.1016/j.brainres.2009.07.078

[50] Bennett SA, Pappas BA, Stevens WD, Davidson CM, Fortin T, Chen J. Cleavage of amyloid precursor protein elicited by chronic cerebral hypoperfusion. Neurobiolology of Aging. 2000;**21**(2):207-214. DOI: 10.1016/S0197-4580(00)00131-7

[51] Obadia N, Lessa MA, Daliry A, Silvares RR, Gomes F, Tibiriçá E, et al. Cerebral microvascular dysfunction in metabolic syndrome is exacerbated by ischemia–reperfusion injury. BMC Neuroscience. 2017;**18**(1):67. DOI: 10.1186/s12868-017-0384-x

[52] Lapi D, Mastantuono T, Sapio D, Paterni M, Colantuoni A. Pial microvascular responses induced by transient bilateral common carotid artery occlusion in Zucker rats. Clinical Hemorheology and Microcirculation. 2013;**54**(4):415-429. DOI: 10.3233/CH-131763

[53] Park JH, Ahn JH, Song M, Kim H, Park CW, Park YE, et al. A 2-min transient ischemia confers cerebral ischemic tolerance in non-obese gerbils, but results in neuronal death in obese gerbils by increasing abnormal mTOR activation-mediated oxidative stress and Neuroinflammation. Cell. 2019;**8**(10):1126. DOI: 10.3390/cells8101126

[54] Ahn JH, Shin MC, Kim DW, Kim H, Song M, Lee TK, et al. Antioxidant properties of Fucoidan alleviate acceleration and exacerbation of hippocampal neuronal death following transient global cerebral ischemia in high-fat diet-induced obese gerbils. International Journal of Molecular Sciences. 2019;**20**(3):554. DOI: 10.3390/ijms20030554

[55] Song M, Ahn JH, Kim H, Kim DW, Lee TK, Lee JC, et al. Chronic high-fat diet-induced obesity in gerbils increases pro-inflammatory cytokines and mTOR activation, and elicits neuronal death in the striatum following brief transient ischemia. Neurochemistry International. 2018;**121**:75-85. DOI: 10.1016/j.neuint.2018.09.009

[56] Yan BC, Park JH, Ahn JH, Kim IH, Lee JC, Yoo KY, et al. Effects of high-fat diet on neuronal damage, gliosis, inflammatory process and oxidative stress in the hippocampus induced by transient cerebral ischemia. Neurochemical Research. 2014;**39**(12):2465-2478. DOI: 10.1007/s11064-014-1450-8

[57] Park S, Kim DS, Kang S, Kwon DY. Ischemic hippocampal cell death induces glucose dysregulation by attenuating glucose-stimulated insulin secretion which is exacerbated by a high fat diet. Life Sciences. 2011;**88**(17-18):766-773. DOI: 10.1016/j.lfs.2011.02.021

[58] Chantler PD, Shrader CD, Tabone LE, d'Audiffret AC, Huseynova K, Brooks SD, et al. Cerebral cortical microvascular rarefaction in metabolic syndrome is dependent on insulin resistance and loss of nitric oxide bioavailability. Microcirculation. 2015;**22**(6):435-445. DOI: 10.1111/micc.12209

[59] Moon SM, Choi GM, Yoo DY, Jung HY, Yim HS, Kim DW, et al. Differential effects of pioglitazone in the hippocampal CA1 region following transient forebrain ischemia in low-and high-fat diet-fed gerbils. Neurochemical Research. 2015;**40**(5):1063-1073. DOI: 10.1007/s11064-015-1568-3

[60] Estato V, Nascimento A, Antunes B, Gomes F, Coelho L, Rangel R, et al. Cerebral microvascular dysfunction and inflammation are improved by centrally acting antihypertensive drugs in metabolic syndrome. Metabolic Syndrome and Related Disorders. 2017;**15**(1):26-35. DOI: 10.1089/met.2016.0085

[61] Nascimento AR, Machado MV, Gomes F, Vieira AB, Gonçalves-de-Albuquerque CF, Lessa MA, et al. Central sympathetic modulation reverses microvascular alterations in a rat model of high-fat diet-induced metabolic syndrome. Microcirculation. 2016;**23**(4):320-329. DOI: 10.1111/micc.12280

[62] Brooks SD, DeVallance E, d'Audiffret AC, Frisbee SJ, Tabone LE, Shrader CD, et al. Metabolic syndrome impairs reactivity and wall mechanics of cerebral resistance arteries in obese Zucker rats. American Journal of Physiology. Heart and Circulatory Physiology. 2015;**309**(11):H1846-H1859. DOI: 10.1152/ajpheart.00691.2015

[63] Estato V, Obadia N, Carvalho-Tavares J, Freitas FS, Reis P, Neto HCF, et al. Blockade of the renin–angiotensin system improves cerebral microcirculatory perfusion in diabetic hypertensive rats.

Microvascular Research. 2013;**87**:41-49. DOI: 10.1016/j.mvr.2013.02.007

[64] Zuloaga KL, Johnson LA, Roese NE, Marzulla T, Zhang W, Nie X, et al. High fat diet-induced diabetes in mice exacerbates cognitive deficit due to chronic hypoperfusion. Journal of Cerebral Blood Flow & Metabolism. 2016;**36**(7):1257-1270. DOI: 10.1177/0271678X15616400

[65] Sweeney P, Park H, Baumann M, Dunlop J, Frydman J, Kopito R, et al. Protein misfolding in neurodegenerative diseases: Implications and strategies. Translational Neurodegeneration. 2017;**6**(1):6. DOI: 10.1186/s40035-017-0077-5

Chapter 8

Neuroprotective and Neurorestorative Properties of Copolymer-1: Its Immunomodulating Effects on Ischemic Stroke

María Yolanda Cruz Martínez,
Melanie Tessa Saavedra Navarrete and
José Juan Antonio Ibarra Arias

Abstract

Stroke is a pathology of great relevance worldwide as it currently occupies the second motif of death and the third reason of disability. Although exits some therapies that are used successfully in the clinic, a very high percentage of patients do not have the opportunity to benefit from them; therefore, it is imperative to propose other alternatives that may favor more patients. In this chapter, we briefly review the inflammatory response induced by stroke and also its deleterious and protective effects. We will describe the characteristics of copolymer-1 and the effects that this compound has shown in models of cerebral ischemia.

Keywords: cerebral ischemia, copaxone, neurogenesis, protective autoimmunity, neuroregeneration, neuroprotection

1. Introduction

Cerebral ischemia is the main disorder of cerebrovascular diseases; currently, according to data from the World Health Organization, it is the second main cause of death worldwide [1] and the third principal cause of disability. In the last 40 years alone, the incidence of this condition has more than doubled in people from low and middle-revenue countries [2].

The increment in the incidence of this condition is due to increased risk factors as diabetes mellitus, hypertension, obesity, hyperlipidemia, and increased longevity of the population [3]. These factors allow the development of atherosclerosis, which is the main cause of ischemia [4]; thereby, it is considered that for the coming years this scenario will be maintained while strategies to reduce these factors are progressing.

Stroke is distinguished by the brusque reduction of blood flow; therefore, the levels of oxygen and glucose are also reduced significantly, to the point of altering the metabolic activities of the neural tissue [5]. As a consequence of the latter, the low production of ATP and the acidification of the environment induce the depolarization of the membranes causing the intracellular increase of Ca^{2+} that is added to the one released by the endoplasmic reticulum and mitochondria [6].

Neuronal depolarization causes the release of glutamate which, when bound to its ionotropic N-methyl-D-aspartate (NMDA) and -amino-3-hydroxy-5-methyl-4-isoxazolpropionic (AMPA) receptors, achieves greater depolarization and, as a consequence, conditions of excitotoxicity [7]. These conditions are coupled with the production of free radicals [8] and lead to cell death by the activation of molecules that induce necrosis and apoptosis [9].

Along with the lesion caused by the decrease in blood flow, the immune response is added to the events involved in both the detriment of the tissue and its protection.

2. Immunological response in stroke

Inflammation is usually present before the development of arterial obstruction that gives rise to the ischemic event. The development of atherosclerosis is accompanied by the production of oxygen free radicals (ROS), expression of cell adhesion molecules, and production of proinflammatory cytokines as IL-1β and tumor necrosis factor-α (TNF-α) by endothelial cells [10].

Shortly after occlusion, endothelial cells express a greater amount of intercellular adhesion molecules (ICAM), deposition of mannose binding lectin molecules that trigger activation of the complement pathway [11], producing higher amounts of ROS. The overproduction of ROS activates the prostaglandin pathway that stimulates the production of matrix metalloproteinases (MMP) that even though degrading constituents of the extracellular matrix, reshape the vascular endothelium seeking to protect of the blood brain barrier (BBB) [12].

The release of chemokines such as CCL2 allows endothelial permeability [13], leading to the translocation of P-selectin from Weibel-Palade bodies, as well as the expression of ICAM-1 and vascular cell adhesion molecule (VCAM)-1 and E-selectin, on the endothelial surface [14]. Theses phenomena, together with the damage of the extracellular matrix facilitate the extravasation of macromolecules and water, which causes the development of vasogenic edema [15]. Peripheral immune cells then enter the injured cerebral parenchyma [16] facilitating the loss of the integrity of the BBB.

Neutrophils are the first leukocytes that migrate to the cerebral parenchyma; they have been detected since the first hour after ischemia and reach their maximum peak in 1–3 days [17]. In the clinic, it has been observed that the higher blood neutrophil count is associated with higher infarction volumes in patients with acute stroke [18].

The second cell type that enters the neural tissue are monocytes, these infiltrate within 24 h of the onset of the ischemic event reaching its peak on day 3 [19]; their differentiation process toward macrophages and their activation will be determined by the molecular environment to which they arrive. This process is similar to that experienced by T lymphocytes, which reach the parenchyma 24–96 h post-ischemia [20].

At the same time, the cells of the injured cerebral parenchyma release damage associated molecular patterns (DAMPs) that activate the microglia. Depending on the activation environment, the microglia can acquire a proinflammatory (M1) or anti-inflammatory (M2) phenotype [21]. In the M1 phenotype, the microglia acquires phagocytic capacity, produces NO, free radicals, and proinflammatory cytokines (e.g. TNF-α, IL-12 and IL-6) [22]. Some regions in the ischemic penumbra present an activation of M2 microglia distinguished by the production of anti-inflammatory and repair molecules, such as insulin growth factor 1 (IGF-1), IL-10, and arginase 1 [23].

Some researchers suggest that the M2 phenotype is initially activated during the acute phase in the peripheral zone to the infarction [24], since it has been determined that the levels of IL-10, TGF-β, and CD206 increase from the first day after the lesion and reach the maximum point between 4 and 6 days, possibly trying to keep the viability of tissue. In addition, TGF-β induces the anti-inflammatory phenotype of microglia, related with enhanced proliferation and neuroprotection [25, 26].

In contrast, some authors suggest that the first response is proinflammatory [27], due to the loss of regulatory mechanisms; when a stroke occurs there is an important activation of the M1 microglial phenotype [28].

Although contradictory, both positions could be correct. The fact is that, M1 and M2 phenotypes actively participate in the response observed after ischemic event; however, in normal conditions, there is an important prevalence of the M1 phenotype leading the response to a proinflammatory reaction that, instead of helping, promotes more damage.

On the other hand, perivascular macrophages and monocytes of peripheral origin that arrive at the injured parenchyma induce the synthesis of chemokines like CXCL1 and CXCL2, which are fundamental for recruiting more neutrophils to the injury site [29, 30]. The dendritic cells (DC) present a greater expression of the major histocompatibility complex II (MHCII) and the co-stimulant molecule CD80. This causes an important enhance in the interaction of T cells around and within the damaged areas inducing then a stronger immune response [31].

When T lymphocytes are activated by antigen-presenting cells (APCs) toward a Th1 phenotype, the secretion of proinflammatory cytokines like as IFN-γ, TNF, and LT-α [lymphotoxin] increases. This cytokine profile, intensify proinflammatory response and thereby, tissue damage. Contrarily, when T cells are activated toward a Th2 phenotype they produce anti-inflammatory cytokines such as IL-4 and IL-10 [32]. These cytokines have been associated with tissue protection mechanisms and even increased neurogenesis. This immune response that exerts protective effects and limits the damage caused by ischemia [19] can be stimulated by immunomodulatory molecules such as copolymer-1.

3. Copolymer-1

Copolymer-1 [Cop-1], also known as glatiramer acetate (GA) or copaxone [trade name], is a blend of peptides formed by random sequences of four amino acids: glutamic acid, lysine, alanine, and tyrosine; these have a variable length from 45 to 200 amino acid residues and a molecular weight of 4000–9000 Da [33].

Cop-1 was originally synthesized from mylelin basic protein (MBP) to identify the precise immunogenic sequence and provoke experimental autoimmune encephalomyelitis (EAE), an animal model of multiple sclerosis (MS); however, it did not present encephalitogenic characteristics [34]; on the contrary, it has suppressive and protective effects on EAE [35]. In the clinic, copaxone is able to diminish the relapse rate and improve the disability of patients with relapsing-remitting MS [36]. Copaxone obtained its approvement by the Food and Drugs Administration [FDA] of U.S.A. in 1996 and in Europe in 2001 [33].

At this time, the exact mechanism by which Cop-1 exerts its protective effects is not known at all. Studies carried out in EAE suggest that Cop-1 has greater affinity for the MHCII binding site of APC when competing with peptide complexes derived from the MBP, specifically with the epitope 82–100 [37]. This competition may also be present among the complexes for the TCR binding site of the lymphocytes [38] that, when activated, induces a Th2 response [39].

The Cop-1 response is distinguished by increased synthesis of IL-4, IL-5, IL-10, IL-13, and TGF-β [33, 40–43]. Cop-1 has also been observed to increase the presence of regulatory T lymphocytes [44] and regulatory CD8+ T lymphocytes in patients with multiple sclerosis [45, 46].

Another important effect of copolymer-1 is the production of growth factors, among which stand out; the brain derived neurotrophic factor [BDNF] [47, 48], IGF-1, [49] and neurotrophins NT-3 and NT-4 [47]. It is known that, in addition to inducing neuroprotection and neurorestoration, these growth factors are related to mechanisms such as memory and learning.

The molecular basis by which Cop-1 exerts its neuroprotective effect has been evaluated in several *in-vitro* assays. The most explanatory results have been obtained in the analysis of the effect of Cop-1 on APC such as monocytes, microglia, and astrocytes.

It has been showed that through the blockade of the nuclear factor kappa B [NF-kB], Cop-1 reduces the expression of the chemokine CCL5 [RANTES], which is upregulated by the presence of IL-1β [50] and TNF-α in human astroglial cells [51]. A similar effect has also been observed on the monocyte chemotactic protein-1 [MPC-1] and adhesion molecules VCAM-1 and selectin E in endothelial cells as well as COX2 and iNOS [52].

It has also been observed that Cop-1 induces differentiation of type II monocytes independently of the binding of Cop-1 to MHCII. Weber et al. demonstrated that this differentiation is due to the fact that Cop-1 reduces the phosphorylation of the transcription factor STAT-1 by stimulating the expression of IL-10 and TGF-β [53].

On the other hand, it has also been observed that Cop-1 has a direct effect on glial cells [microglia and astrocytes] which are activated in conjunction with T cells reducing STAT-1 and STAT-3 phosphorylation through increased expression of cytokine signaling suppressor (SOCS-1) and independently of IFNϒR, accompanied by a reduction of IL-12 by CD4+ T lymphocytes [54].

Even though the molecular pathways by which Cop-1 acts are not yet completely established, the microenvironment induced by this compound is capable of allowing neuroprotection since it reduces the deleterious scenario that leads to neural death. Additionally, the new conditions could facilitate tissue restoration through the synthesis of growth factors.

4. The effect of copolymer-1 on inflammatory diseases

The beneficial effects showed by copaxone in patients with MS, even though the knowledge of its immunomodulatory mechanisms is partial, encouraged the evaluation of its effect in other experimental models.

In the model of optic nerve lesion—which tries to reproduce the characteristics of secondary degeneration—Cop-1 demonstrated an interesting neuroprotective effect. Kipnis et al. [55] evaluated the effect of adoptive anti-Cop-1 T cell transfer and immunization with Cop-1 immediately after causing optic nerve contusion in Lewis rats; their results were very encouraging as they observed reduction in axonal degeneration, accumulation of T lymphocytes in injured areas and obtained a significant increase in IL-10 and BDNF *in-vitro*. In contrast, using a model of axon transection of the optic nerve, Blair and coworkers [56] found no beneficial effects of Cop-1. The difference in the results may be due to the different inflammatory response evoked by the type of injury (contusion or transection). Inflammation is more pronounced after contusion as compared to the one observed after a transection. It should be an issue to be studied by future investigations.

Parkinson's disease presents gradual reduction of dopaminergic neurons in the region of the substantia nigra and the striatum in the brain, it is not known the reason that causes the death of these neurons, but the pathology is characterized by a significant increase in oxidative stress, mitochondrial dysfunction, neuroinflammation, and cell death [57]. Patients with PD present an increase in TNF-β, IL-1β, and IL-6 and other inflammatory cytokines resulting from the activation of the macrophages and microglia towards a proinflammatory phenotype capable of releasing NO and superoxide radicals that further damage neural tissue facilitating disease progression [58].

In the traditional model to induce Parkinson's disease in mice [induction by 1-1-methyl-1,2,3,6-tetrahydropyridine], it was observed that Cop-1 reduces the degeneration of dopaminergic cells. This effect is achieved since Cop-1 induces the up-regulation in the protein expression of tyrosine hydroxylase [59, 60]. Additionally, it has been reported an increase in glial cell-derived neurotrophic factor (GDNF), reduction of activated microglia markers, and restoration of BDNF [61]. Based in these findings, several research groups consider COP-1 as a pharmacological alternative for this pathology which should be deeply studied [62].

Copolimer-1 has also been tested in models of Alzheimer's disease (AD). AD is a pathology that produces deposits of the β-amyloid protein, dystrophic neurites, loss of synapses and neurons, and elevated gliosis [63]. From the early stages of the pathology, it has been observed microgial activation toward a M2 neuroprotective phenotype that is modified as the disease progresses [64]. In advanced stages, a proinflammatory microenvironment characterized by the presence of cytokines such as IL-1β, TNF-α, IL-6 has been reported [65].

After Cop-1 administration, microglia modulation toward a M2 phenotype is observed, in such a way as to promote neuronal survival and neural tissue repair in AD models [66]. Butovsky and coworkers showed that Cop-1 immunizations lead to enhanced infiltration of monocyte-derived macrophages into neural tissue with an anti-inflammatory profile expressing minor levels of TNF-α and high levels of IL-10, TGF-β1, and IGF1. In this scenario, phagocytosis of preformed fibrillar amyloid-β by bone marrow-derived macrophages increased dramatically after the administration of Cop-1. Also, to demonstrate benefits on the preservation of cognitive function, the investigation showed an important synaptic protection, plaque removal, restriction of astrogliosis, and modulation of the immune molecular environment [67, 68].

Another pathology that evidenced the beneficial effects produced by Cop-1 is amyotrophic lateral sclerosis (ALS). This is a neurodegenerative disease known by the progressive depletion of the upper and lower motor neurons [69]. During pathogenesis, glutamate excitotoxicity, structural and functional anomalies of mitochondria, damaged axonal structure, and oxidative stress conducted by free radicals are strongly observed [70].

In this case, Angelov and colleagues showed—in mouse models—that the administration of Cop-1 promotes the survival of motor neurons [71].

The beneficial effects of Cop-1 on ALS have been assessed in a Phase II trial conducted by Mosley. This investigation evaluated the cytokine response of ALS patients treated with copaxone and showed that copaxone is capable of inducing a temporary change in cytokines from Th1 to Th2 phenotype [72].

Copaxone is also tested in other pathologies at clinical settings. For instance, a phase III study on optic neuritis is now being conducted to evaluate the thickness of the layer of nerve fiber of the retina after 6 months of treatment. The results of this study have not been published. Finally, copaxone has been tested in Crohn's disease and various types of carcinomas, studies where copaxone is in evaluation processes [73].

The ability of Cop-1 to modify the proinflammatory milieu and to stimulate the production of growth factors encourages the idea of testing this compound on other pathologies with characteristics of secondary degeneration caused by inflammation. In line with this, the use of Cop-1 after stroke envisions an optimistic result.

5. Effect of copolymer-1 on stroke

As copolymer-1 has been shown to have beneficial effects in various models where neuroinflammation is a detrimental determinant, our group decided to evaluate its neuroprotective effect on cerebral ischemia. For this purpose, we used the median transient cerebral artery obstruction (tMCAO) model. Sprague-Dawley male rats were used. After being subjected to ischemia for 90 min, the rats were immunized in the interscapular region with a dose of 200 μg of Cop-1.

In the first study, the animals were evaluated for neurological deficit at day 1 and day 7 post-ischemia using the Zea Longa scale [74]. Then, a histological analysis was performed using hematoxylin and eosin staining to determine neuroprotection. The results indicated that Cop-1 is able to avoid up to 85.1% increase in infarct size (4.8 ± 1.5 for Cop-1 vs. 32.2 ± 8 for control group; $p = 0.004$ mean ± SD; **Figure 1A**) and is able to reduce neurological deficit on day 7 post-ischemia.

This neuroprotective effect may be due to the reduction of the proinflammatory cytokines TNF-α and IL-1β and the increase of IL-4, as was observed by the Manguin group in a model of ischemia in diabetic mice [75]. Additionally, the production of neurotrophic factors—known to be implicated in the processes of neural survival and proliferation of neuron precursor cells—could also be involved [76].

On the other hand, recovery from neurological deficit can be achieved by diverse mechanisms; for instance, neuroprotection exerted by Cop-1 could be limiting tissue damage caused by inflammation, this could allow the proper functioning of remaining neuronal connections. Functional recovery could also be the result of neurogenesis induced by Cop-1. Neurogenesis is a phenomenon that can replace neurons that died during the ischemic insult by allowing the substitution of neuronal circuits and thus neurorestoration.

Our study provided evidences about the neuroprotective effect of Cop-1; however, the fact that Cop-1-induced T cells are able to produce neurotrophic factors, led us to think that, it was imperative to investigate if behind the clinical recovery there was also a possible neurogenesis phenomenon.

In the following study, we evaluated whether Cop-1 induces neurogenesis in the two neurogenic niches of the adult brain: in the subventricular (SVZ) and the

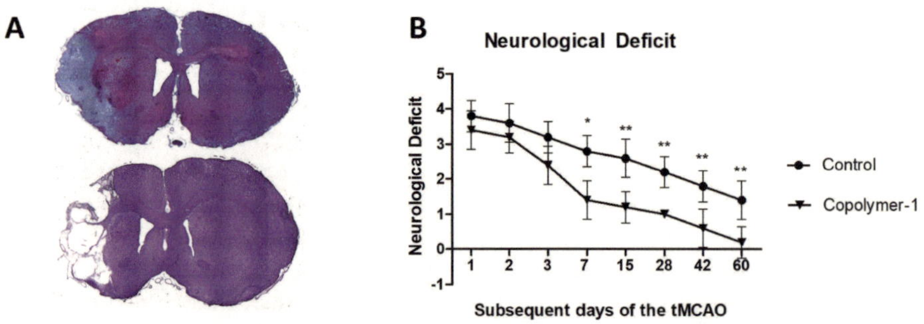

Figure 1.
Neuroprotective effect of the copolymer-1. (A) Infarction size reduction. (B) Effect of the copolymer-1 on the neurological deficit. n = 8. Each bar represents mean ± SEM. Two-way repeated measure ANOVA. Sidak's post hoc multiple comparisons test. $^{*}p < 0.05$; $^{**}p < 0.0$.

subgranular zone of the dentate hippocampus gyrus (SGZ) [77]. To accomplish the evaluation, we performed an immunofluorescence technique using a double marking of 5-bromo-2′-deoxyuridine (BrdU) and doublecortin (Dcx) at 7 and 60 days after ischemia.

The results were very encouraging, the neurological recovery caused by Cop-1 was observed from day 7 post-ischemia as in the first experiment [78] and was improving even in the chronic phase at 60 days (**Figure 1B**). The number of neuroblasts in the groups treated with Cop-1 was significantly higher in the two neurogenic niches at both 7 and 60 days in the SVZ and SGZ (**Figure 2**). This neurogenic phenomenon correlated with the clinical recovery of treated rats. Simultaneously, an important increase of NT-3 was observed in the area of the ischemic penumbra [79].

Cop-1-induced neurogenesis has been evaluated in other animal models such as EAE [47], Alzheimer [66], and recently in the model of permanent cerebral ischemia in diabetic male mice C57Bl6 [75]. Regarding the latter, it is important to mention that, in a previous experiment carried out by the same group, they did not observe improvement in the neurological function nor reduction in the volume of the infarction. These findings could be the result of the use of inappropriate evaluation techniques [80] as in their most recent study, they observed a reduction in infarct size of up to 30–40% and an increase in neurogenesis 7 days after permanent ischemia in the SVZ. In addition, they found a reduction of proinflammatory cytokines such as TNF-α, IL-1β, and a significant increase of IL-4 and IL-10 [75].

Neurogenesis is a mechanism widely regulated by signals that stimulate the stem cells of neurogenic niches [81]; many of these signals are produced by the choroid plexus (CP), which is a complex structure of cells considered an interface that mediates communication between the immune system and the cerebral parenchyma [82]. Therefore, trying to analyze the mechanism by which Cop-1 induces neurogenesis, we evaluate whether Cop-1 modifies the microenvironment of CP, 14 days after tMCAO.

In the third investigation, we evaluated neurological recovery—which was observed according to our previous experiments [78, 79], neurogenesis and the expression of proinflammatory (IL-1β, TNF-α, INF-ϒ, and IL-17) and anti-inflammatory cytokines (IL-4 and IL-10) as well as the concentration of growth factors (BDNF, NT-3 and IGF-1) at the CP (**Figure 3**).

In this experiment, we again proved a significant increase of neurogenesis in the groups treated with Cop-1 in both, the SVZ and SGZ [83]. This data was similar to that previously reported [79]. As for the expression of proinflammatory cytokines, we only found significant differences in the expression of IL-17, which was observed reduced in the groups treated with Cop-1. With respect to anti-inflammatory cytokines, only IL-10 was significantly increased. In this investigation, we also found a significant increase of growth factors (BDNF, NT-3, and IGF-1) in the CP [83].

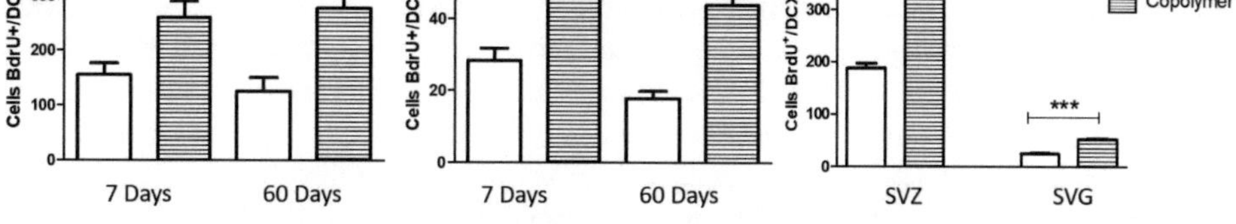

Figure 2.
*Effect of copolymer-1 on neurogenesis at 7, 14, and 60 days. (A) Neurogenesis in SVZ at 7 and 60 days. (B) Neurogenesis in SGZ at 7 and 60 days. (C) Neurogenesis in SVZ and SGZ at 14 days. n = 8 in A and B. n = 5 in C. Each bar represents mean ± SEM. Two-tailed Mann-Whitney U test. Dunn's post hoc multiple comparison test. *p < 0.05, **p < 0.01, ***p < 0.001. SVZ: Subventricular zone and SGZ: Subgranular zone.*

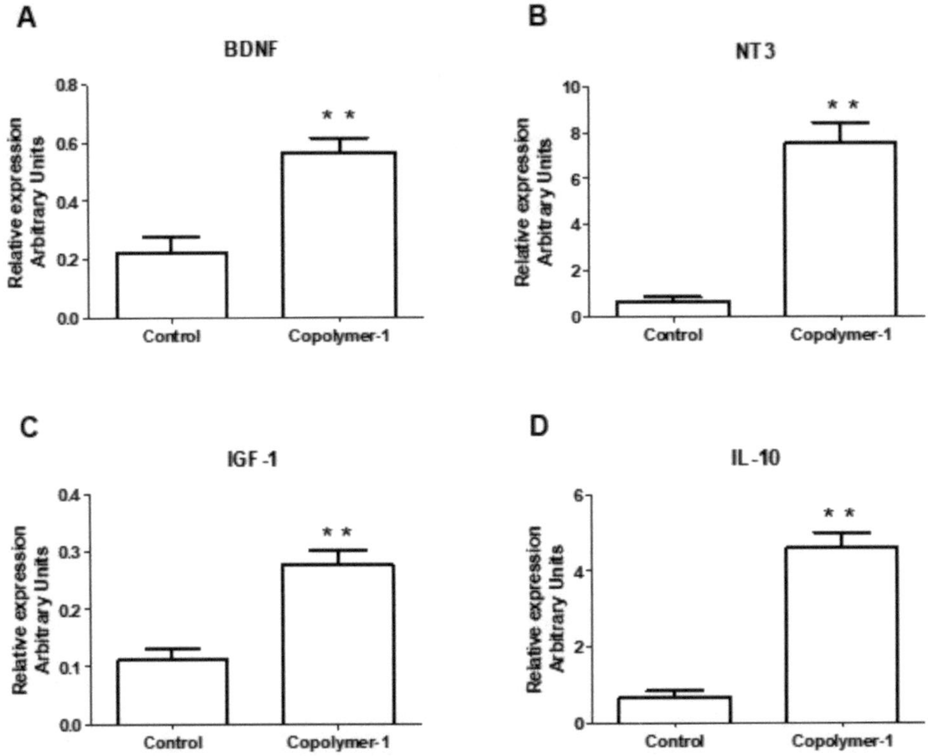

Figure 3.
*Effect of the copolymer-1 on the expression of growth factors and IL-10. Gene expression of: (A) BDNF; (B) NT-3; (C) IGF-1; and (D) IL-10. Bars represent mean ± SEM of 5 rats from each group. *p < 0.05, **p < 0.001. Mann-Whitney U test. Dunn's post hoc multiple comparison test.*

Both growth factors and IL-10 have been reported to be directly involved in the stimulation of SVZ and SGZ stem cells; specifically, IL-10 has been observed to induce stem cell proliferation but not differentiation in primary cultures [84]. Moreover, IL-10 has immunomodulatory capacity as it inhibits the synthesis and release of proinflammatory cytokines such as TNF-α, IL-6, and IL-1β that are known to affect neurogenesis [85]. Moreover, growth factors such as NT-3 maintain viable stem cells from neurogenic niches facilitating plasticity [86]. BDNF promotes the proliferation and survival of neuroblasts [87] and IGF-1 promotes stem cell differentiation and migration of neuroblasts [88]. Therefore, this investigation allowed to demonstrate that Cop-1 is capable of raising the expression of IL-10 and growth factors, which have beneficial effects on neurogenesis.

In order to know if Cop-1 modulates the number of leukocytes in CP and to know if these intervene in the synthesis and release of growth factors and IL-10, we evaluated the cell types present in the cerebrospinal fluid in animals submitted to tMCAO and Cop-1 therapy. The results showed a significant increment in CD8+ T cells, which positively linked with the increase in growth factors and IL-10 [unpublished data].

The increase in CD8+ T lymphocytes has been observed as an effect of copaxone immunization in patients with MS [46]. In addition, experiments performed in the EAE model have considered these cells indispensable for the development of the beneficial effect of Cop-1 [89]. However, it is necessary to identify the nature of these cells and whether the type of CD8 T lymphocytes is of a regulatory phenotype.

Finally, the combination of Cop-1 with other strategies like polyunsaturated fatty acids has shown optimistic results as together, they have a greater capacity to significantly reduce the size of the infarction in the tMCAO model [unpublished data].

6. Conclusion

The existing evidence of the effect of Cop-1 in the tMCAO model has been very encouraging, as it shows a significant neurological recovery. This beneficial effect could be caused by modulatory mechanisms that allow the increase of IL-4 and the reduction of TNF-α and IL-1β at the lesion site, promoting then neuroprotection. Additionally, neurological recovery could also be reinforced by the changes induced by Cop-1 at the CP as the increase of IL-10 and growth factors in this site stimulate neurogenesis after ischemia. We consider that more investigations are needed in order to analyze in greater detail the mechanism by which Cop-1 acts so that in the medium term, it may be considered as a pharmacological alternative for patients suffering from a cerebrovascular event.

Author details

María Yolanda Cruz Martínez, Melanie Tessa Saavedra Navarrete and José Juan Antonio Ibarra Arias*
Centro de Investigación en Ciencias de la Salud (CICSA), Facultad de Ciencias de la Salud, Universidad Anáhuac México, Estado de México, Mexico

*Address all correspondence to: jose.ibarra@anahuac.mx

References

[1] OMS. Top 10 causas de muerte. Datos del observatorio mundial de la salud [GHO]. 2018. Available from: http://www.who.int/en/news-room/fact-sheets/detail/the-top-10-causes-of-death

[2] OMS. Noncommunicable Diseases. World Health Organization [Internet]. 2018. Available from: https://www.who.int/nmh/publications/ncd-profiles-2018/en/ [Accessed: 03 November 2019]

[3] Boehme AK, Esenwa C, Elkind MS. Stroke risk factors, genetics, and prevention. Circulation Research. 2017;**120**(3):472-495

[4] Banerjee C, Chimowitz MI. Stroke caused by atherosclerosis of the major intracranial arteries. Circulation Research. 2017;**120**(3):502-513. DOI: 10.1161/circresaha.116.308441

[5] Su YC, Lim SN, Yang FY, Lin SK. Evaluation of cerebral blood flow in acute ischemic stroke patients with atrial fibrillation: A sonographic study. Journal of the Formosan Medical Association. 2017;**116**(4):287-294

[6] Gerkau NJ, Rakers C, Petzold GC, Rose CR. Differential effects of energy deprivation on intracellular sodium homeostasis in neurons and astrocytes. Journal of Neuroscience Research. 2017;**95**(11):2275-2285. DOI: 10.1002/jnr.23995

[7] Borah M, Dhar S, Gogoi DM, Ruram AA. Association of serum calcium levels with infarct size in acute ischemic stroke: Observations from Northeast India. Journal of Neurosciences in Rural Practice. 2016;**7**(Suppl 1):S41-SS5. DOI: 10.4103/0976-3147.196461

[8] Shirley R, Ord EN, Work LM. Oxidative stress and the use of antioxidants in stroke. Antioxidants. 2014;**3**(3):472-501. DOI: 10.3390/antiox3030472

[9] Guo P, Jin Z, Wu H, Li X, Ke J, Zhang Z, et al. Effects of irisin on the dysfunction of blood-brain barrier in rats after focal cerebral ischemia/reperfusion. Brain and Behavior: A Cognitive Neuroscience Perspective. 2019;**9**(10):e01425. DOI: 10.1002/brb3.1425

[10] Zmyslowski A, Szterk A. Current knowledge on the mechanism of atherosclerosis and pro-atherosclerotic properties of oxysterols. Lipids in Health and Disease. 2017;**16**(1):188. DOI: 10.1186/s12944-017-0579-2

[11] Orsini F, Fumagalli S, Csaszar E, Toth K, De Blasio D, Zangari R, et al. Mannose-binding lectin drives platelet inflammatory phenotype and vascular damage after cerebral ischemia in mice via IL [interleukin]-1alpha. Arteriosclerosis, Thrombosis, and Vascular Biology. 2018;**38**(11):2678-2690. DOI: 10.1161/atvbaha.118.311058

[12] Abdelnaseer MM, Elfauomy NM, Esmail EH, Kamal MM, Elsawy EH. Matrix metalloproteinase-9 and recovery of acute ischemic stroke. Journal of Stroke and Cerebrovascular Diseases. 2017;**26**(4):733-740. DOI: 10.1016/j.jstrokecerebrovasdis.2016.09.043

[13] Dimitrijevic OB, Stamatovic SM, Keep RF, Andjelkovic AV. Effects of the chemokine CCL2 on blood-brain barrier permeability during ischemia-reperfusion injury. Journal of Cerebral Blood Flow and Metabolism. 2006;**26**(6):797-810. DOI: 10.1038/sj.jcbfm.9600229

[14] Zhang H, Park JH, Maharjan S, Park JA, Choi KS, Park H, et al. Sac-1004, a vascular leakage blocker, reduces cerebral ischemia-reperfusion injury

by suppressing blood-brain barrier disruption and inflammation. Journal of Neuroinflammation. 2017;**14**(1):122. DOI: 10.1186/s12974-017-0897-3

[15] Krueger M, Mages B, Hobusch C, Michalski D. Endothelial edema precedes blood-brain barrier breakdown in early time points after experimental focal cerebral ischemia. Acta Neuropathologica Communications. 2019;7(1):17. DOI: 10.1186/s40478-019-0671-0

[16] Shi Y, Zhang L, Pu H, Mao L, Hu X, Jiang X, et al. Rapid endothelial cytoskeletal reorganization enables early blood-brain barrier disruption and long-term ischaemic reperfusion brain injury. Nature Communications. 2016;**7**:10523. DOI: 10.1038/ncomms10523

[17] Chu HX, Kim HA, Lee S, Moore JP, Chan CT, Vinh A, et al. Immune cell infiltration in malignant middle cerebral artery infarction: Comparison with transient cerebral ischemia. Journal of Cerebral Blood Flow and Metabolism. 2014;**34**(3):450-459. DOI: 10.1038/jcbfm.2013.217

[18] Planas AM. Role of immune cells migrating to the ischemic brain. Stroke. 2018;**49**(9):2261-2267. DOI: 10.1161/strokeaha.118.021474

[19] Gliem M, Schwaninger M, Jander S. Protective features of peripheral monocytes/macrophages in stroke. Biochimica et Biophysica Acta. 2016;**1862**(3):329-338. DOI: 10.1016/j.bbadis.2015.11.004

[20] Stubbe T, Ebner F, Richter D, Engel O, Klehmet J, Royl G, et al. Regulatory T cells accumulate and proliferate in the ischemic hemisphere for up to 30 days after MCAO. Journal of Cerebral Blood Flow and Metabolism. 2013;**33**(1):37-47. DOI: 10.1038/jcbfm.2012.128

[21] Gülke E, Gelderblom M, Magnus T. Danger signals in stroke and their role on microglia activation after ischemia. Therapeutic Advances in Neurological Disorders. 2018;**11**:1756286418774254. DOI: 10.1177/1756286418774254

[22] Barakat R, Redzic Z. The role of activated microglia and resident macrophages in the neurovascular unit during cerebral ischemia: Is the jury still out? Medical Principles and Practice. 2016;**25**(Suppl 1):3-14. DOI: 10.1159/000435858

[23] Anttila JE, Whitaker KW, Wires ES, Harvey BK, Airavaara M. Role of microglia in ischemic focal stroke and recovery: Focus on toll-like receptors. Progress in Neuro-Psychopharmacology & Biological Psychiatry. 2017;**79**(Pt A):3-14. DOI: 10.1016/j.pnpbp.2016.07.003

[24] Hu X, Li P, Guo Y, Wang H, Leak RK, Chen S, et al. Microglia/macrophage polarization dynamics reveal novel mechanism of injury expansion after focal cerebral ischemia. Stroke. 2012;**43**(11):3063-3070. DOI: 10.1161/strokeaha.112.659656

[25] Perego C, Fumagalli S, De Simoni MG. Temporal pattern of expression and colocalization of microglia/macrophage phenotype markers following brain ischemic injury in mice. Journal of Neuroinflammation. 2011;**8**:174. DOI: 10.1186/1742-2094-8-174

[26] Patel AR, Ritzel R, McCullough LD, Liu F. Microglia and ischemic stroke: A double-edged sword. International Journal of Physiology, Pathophysiology and Pharmacology. 2013;**5**(2):73-90

[27] Lan X, Han X, Li Q, Yang QW, Wang J. Modulators of microglial activation and polarization after intracerebral haemorrhage. Nature Reviews. Neurology. 2017;**13**(7):420-433. DOI: 10.1038/nrneurol.2017.69

[28] Zhao SC, Ma LS, Chu ZH, Xu H, Wu WQ, Liu F. Regulation of microglial activation in stroke. Acta Pharmacologica

Sinica. 2017;**38**(4):445-458. DOI: 10.1038/aps.2016.162

[29] Jickling GC, Liu D, Ander BP, Stamova B, Zhan X, Sharp FR. Targeting neutrophils in ischemic stroke: Translational insights from experimental studies. Journal of Cerebral Blood Flow and Metabolism. 2015;**35**(6):888-901. DOI: 10.1038/jcbfm.2015.45

[30] Enzmann G, Kargaran S, Engelhardt B. Ischemia-reperfusion injury in stroke: Impact of the brain barriers and brain immune privilege on neutrophil function. Therapeutic Advances in Neurological Disorders. 2018;**11**:1-15. DOI: 10.1177/1756286418794184

[31] Rayasam A, Hsu M, Kijak JA, Kissel L, Hernandez G, Sandor M, et al. Immune responses in stroke: How the immune system contributes to damage and healing after stroke and how this knowledge could be translated to better cures? Immunology. 2018;**154**(3):363-376. DOI: 10.1111/imm.12918

[32] Brait VH, Arumugam TV, Drummond GR, Sobey CG. Importance of T lymphocytes in brain injury, immunodeficiency, and recovery after cerebral ischemia. Journal of Cerebral Blood Flow and Metabolism. 2012;**32**(4):598-611. DOI: 10.1038/jcbfm.2012.6

[33] Prod'homme T, Zamvil SS. The evolving mechanisms of action of glatiramer acetate. Cold Spring Harbor Perspectives in Medicine. 2019;**9**:1-16. DOI: 10.1101/cshperspect.a029249

[34] Scheindlin S. Copolymer 1: An off-beat drug development story. Molecular Interventions. 2004;**4**(1):6-9. DOI: 10.1101/cshperspect.a029249

[35] Aharoni R, Teitelbaum D, Sela M, Arnon R. Copolymer 1 induces T cells of the T helper type 2 that crossreact with myelin basic protein and suppress experimental autoimmune encephalomyelitis. Proceedings of the National Academy of Sciences of the United States of America. 1997;**94**(20):10821-10826. DOI: 10.1073/pnas.94.20.10821

[36] Johnson KP, Brooks BR, Cohen JA, Ford CC, Goldstein J, Lisak RP, et al. Copolymer 1 reduces relapse rate and improves disability in relapsing-remitting multiple sclerosis: Results of a phase III multicenter, double-blind placebo-controlled trial. The copolymer 1 multiple sclerosis study group. Neurology. 1995;**45**(7):1268-1276. DOI: 10.1212/wnl.45.7.1268

[37] Aharoni R, Teitelbaum D, Arnon R, Sela M. Copolymer 1 acts against the immunodominant epitope 82-100 of myelin basic protein by T cell receptor antagonism in addition to major histocompatibility complex blocking. Proceedings of the National Academy of Sciences of the United States of America. 1999;**96**(2):634-639. DOI: 10.1073/pnas.94.20.10821

[38] Fridkis-Hareli M, Santambrogio L, Stern JN, Fugger L, Brosnan C, Strominger JL. Novel synthetic amino acid copolymers that inhibit autoantigen-specific T cell responses and suppress experimental autoimmune encephalomyelitis. The Journal of Clinical Investigation. 2002;**109**(12):1635-1643. DOI: 10.1172/jci15402

[39] Gran B, Tranquill LR, Chen M, Bielekova B, Zhou W, Dhib-Jalbut S, et al. Mechanisms of immunomodulation by glatiramer acetate. Neurology. 2000;**55**(11):1704-1714. DOI: 10.1212/wnl.55.11.1704

[40] Aharoni R, Kayhan B, Eilam R, Sela M, Arnon R. Glatiramer acetate-specific T cells in the brain express T helper 2/3 cytokines and brain-derived neurotrophic factor in situ. Proceedings of the National Academy of Sciences

of the United States of America. 2003;**100**(24):14157-14162. DOI: 10.1073/pnas.2336171100

[41] Aharoni R. Immunomodulation neuroprotection and remyelination—The fundamental therapeutic effects of glatiramer acetate: A critical review. Journal of Autoimmunity. 2014;**54**: 81-92. DOI: 10.1016/j.jaut.2014.05.005

[42] Duda PW, Schmied MC, Cook SL, Krieger JI, Hafler DA. Glatiramer acetate [copaxone] induces degenerate, Th2-polarized immune responses in patients with multiple sclerosis. The Journal of Clinical Investigation. 2000;**105**(7):967-976. DOI: 10.1172/jci8970

[43] Sheremata W, Campos Y. Mechanisms of action of glatiramer acetate in the treatment of multiple sclerosis. In: Campos Y, editor. Multiple Sclerosis: A Mechanistic View. 1st ed. Elsevier Inc.; 2015. pp. 339-363. DOI: 10.1016/B978-0-12-800763-1.00014-2

[44] Spadaro M, Montarolo F, Perga S, Martire S, Brescia F, Malucchi S, et al. Biological activity of glatiramer acetate on Treg and anti-inflammatory monocytes persists for more than 10 years in responder multiple sclerosis patients. Clinical Immunology. 2017;**181**:83-88. DOI: 10.1016/j.clim.2017.06.006

[45] Sinha S, Boyden AW, Itani FR, Crawford MP, Karandikar NJ. CD8[+] T-cells as immune regulators of multiple sclerosis. Frontiers in Immunology. 2015;**6**:619. DOI: 10.3389/fimmu.2015.00619

[46] Karandikar NJ, Crawford MP, Yan X, Ratts RB, Brenchley JM, Ambrozak DR, et al. Glatiramer acetate [copaxone] therapy induces CD8[+] T cell responses in patients with multiple sclerosis. The Journal of Clinical Investigation. 2002;**109**(5):641-649. DOI: 10.1172/jci14380

[47] Aharoni R, Arnon R, Eilam R. Neurogenesis and neuroprotection induced by peripheral immunomodulatory treatment of experimental autoimmune encephalomyelitis. The Journal of Neuroscience. 2005;**25**(36):8217-8228. DOI: 10.1523/jneurosci.1859-05.2005

[48] Blanco Y, Moral EA, Costa M, Gomez-Choco M, Torres-Peraza JF, Alonso-Magdalena L, et al. Effect of glatiramer acetate [copaxone] on the immunophenotypic and cytokine profile and BDNF production in multiple sclerosis: A longitudinal study. Neuroscience Letters. 2006;**406**(3):270-275. DOI: 10.1016/j.neulet.2006.07.043

[49] Skihar V, Silva C, Chojnacki A, Doring A, Stallcup WB, Weiss S, et al. Promoting oligodendrogenesis and myelin repair using the multiple sclerosis medication glatiramer acetate. Proceedings of the National Academy of Sciences of the United States of America. 2009;**106**(42):17992-17997. DOI: 10.1073/pnas.0909607106

[50] Li QQ, Burt DR, Bever CT. Glatiramer acetate inhibition of tumor necrosis factor-alpha-induced RANTES expression and release from U-251 MG human astrocytic cells. Journal of Neurochemistry. 2001;**77**(5):1208-1217. DOI: 10.1046/j.1471-4159.2001.00327.x

[51] Li QQ, Bever CT. Glatiramer acetate blocks interleukin-1-dependent nuclear factor-kappaB activation and RANTES expression in human U-251 MG astroglial cells. Brain Research. Molecular Brain Research. 2001;**87**(1):48-60. DOI: 10.1016/s0169-328x[00]00282-5

[52] Wei G, Zhang X, Su Z, Li X. Glatiramer acetate [GA] prevents TNF-alpha-induced monocyte adhesion to primary endothelial cells through interfering with the NF-kappaB pathway. Biochemical and Biophysical Research

Communications. 2015;**457**(1):101-105. DOI: 10.1016/j.bbrc.2014.12.070

[53] Weber MS, Prod'homme T, Youssef S, Dunn SE, Rundle CD, Lee L, et al. Type II monocytes modulate T cell-mediated central nervous system autoimmune disease. Nature Medicine. 2007;**13**(8):935-943. DOI: 10.1038/nm1620

[54] Ahn YH, Jeon SB, Chang CY, Goh EA, Kim SS, Kim HJ, et al. Glatiramer acetate attenuates the activation of CD4[+] T cells by modulating STAT1 and -3 signaling in glia. Scientific Reports. 2017;**7**:40484. DOI: 10.1038/srep40484

[55] Kipnis J, Yoles E, Porat Z, Cohen A, Mor F, Sela M, et al. T cell immunity to copolymer 1 confers neuroprotection on the damaged optic nerve: Possible therapy for optic neuropathies. Proceedings of the National Academy of Sciences of the United States of America. 2000;**97**(13):7446-7451. DOI: 10.1073/pnas.97.13.7446

[56] Blair M, Pease ME, Hammond J, Valenta D, Kielczewski J, Levkovitch-Verbin H, et al. Effect of glatiramer acetate on primary and secondary degeneration of retinal ganglion cells in the rat. Investigative Ophthalmology & Visual Science. 2005;**46**(3):884-890. DOI: 10.1167/iovs.04-0731

[57] Dionisio PA, Oliveira SR, Gaspar MM, Gama MJ, Castro-Caldas M, Amaral JD, et al. Ablation of RIP3 protects from dopaminergic neurodegeneration in experimental Parkinson's disease. Cell Death & Disease. 2019;**10**(11):840. DOI: 10.1038/s41419-019-2078-z

[58] Kim YS, Joh TH. Microglia, major player in the brain inflammation: Their roles in the pathogenesis of Parkinson's disease. Experimental & Molecular Medicine. 2006;**38**(4):333-347. DOI: 10.1038/emm.2006.40

[59] Benner EJ, Mosley RL, Destache CJ, Lewis TB, Jackson-Lewis V, Gorantla S, et al. Therapeutic immunization protects dopaminergic neurons in a mouse model of Parkinson's disease. Proceedings of the National Academy of Sciences of the United States of America. 2004;**101**(25):9435-9440. DOI: 10.1073/pnas.0400569101

[60] Laurie C, Reynolds A, Coskun O, Bowman E, Gendelman HE, Mosley RL. CD4+ T cells from copolymer-1 immunized mice protect dopaminergic neurons in the 1-methyl-4-phenyl-1,2,3,6-tetrahydropyridine model of Parkinson's disease. Journal of Neuroimmunology. 2007;**183**(1-2): 60-68. DOI: 10.1016/j.jneuroim.2006.11.009

[61] Churchill MJ, Cantu MA, Kasanga EA, Moore C, Salvatore MF, Meshul CK. Glatiramer acetate reverses motor dysfunction and the decrease in tyrosine hydroxylase levels in a mouse model of Parkinson's disease. Neuroscience. 2019;**414**:8-27. DOI: 10.1016/j.neuroscience.2019.06.006

[62] von Euler Chelpin M, Vorup-Jensen T. Targets and mechanisms in prevention of Parkinson's disease through immunomodulatory treatments. Scandinavian Journal of Immunology. 2017;**85**(5):321-330. DOI: 10.1111/sji.12542

[63] Wyss-Coray T, Rogers J. Inflammation in Alzheimer disease—A brief review of the basic science and clinical literature. Cold Spring Harbor Perspectives in Medicine. 2012;**2**(1):a006346. DOI: 10.1101/cshperspect.a006346

[64] Fan Z, Brooks DJ, Okello A, Edison P. An early and late peak in microglial activation in Alzheimer's disease trajectory. Brain. 2017;**140**(3):792-803. DOI: 10.1093/brain/aww349

[65] Dani M, Wood M, Mizoguchi R, Fan Z, Walker Z, Morgan R, et al. Microglial activation correlates in vivo with both tau and amyloid in Alzheimer's disease. Brain. 2018;**141**(9):2740-2754. DOI: 10.1093/brain/awy188

[66] Butovsky O, Koronyo-Hamaoui M, Kunis G, Ophir E, Landa G, Cohen H, et al. Glatiramer acetate fights against Alzheimer's disease by inducing dendritic-like microglia expressing insulin-like growth factor 1. Proceedings of the National Academy of Sciences of the United States of America. 2006;**103**(31):11784-11789. DOI: 10.1073/pnas.0604681103

[67] Butovsky O, Talpalar AE, Ben-Yaakov K, Schwartz M. Activation of microglia by aggregated beta-amyloid or lipopolysaccharide impairs MHC-II expression and renders them cytotoxic whereas IFN-gamma and IL-4 render them protective. Molecular and Cellular Neurosciences. 2005;**29**(3):381-393. DOI: 10.1016/j.mcn.2005.03.005

[68] Koronyo Y, Salumbides BC, Sheyn J, Pelissier L, Li S, Ljubimov V, et al. Therapeutic effects of glatiramer acetate and grafted CD115[+] monocytes in a mouse model of Alzheimer's disease. Brain. 2015;**138**(Pt 8):2399-2422. DOI: 10.1093/brain/awv150

[69] Morrice JR, Gregory-Evans CY, Shaw CA. Animal models of amyotrophic lateral sclerosis: A comparison of model validity. Neural Regeneration Research. 2018;**13**(12):2050-2054. DOI: 10.4103/1673-5374.241445

[70] Zarei S, Carr K, Reiley L, Diaz K, Guerra O, Altamirano PF, et al. A comprehensive review of amyotrophic lateral sclerosis. Surgical Neurology International. 2015;**6**:171. DOI: 10.4103/2152-7806.169561

[71] Angelov DN, Waibel S, Guntinas-Lichius O, Lenzen M, Neiss WF, Tomov TL, et al. Therapeutic vaccine for acute and chronic motor neuron diseases: Implications for amyotrophic lateral sclerosis. Proceedings of the National Academy of Sciences of the United States of America. 2003;**100**(8):4790-4795. DOI: 10.1073/pnas.0530191100

[72] Mosley RL, Gordon PH, Hasiak CM, Van Wetering FJ, Mitsumoto H, Gendelman HE. Glatiramer acetate immunization induces specific antibody and cytokine responses in ALS patients. Amyotrophic Lateral Sclerosis. 2007;**8**(4):235-242. DOI: 10.1080/17482960701374601

[73] Clinical Trials. Glatiramer Acetate. 2019. Available from: https://clinicaltrials.gov/ct2/results?cond=&term=glatiramer+acetate&cntry=&state=&city=&dist

[74] Longa EZ, Weinstein PR, Carlson S, Cummins R. Reversible middle cerebral artery occlusion without craniectomy in rats. Stroke. 1989;**20**(1):84-91. DOI: 10.1161/01.str.20.1.84

[75] Mangin G, Poittevin M, Charriaut-Marlangue C, Giannesini C, Merkoulova-Rainon T, Kubis N. Glatiramer acetate reduces infarct volume in diabetic mice with cerebral ischemia and prevents long-term memory loss. Brain, Behavior, and Immunity. 2019;**80**:315-327. DOI: 10.1016/j.bbi.2019.04.009

[76] Mirzadeh Z, Merkle FT, Soriano-Navarro M, Garcia-Verdugo JM, Alvarez-Buylla A. Neural stem cells confer unique pinwheel architecture to the ventricular surface in neurogenic regions of the adult brain. Cell Stem Cell. 2008;**3**(3):265-278. DOI: 10.1016/B978-0-12-800763-1

[77] Winner B, Winkler J. Adult neurogenesis in neurodegenerative diseases. Cold Spring Harbor Perspectives

in Biology. 2015;7(4):a021287. DOI: 10.1101/cshperspect.a021287

[78] Ibarra A, Avendano H, Cruz Y. Copolymer-1 [cop-1] improves neurological recovery after middle cerebral artery occlusion in rats. Neuroscience Letters. 2007;**425**(2):110-113. DOI: 10.1016/j.neulet.2007.08.038

[79] Cruz Y, Lorea J, Mestre H, Kim-Lee JH, Herrera J, Mellado R, et al. Copolymer-1 promotes neurogenesis and improves functional recovery after acute ischemic stroke in rats. PLoS One. 2015;**10**(3):e0121854. DOI: 10.1371/journal.pone.0121854

[80] Poittevin M, Deroide N, Azibani F, Delcayre C, Giannesini C, Levy BI, et al. Glatiramer acetate administration does not reduce damage after cerebral ischemia in mice. Journal of Neuroimmunology. 2013;**254**(1-2):55-62. DOI: 10.1016/j.jneuroim.2012.09.009

[81] Faigle R, Song H. Signaling mechanisms regulating adult neural stem cells and neurogenesis. Biochimica et Biophysica Acta. 2013;**1830**(2):2435-2448. DOI: 10.1016/j.bbagen.2012.09.002

[82] Baruch K, Schwartz M. CNS-specific T cells shape brain function via the choroid plexus. Brain, Behavior, and Immunity. 2013;**34**:11-16. DOI: 10.1016/j.bbi.2013.04.002

[83] Cruz Y, Garcia EE, Galvez JV, Arias-Santiago SV, Carvajal HG, Silva-Garcia R, et al. Release of interleukin-10 and neurotrophic factors in the choroid plexus: Possible inductors of neurogenesis following copolymer-1 immunization after cerebral ischemia. Neural Regeneration Research. 2018;**13**(10):1743-1752. DOI: 10.4103/1673-5374.238615

[84] Pereira L, Font-Nieves M, Van den Haute C, Baekelandt V, Planas AM, Pozas E. IL-10 regulates adult neurogenesis by modulating ERK and STAT3 activity. Frontiers in Cellular Neuroscience. 2015;**9**:57. DOI: 10.3389/fncel.2015.00057

[85] Cunha C, Brambilla R, Thomas KL. A simple role for BDNF in learning and memory? Frontiers in Molecular Neuroscience. 2010;**3**:1. DOI: 10.3389/neuro.02.001.2010

[86] Delgado AC, Ferron SR, Vicente D, Porlan E, Perez-Villalba A, Trujillo CM, et al. Endothelial NT-3 delivered by vasculature and CSF promotes quiescence of subependymal neural stem cells through nitric oxide induction. Neuron. 2014;**83**(3):572-585. DOI: 10.1016/j.neuron.2014.06.015

[87] Snapyan M, Lemasson M, Brill MS, Blais M, Massouh M, Ninkovic J, et al. Vasculature guides migrating neuronal precursors in the adult mammalian forebrain via brain-derived neurotrophic factor signaling. The Journal of Neuroscience. 2009;**29**(13):4172-4188. DOI: 10.1523/jneurosci.4956-08.2009

[88] Yuan H, Chen R, Wu L, Chen Q, Hu A, Zhang T, et al. The regulatory mechanism of neurogenesis by IGF-1 in adult mice. Molecular Neurobiology. 2015;**51**(2):512-522. DOI: 10.1007/s12035-014-8717-6

[89] Tyler AF, Mendoza JP, Firan M, Karandikar NJ. CD8[+] T cells are required for glatiramer acetate therapy in autoimmune demyelinating disease. PLoS One. 2013;**8**(6):e66772. DOI: 10.1371/journal.pone.0066772

Chapter 9

Trends in Neuroprotective Strategies after Spinal Cord Injury: State of the Art

Roxana Rodríguez-Barrera, Marcela Garibay-López and Antonio Ibarra

Abstract

Spinal cord injury (SCI) is an important pathology leading to possibly fatal consequences. The most common repercussions are those affecting motor and sensitivity skills. SCI-damage occurs in its first phase—as a result of the lesion mechanism (contusion, compression, transection, and primary lesion). After this primary damage, there is a second phase with further deleterious effects on neural degeneration and tissue restoration. At the moment, several investigation groups are working on developing therapeutic strategies to induce neuroprotection. This chapter pretends to introduce the reader to a wide range of these therapies, particularly those with promising results and tested in preclinical and clinical studies. In the first section, physiopathology of SCI will be addressed. Afterwards, the chapter will review neuroprotective strategies such as cyclooxygenase, calpain, and apoptosis inhibitors. Finally, the effect of immunophilin ligands, neural-derived peptides, antioxidants, hypoglycemic agent, gonadal hormones, Na channel blockers, and transplant of cultured cells will also be reviewed.

Keywords: neuroprotection, SCI, therapies, acute phase

1. Introduction

Spinal cord injury (SCI) can be defined as damage to the spinal cord (SC). It causes anatomical and physiological changes that result in permanent or temporary alterations in its function [1]. The injury causes ionic deregulation, edema, ischemia, bleeding, free radicals production, and a generalized inflammatory response that will cause partial or total loss of sensitive and motor function below the site of injury [2, 3].

In the United States, there are around 17,500 new cases of SCI per year, with an approximate prevalence of 280,000 people [4]. SCI is found most frequently in men (79.8%) than women (20.2%) and the age distribution reflects a bimodal performance with a peak between 15 and 29 years of age and another one on ages above 50 years [4–6]. Traffic accidents are the main cause of traumatic SCI (38%), and they are most prevalent in young people. The low impact accidents like falls are the second cause of SCI (31%), and they are more common among people older than 60 years old [5]. In Mexico, the estimated annual incidence of SCI is about 18.1 per million inhabitants. Statistically, the number of people involved rises each year [7].

2. Pathophysiology

The Spinal Cord Injury could be divided by its etiology in traumatic and nontraumatic. The traumatic type is caused by physical damage (traffic accident, sportive, and fall), whereas nontraumatic is occasioned by an illness/sickness, such as tumors, infections or degenerative diseases which directly affect the SC [8]. In addition, SCI can be divided into primary and secondary injury [1, 9].

Primary injury is caused at the moment of physical damage and leads to irreversible affection on gray matter during the first hour post-lesion. There are three main mechanisms of injury: contusion, when there is not a visible alteration in its morphology, producing a necrotic region at the injury area; laceration or transection, when there is an extreme trauma or penetration, affecting SC conduction of nervous impulses depending on whether the tissue is partial or totally transected; compression from vertebral fractures leading ischemic damage in the area where blood flow was disrupted [10, 11].

After injury, superficial blood vessels undergo to vasospasm which provokes damage in the microvasculature of gray matter [12]. Reduction in the perfusion has two important implications: hypoxia and ischemia; which may involve to neurogenic shock characterized by arterial hypotension, bradycardia, arrhythmia, and intraparenchymal hemorrhage that causes neuronal death by necrosis. Afterwards, primary injury provokes the rupture of blood brain barrier and a cascade of destructive secondary phenomena leading to a further damage in SC and neurological dysfunction [1, 13]. Therefore, the primary lesion results in the development of a succession of cellular and molecular changes that alter gene expression patterns, which are processes that are already part of the secondary injury [11, 12]. During the acute phase, injury to the blood vessels and severe hemorrhages cause massive influx of inflammatory cells, cytokines, and vasoactive peptides. This phase is almost characterized by ionic deregulation that leads to edema, thus interrupting the conduction of nerve impulses. Following, subacute phase involves a sequence of events like ischemia, vasospasm, thrombosis, inflammatory response, free radicals (FR) production, lipid peroxidation (LPO), and activation of autoimmune responses causing apoptosis. The huge inflammatory responses after the acute and subacute phase, together with the disruption of the blood-brain barrier (BBB), contribute to the progressively swelling of the SC. This generalized edema may increase the mechanical pressure of the SC, aggravating the injury [1, 11, 14].

To counteract all these acute effects after SCI, neuroprotective strategies have been investigated to rapidly intervene decreasing the neuronal death occurring after damage mechanisms. Many pharmacological and nonpharmacological therapies have been developed, and others are still under investigation, this in order to improve the quality of life of patients.

3. Neuroprotective therapy after acute SCI

As we review previously, SCI leads to motor and sensory dysfunction, first with the primary mechanical injury and then with the complex cascade of secondary damaging events [15]. For several years, basic science, preclinical, and clinical studies are focused in overcoming elements involved in accurate recovery from SCI [1]. An ideal neuroprotective therapy must reduce neurological symptoms including degenerative changes; starting from there, we can discriminate between potential clinical therapies, which could have a better effect [16]. While these therapies are being searched, there are many preclinical and clinical investigations exploring pharmacological and nonpharmacological treatments.

3.1 Preclinical pharmacological therapies

This range of therapeutic approaches includes: ionic channel blockers, inhibitors of NMDA and AMPA-kainate receptors, inhibitors of FR and LPO, anti-apoptotic drugs, calpain inhibitors, immunosuppressive or immunomodulatory drugs, immunophilin ligands, immunomodulatory peptides, hypoglycemic agents, and gonadal hormones.

3.1.1 Ionic channel blockers

3.1.1.1 Sodium

3.1.1.1.1 Tetrodotoxin

Tetrodotoxin (TTX) is a low-molecular-weight guanidine neurotoxin that acts as a specific blocker of voltage-gated sodium (NaV) channel [17]. TTX has neuroprotective properties by blocking NaV channels, preventing neuronal death by diminishing depolarization, cellular Na^+/Ca^{+2} exchange, and neuronal glutamate release [18].

The beneficial effects of TTX in preclinical studies include a reduction of white matter loss after SCI [17–19], promoting a motor function restoration. The effect of TTX is time-dependent [20]. The administration of TTX 15 minutes after a SCI helps to restore the function of hindlimbs [21]. Despite these promissory effects, there are some limitations for the use of TTX in patients, one of them is its toxicity. This may appear as a consequence of its systemic distribution and it can involve the blocking of diaphragmatic nerves ending in respiratory tract paralysis [17]. Even with previous findings, current studies are needed to improve its use in SCI.

3.1.1.1.2 Riluzole

Riluzole is a benzothiazole anticonvulsant drug with neuroprotective effects in the SCI [22]. One of the mechanisms by which riluzole operates is the inhibition in the presynaptic terminals of glutamate, and this helps to limit the glutamate-induced toxicity [23]. In addition, riluzole blocks the NaV-gated channels, avoiding swelling and neuronal acidosis. Riluzole blocks the entry of H+ to the neurons through the Na^+/H^+ exchanger; this prevents the Ca^{+2} from inducing the release of glutamate and excitotoxicity [22]. Investigations have shown that the interruption of events associated with glutamate release on the presynaptic space by reducing Ca^{+2} influxes provokes a glutamate-mediated LPO reduction [23, 24]. Administration of riluzole within 12 hours of SCI was well tolerated and suggests that it may have a beneficial effect on motor outcome [25].

3.1.1.2 Calcium

3.1.1.2.1 Nimodipine

Nimodipine is a dihydropyridinic Ca^{+2} channel antagonist that boosts the brain's blood flow, without compromising metabolism [26, 27]. It reduces malondialdehyde (MDA) levels, ED-1 markers for activated macrophages and myeloperoxidase (MPo). Studies have shown that nimodipine helps reducing FR, oxidative damage, resulting in the reduction of the damaged area and the infiltration of the inflammatory cells to the region, allowing SCI restoration [26]. Furthermore, the effect of inhibiting Ca^{+2} flux by nimodipine reduces apoptosis and tissue damage after SCI, increasing cell viability [27].

3.1.2 Inhibitors of NMDA and AMPA-kainate receptors

3.1.2.1 Memantine

Memantine is a noncompetitive N-methyl-D-aspartate (NMDA) receptor antagonist, which through the inhibition of hypoxic or ischemic damage/necrosis helps to prevent the secondary damage in SCI [28, 29]. The use of an NMDA antagonist limits neuronal glutamate exposure caused by excitatory amino acid neurotransmitters [29]. The use of memantine with anti-apoptotic agents like Q-VD-OPh boosts the neuroprotective effect through the reduction in apoptosis and necrosis mechanisms. Moreover, it provides better clinical and histological outcomes by limiting neuronal necrosis [28, 29].

3.1.2.2 Gacyclidine

Gacyclidine is a noncompetitive NMDA antagonist that is able to reduce the extension of ischemic lesions in SCI. It has been proven that gacyclidine is efficient in enhancing the functional and histological condition of the injury, but their neuroprotective effects are time and dose-dependent [30, 31].

3.1.2.3 NBQX (2,3-dihydroxy-6-nitro-7-sulfamoylbenzoquinoxaline)

NBQX is an AMPA/kainate antagonist that during acute SCI improves mitochondrial function and diminishes reactive oxygen species (ROS) formation as well as LPO production [32, 33]. The treatment with NBQX reduces white matter loss following SCI. Further studies are needed to know more about its efficacious effects in acute SCI.

3.1.3 Inhibitors of free radicals and lipid peroxidation

3.1.3.1 Polyunsaturated fatty acids (PUFAs)

Omega-3 polyunsaturated fatty acids (ω-3 PUFAs) are structural compounds of the phospholipid membrane. They produce beneficial effects in neurodegenerative diseases by its anti-inflammatory, antioxidant, and membrane stabilizing properties [34]. ω-3 PUFAs, particularly docosahexaenoic acid (DHA), exert profound anti-inflammatory effects on the central nervous system (CNS), confer significant protection to the white matter, and help to increase neurite growth and synapse formation. DHA acts on cyclooxygenases (COX), cytosolic phospholipase A2 (cPLA2), and nuclear factor kappa-light-chain-enhancer of activated B cells (NF-kB) [35, 36]. Deficiencies of lipids affect neural responses in CNS injuries, and this must predispose nerve cells to dysfunction [37]. According to previous findings, there are some investigations (**Table 1**) that have previously shown the effects of PUFAs in preclinical models.

3.1.3.2 Glutathione

Glutathione (GSH) is a tripeptide compound constituted by glutamine, glycine, and cysteine. The reduced form of GSH is glutathione-monoethyl-ester (GSHE), which is an endogenous, rechargeable antioxidant. Besides its anti-oxidant functions, GSHE plays a role in regulation of apoptosis, and it is important for

Treatment outcome	Ref.
α-linolenic acid (ALA) and DHA reduce lesion size and increase motor recovery and neuronal survival.	[34]
DHA reduces microglia activation in both ventral and dorsal horns and increases motor recovery, promoting beneficial functional effect in SCI.	[38]
ALA, combined with DHA, protects against neuronal necrosis and apoptosis.	[39]
DHA induces a reduction in neutrophil number in SC epicenter. The administration confers histological protection and improves motor recovery.	[40]
Prophylactic therapy with ω-3 has shown a reduction in cellular vulnerability. Supporting functional recovery, there is also an increase in levels of protein kinase B/Akt and CREB.	[37, 41]
DHA plus rehabilitation enhance a functional, anatomical, and synaptic plasticity in cervical SCI.	[42]

Table 1.
Polyunsaturated fatty acids in spinal cord injury.

cellular defense against ROS [43, 44]. Some studies have reported that GSHE diminishes SC LPO after SCI, while also acting as a vasodilator under conditions of oxidative stress [44, 45]. In addition, GSHE plays an anti-excitotoxic role by inhibiting the binding ligands to ionotropic glutamate receptors under redox modulation, which have been involved in excitotoxicity after SCI. As a consequence of the reduction of GSH after an injury, there is neuronal loss in the SC, probably due to oxidative stress and mitochondrial dysfunction. Combined therapy of GSHE with A91 resulted in a better motor recovery and axonal sparing associated with a higher axonal myelination [46]. The use of GSHE could be an interesting alternative for SCI therapy; however, it should be strongly evaluated before its use in clinical trials.

3.1.4 Anti-apoptosis therapy

3.1.4.1 Zdevd-fmk

Caspase inhibitor Z-DEVD-fmk is a selective caspase-3 inhibitor that also has anti-inflammatory properties. Anti-apoptosis compounds are used to block apoptotic cell death but also to inhibit cytokine production. Treatment of SCI with z-DEVD reduces secondary tissue damage, ischemic injury, preserves motor function, and provides neuroprotection via the inhibition of cell death in all of cell types in the SC [47, 48]. Low doses of z-DEVD-fmk combined with basic fibroblast growth factor (bFGF) reduce neurological deficit in ischemia, therefore providing neuroprotection [49].

3.1.4.2 z-LEHD-fmk

Caspase inhibitor z-LEHD-fmk acts as a selective caspase-9 inhibitor with anti-apoptotic properties. This drug helps decreasing levels of apoptosis biochemical markers, reducing lesion size and remaining active during treatment to maintain its therapeutic effect. Treatment with z-LEHD-fmk helps to prevent apoptosis in a variety of cell types like neurons, astrocytes, oligodendrocytes, and microglia populations [50]. Further studies are needed to understand more about its effects and benefits in acute SCI.

3.1.5 Calpain inhibitors

Calpains belong to the family of calcium-dependent nonlysosomal cysteine proteases, which can be found expressed through the CNS. They are involved in neurodegeneration, degradation of cytoskeleton, and apoptosis via caspase-3 due to its proteolytic activities, in SCI. The influx of Ca^{+2} stimulates Ca^{+2}-dependent enzymes, within them are calpains, which seem to play a role in proteolysis by contributing to apoptosis in CNS cells. The cell death decreases mRNA expression and transcription of myelin basic protein (MBP) and proteolipid protein (PLP), which are axonal neurofilament proteins [49, 51, 52]. The administration of a calpain inhibitor such as E-64-d (1 mg/kg) to injured rats blocks apoptosis and helps to re-establish MBP and PLP genes [51]. The administration of other calpain inhibitors such as SJA 6017 and calpeptin has demonstrated their ability to induce neuroprotection after SCI [53, 54]. Despite the study efforts and the promising therapeutic effects for functional neuroprotection, there are no clinical trials testing these drugs, so further studies are needed for the use of calpain inhibitors in patients.

3.1.6 Immunosuppressive or immunomodulatory drugs.

3.1.6.1 Inhibitors of cyclooxygenase

3.1.6.1.1 Indomethacin

Indomethacin, a nonsteroidal anti-inflammatory (NSAID) drug, acts as a nonselective cyclooxygenase inhibitor. It has shown that it inhibits the synthesis of prostaglandins and ameliorates the effects of secondary injuries like tissue necrosis in SCI [55–57]. RhoA is a convergent intracellular pathway that limits axonal growth; its inhibition with indomethacin prevents oligodendrocyte loss and induces myelination across damaged white matter [58]. Nevertheless, the administration of nonselective cyclooxygenase inhibitors is a controversial issue since these compounds could inhibit platelet aggregation and may produce gastrointestinal ulceration [55]. Moreover, there is evidence that a single injection of indomethacin in SCI had a minimal effect on functional recovery and anatomical repair [57].

3.1.6.1.2 Meloxicam

Meloxicam is a drug derived from enolic acid, which inhibits prostaglandin biosynthesis under inflammatory conditions via the inhibition of COX-2. It has minimal gastric toxicity. Meloxicam has shown to reduce SCI-induced oxidative stress and exert neuroprotection by inhibiting LPO, GSH depletion, and DNA fragmentation [59, 60]. Despite these interesting results, meloxicam has not been further studied. Therefore, more studies are needed to know about its clinical management in SCI.

3.1.7 Immunophilin ligands

3.1.7.1 Cyclosporine A

Cyclosporine A (CsA) is an immunosuppressant agent compound formed by 11 amino cyclic peptides, and it is obtained from *Tolypocladium inflatum*. CsA inhibits T-helper lymphocytes, cytotoxic and inflammatory responses in macrophages, inducible nitric oxide synthase (iNOs) expression avoiding the formation of nitric oxide (NO)-derived cytotoxic species, Cox-2 mRNA accumulation, tumor necrosis factor (TNFα) production and reduces cytokines and interleukins production (IL-1, IL-2, and IL-6). Also, CsA reduced the apoptosis of SC cells and increased the protein expression levels of cyclophilin-D (Cyp-D) and apoptosis-inducing factor (AIF) [61, 62]. This compound is capable of inducing motor recovery after SCI [63].

3.1.7.2 Tacrolimus

Tacrolimus or FK506 is an immunosuppressant macrolide drug, isolated from *Streptomyces tsukubaensis*, and it is approved by The Food and Drug Administration (FDA) [64, 65]. An indirect neuroprotective effect results from its immunosuppressant action on T-cells that infiltrate SCI, and this action modulates inflammation. On the other hand, FK506 inhibits caspase-3 and NF-kB, improving functional recovery with the increase of rostral axonal sparing and oligodendroglial survival [66, 67]. Additionally, this compound is capable of reducing FR and thereby LPO. These neuroprotective effects improve if the administration of FK506 is during the first 30 min after injury [65]. The studies suggest that FK506 might be a good drug for treating SCI in humans.

3.1.8 With neural derived peptides

Immunization with neural derived peptides (INDP) such as A91, a peptide derived from the 87–99 immunogenic sequence of myelin basic protein has shown to induce neuroprotection and motor recovery after SCI [68]. Its mechanism of action is related to the activation of T-lymphocytes inducing an anti-inflammatory Th2 response that allows microglia to differentiate into a M2 phenotype. Th2 response is capable of producing brain-derived neurotrophic factor (BDNF), a molecule strongly related to tissue protection [69]. INDP has shown that anti-A91 T-lymphocytes promote tissue protection by inhibiting the expression of iNOS, reducing ON production [68] and decrease LPO after SCI [70]. On the other hand, it has been shown that all these beneficial effects contribute to the preservation of neural tissue by preventing apoptosis [71], the survival of neurons in rubrospinal tract [72] and promoting a better neurological recovery in models of SCI [46]. Studies suggest that A91 might be an immune modulating treatment for SCI.

3.1.9 Metformin

Metformin is a hypoglycemic agent used for therapy of type 2 diabetes mellitus; it is an AMP-activated protein kinase (AMPK) agonist. Metformin also acts through signaling pathway of mTOR and p70S6K causing an inhibition of apoptosis and inflammation. This drug is also capable of stimulating autophagy and reducing expression of NF-kB-mediated inflammation [73, 74]. Studies indicate that long-term use of metformin has been proved effective as a pharmacological treatment for some CNS disorders like Parkinson's disease, Huntington's disease, and ischemic brain injury. Using a rat model of traumatic SCI, the administration of metformin helps restoring the dysfunctional autophagy-lysosome pathways providing neuroprotection, decreasing neuronal death and mitigating apoptosis [75, 76]. The immediate administration of metformin after the injury showed diminishing complications, reflecting a decrease on histopathological signs of neuroinflammation, including TNFα and IL-1β inflammatory cytokines in the SC [73]. Although these outcomes are promising, subsequent studies are required to determine the risk ad optimal doses for the use of metformin on clinical studies.

3.1.10 Gonadal hormones

Androgens and estrogens are multi-active steroidal hormones that have neuroprotective effects in neural injuries; both testosterone and estradiol improve safeguard against apoptosis and promote motor and sensitive recovery. Also, reduce inflammation and FR generation and have been involved in regulating the expression of cytoskeletal proteins, promoting them as an increasing in neurite outgrowth [77, 78]. Studies in rats treated with estradiol have shown a reduction in the lesion size, an increase in white matter sparing, and an improving in motor function [77, 79, 80]. On the other hand, testosterone has shown to exert similar but not identical effects; it is neuroprotective against apoptosis in oxidative stress [77, 78]. A study with young adult female rats implanted with testosterone-filled silastic capsules reported regressive changes in motoneuron and muscle morphology after a SCI providing the possibility of improving motor function [81]. A study with administration of progesterone in rats improves neurological deficits and reduces inflammatory response. Prevents degeneration of motor neurons and reestablishes proliferation and differentiation of oligodendrocytes [82]. At the moment, investigations on the field conclude that gonadal hormones could be an effective alternative after SCI.

3.2 Clinical pharmacological therapies

Methylprednisolone, minocycline, GM-1-ganglioside, and glyburide are some of the most investigated pharmacological therapies in clinical settings.

3.2.1 Methylprednisolone

Methylprednisolone (MP) is a synthetic glucocorticoid, with anti-inflammatory and anti-oxidant effects [83, 84]. MP blocks the inflammatory cascade and disrupts neuron regeneration by inhibiting immunological cells [85, 86]. The potential neuroprotective effects of MP have been reported especially in the acute phase of SCI. According to some investigations, MP is capable of reducing FR production, Ca^{+2} influx, excitotoxicity, and immune-mediated phagocytosis over the course of hypoperfusion of SCI [87]. In addition, MP appears to have effect in apoptosis and autophagy regulation; however, the mechanisms are not clear [84]. While it remains the only option for acute SCI treatment in clinical settings, a debate regarding optimal dose, time of administration, efficacy, and adverse effects has dominated the field for years. There are three National Acute SCI Studies (NASCIS) and other clinical or biomedical investigations, in which the safety and efficacy of MP were assessed (**Table 2**) [88]. Despite the intense investigation, currently there is an important controversy regarding the real utility of this drug.

3.2.2 Minocycline

Minocycline is a second generation tetracycline, a semi-synthetic antibiotic able to cross blood brain barrier, and it can be used to treat rheumatoid arthritis [95, 96]. Minocycline has neuroprotective effects when administered during the acute neural trauma. Current data suggest that minocycline has anti-inflammatory, immunomodulatory, and neuroprotective effects. These beneficial actions are achieved as a result of the inhibition of iNOS matrix metalloproteinases (MMPs), PLA2, TNF-α, caspase-1, and caspase-3. Moreover, minocycline enhances Bcl-2 and thus, reduces apoptosis, also, it decreases p38 mitogen-activated protein kinase (MAPK) phosphorylation and inhibits PARP-1 [97–100]. Other studies report that minocycline can bind to Ca^{+2} and Mg^{+}, reduces reactive astrocytes to increase oligodendrocyte viability in white matter, and inhibits the activation of microglial cells [101, 102]. A multi-center phase II trial was performed to explore the neuroprotective effect of minocycline; however, the results of the study did not establish a real improvement in SCI. Authors suggest further investigations in a multi-center phase III trial [103].

Treatment outcome	Ref.
NASCIS I: Treatment with a dose 1.0 g daily promotes neurological recovery. The morbidity and mortality is increased.	[89]
NASCIS II: Administration of (30 mg/kg intravenous bolus plus 23 hour infusion of 5.4 mg/kg) during the first 8 hours after injury causes neurological recovery seen from 6 weeks after the SCI.	[86]
NASCIS III: Administration within 8 hours from the SCI, should maintain the administration for 48 hours to improve neurological function.	[90]
Combination of riluzole and MP improves functional recovery and tissue sparing. In addition, beneficial effects on oxidative stress were observed.	[91]
MP may cause acute corticosteroid myopathy, at doses recommended by the NASCIS.	[92]
High-dose MP inhibits glucocorticoid receptors as well as having effects in LPO; however, their beneficial effects are independent of LPO inhibition.	[55]
Administration of MP for treatment of SCI is not recommended. There is evidence that high-dose steroids are associated with harmful side effects including death.	[93]
A comparative study of MP vs. A91-immunization showed that A91-immunization has a better efficiency promoting motor recovery. Combining MP with A91-immunization allowed to observe that MP has a transient immunosuppressive effect that eliminated the beneficial actions of A91-immunization.	[94]

Table 2.
Effects of methylprednisolone in spinal cord injury.

3.2.3 GM-1-ganglioside

Gangliosides (GM-1) are sialic acid-containing glycosphingolipids, present in cell membranes of CNS cells, specifically in the external leaflet of plasma membranes. They participate in the repair and maintenance of CNS [104, 105]. A randomized placebo-controlled (Phase II) trial with administration of GM-1 within 24 hours after injury was realized in 37 patients with SCI. The results of this study showed that GM-1 enhances the recovery of neurologic function after 1 year [104]. Further studies should be designed in order to provide more evidence about the efficacy of GM-1.

3.2.4 Glyburide

Glyburide (glibenclamide) is a FDA approved sulfonylurea drug widely used to treat type 2 diabetes; it has the ability to target receptor (SUR1) regulated Ca^{+2} activated [ATP] cation (NCCa-ATP) channels [96, 106]. After SCI, there are small hemorrhagic lesions at the epicenter of gray matter. Glyburide diminishes the progressive hemorrhage necrosis by jamming the interaction between SUR-1 and preforming subunits of NCCa-ATP channels located in endothelial cells. In addition, improves neurological function [107]. Actually, a phase I/II clinical trial is currently under way to test the safety and neuroprotective effectiveness of glyburide in patients with SCI [88].

4. Nonpharmacological therapies (preclinical interventions)

The most common preclinical nonpharmacological therapies in the acute phase of SCI are antioxidants, growth factors, and transplant of cultured cells like neural stem cells (NSCs), bone marrow stem cells (BMSCs), olfactory ensheathing cells (OECs), and Schwann cells (SCs).

4.1 Antioxidants

First damage in the acute phase of injury is generated in membranes, membranes which are susceptible to the attack of ROS and reactive nitrogen species (RNS). ROS are produced in metabolic and physiological processes of cells; however, they are overproduced by inflammatory response. ROS and RNS induce LPO, which leads to demyelinating processes. Among the nonpharmacological therapies to prevent damage from FR are nonenzymatic antioxidants like vitamins.

4.1.1 Vitamins

Vitamins are one of the main natural antioxidants. **Table 3** shows some vitamins and their neuroprotective effect after SCI.

4.1.2 Resveratrol

Resveratrol is a natural polyphenolic compound that has exhibited beneficial health properties as well as antioxidant, anti-inflammatory, and antitumor effects. Resveratrol exerts a neuroprotective effect by regulating apoptosis [118]. Studies have shown that the anti-inflammatory effects of resveratrol are mediated mainly by sirtuin (SIRT) 1 [119, 120]. Resveratrol enhances locomotor recovery [121–123]. Furthermore, resveratrol increases nuclear factor erythroid 2-related factor (Nrf-2) activation, providing antioxidant effects [121]. Further investigation is needed in order to provide more evidence about the efficacy of this treatment.

Treatment	Neuroprotection mechanism	Ref.
Vitamin E	Increases functional recovery. Reduces cavitation and decreases FR, LPO, and glutathione peroxidase and improves functional recovery.	[108–112]
Vitamin C	Stops lipid hydroperoxyides formation and decreases membrane damage. Reduces necrotic tissues and improves functional recovery in rats. Inhibits ROS generation and LPO. Decreases levels of proteins like NF-kB, iNOS, and COX-2. Down-regulates the levels of TNFα and IL-1β. Modulates antioxidant status and MPO activity	[113, 114]
Vitamin C + fluoxetine	Co-treatment with vitamin C + fluoxetine inhibits the blood-SC barrier disruption after SCI. Inhibits capillary fragmentation by reducing mRNA levels of MMP-9. Prevents degradation of tight-junction proteins, inhibits infiltration of neutrophils and macrophages. Inhibits apoptotic cell death and improves functional recovery.	[115]
Vitamin A	Increases the expression of IL-1β, IL-6, and TNFα after SCI. Systemic administration reduces early transcript levels of IL-1β, IL-6, and TNFα. Reduces blood-SC-barrier permeability and improves functional recovery	[116]
	Decreases levels of β-catenin, P120 catenin, occluding, and claudin5. Inhibits endocytoplasmic reticulum stress and caspase-12 expression.	[117]

Table 3.
Vitamins in spinal cord injury.

4.2 Growth factors

The use of growth factors like BDNF, transforming growth factor-β (TGF-β), and insulin-like growth factor-1 (IGF-1) as a therapy to improve morphological and behavioral outcomes after SCI has been topic of study of many investigations.

4.2.1 Brain-derived neurotrophic factor

BDNF exerts a relevant function in the repair of neural tissue and plasticity in CNS [124, 125]. Nevertheless, recent studies have also shown that BDNF is capable of exerting neuroprotective effects. In acute phases of injury, several reports indicate that both, BDNF alone [126, 127] or in any combination [128, 129] has improved functional recovery, neuronal survival, and tissue preservation. Moreover, BDNF has potent antioxidant effects and may be involved in regulation of immune responses after an SCI [130]. BDNF after SCI requires careful selection to consider the location, mode, and time of application after an injury.

4.2.2 Transforming growth factor-β

TGF-β is a pleiotropic molecule with specific key functions in cell differentiation, proliferation, migration, immunosuppression, and extracellular matrix metabolism [131]. TGF-β could also be contributing to neuroprotective mechanisms

Therapy	Neuroprotective effects	Ref.
NSCs	Increase functional recovery. Reduction in neutrophils and M1 macrophages. Downregulation of TNFα, IL-1 β, IL-6, and IL-12. Improve functional recovery and reduce neuronal apoptosis, microglia activation, reduce pro-inflammatory cytokines like TNFα, IL-1β, and IL-6. Improve locomotor and sensory function and increase mRNA expression of BDNF.	[141–144]
BMSCs	Improve locomotor function and tissue protection. Increase the neurotrophic growth factor. Stimulate M2 macrophage activation. Reduce cystic cavities size and suppress glial scar formation.	[145–148]
BMSCs + SCs	Reduce the formation of the glial scar, remyelinate the injured axons, and promote functional recovery	[149]
BMSCs + IGF-1	Induce modulation of inflammatory cytokines and oxidative stress. Increase functional recovery and reduce activation of glial fibrillary acidic protein and increase myelination 4 weeks following SCI.	[150]
BMSCs + OECs	Reduce apoptosis and increase locomotor recovery.	[151]
OECs	Reduce cavity size, increase the neurofilaments sprouting and serotonin axons, and improve functionality.	[152]
OECs + SCs	Diminish astrocyte number, microglia/macrophage infiltration and expression of CCL2 and CCL3.	[153]
SCs	Upregulate the expression of NOS, activate the NO-dependent cyclic-GMP pathway, which enhances neuronal survival. Stimulate the expression of neural growth factor and BDNF. Reduce inflammatory cytokines and ROS.	[154, 155]
SCs + NSCs	Promote neuronal differentiation, increase axonal regeneration/myelination, reduce neuronal loss, and improve functional recovery.	[156]

Table 4.
Stem cell therapy in spinal cord injury.

after SCI since it participates in the regulation of neuronal survival and orchestrates repairing processes in the CNS [132]. It has been previously observed that TGF-β administration reduces microglial activation and increases neuronal survival [133]. The early induction of TGF-β after SCI modulates the acute immune response, the formation of glial scar and improves functional recovery [134].

4.2.3 Insulin-like growth factor-1

IGF-1 belongs to the family of insulin-related peptides, and it is the mediator of the anabolic and mitogenic activity of the growth hormone [135]. Aside from this, IGF-1 acts as a strong antioxidant [136] and pro-survival [137] factor in the CNS since it diminishes caspase-9 and elevates Bcl2 [138]. Experimental studies have shown that IGF-1 reduces edema and the upregulation of iNOS after SCI [139]. In the same way, it has been suggested that IGF-1 and erythropoietin protect against ischemic SCI in rabbits [140]. Therefore, the beneficial properties of IGF-1 make this molecule an interesting neuroprotective strategy in the acute phase of SCI.

4.3 Stem cells

Stem cells have also been the focus of several investigations. **Table 4** summarizes some of the neuroprotective effects exerted by stem cells like NSCs, BMSCs, OECs, and SCs.

5. Nonpharmacological therapies (clinical trials)

Nonpharmacological therapies with clinical studies are hence limited in acute phases of the injury.

5.1 Stem cells neural stem cells

Pilot studies cover the acute phase of SCI.

5.1.1 Neural stem cells

Transplants with human NSCs in phase I/IIa assessed the safety and neurological effects after SCI. Of 19 treated subjects, 17 were sensorimotor complete and two were motor complete and sensory incomplete. They demonstrated that 1 year after cell transplantation, there was no evidence of SC damage, syrinx or tumor formation, neurological deterioration, and exacerbating neuropathic pain or spasticity [157]. Additional studies should be designed in order to afford more evidence about the efficacy of NSCs.

5.1.2 Bone marrow stem cells

Regarding bone marrow stem cells (BMSC), an interesting study reported data from 20 patients with complete SCI who received transplants of BMSC. They showed improvement in motor and sensory functions [158]. In addition, a study with autologous BMSCs in three patients in the sub-acute phase of injury (<6 months of disease) demonstrated that, these cells could be safely administered through intrathecal injection in SCI patients [159]. Other study showed that 45.5% of transplanted patients presented improved neurological function. They showed some degree of improvement in sensitivity and motor function as well as in sexual function. In two patients, neuropathic pain disappeared and bladder and bowel control increased [160]. Nevertheless, more investigation through clinical trials is required with a larger population of patients before further conclusions can be drawn.

5.1.3 Olfactory ensheathing cells

Transplants with autologous OECs in three patients indicated that there were no adverse effects 1 year after transplantation. The neurosurgical process did not lead to any negative sequelae either during the operation or postoperatively. Additionally, they demonstrated the possibility of taking a nasal biopsy and reliably generating enough cells for transplantation within 4 weeks [161]. These observations suggest that autologous transplantation is safe but further researches are needed.

5.1.4 Schwann cells

A Phase I clinical trial with autologous human SCs was conducted to evaluate the safety of transplantation into the injury of six subjects with subacute SCI. There was no evidence of additional SC damage, mass lesion or syrinx formation. They conclude that it is feasible to identify eligible candidates, appropriately obtain informed consent, perform a peripheral nerve harvest to obtain SCs within 5–30 days of injury, and perform intra-spinal transplantation of highly purified autologous SCs within 4–7 weeks of injury [162]. Studies in acute phases using SCs are very few: therefore, more studies are needed in this area.

5.2 Physical therapy

Timing as a specific prognostic factor in rehabilitation results and confirms that early specific rehabilitation treatment is associated with greater improvement. Several studies investigate the early rehabilitation as a therapeutic strategy to improve locomotor function, some of them have even shown physical functional independence [163–165]. Other studies indicated that in acute SCI physical therapy of body weight support on a treadmill and defined overground mobility therapy did not produce different results [166]. Further studies are required to afford conclusive results.

6. Conclusions

In conclusion, there are several pharmacological and nonpharmacological treatments that have been tested in preclinical and clinical phases. However, so far have not yielded fully satisfactory results; even using combined therapies. Further studies are needed in order to identify novel therapeutic targets and strategies that provide a better medical care avoiding complications.

Acknowledgements

We gratefully acknowledge to Universidad Anáhuac México Norte for the support to this chapter.

Conflict of interest

The authors declare no conflict of interest.

Author details

Roxana Rodríguez-Barrera, Marcela Garibay-López and Antonio Ibarra*
Centro de Investigación en Ciencias de la Salud (CICSA), Universidad Anáhuac México Campus Norte, Huixquilucan, Estado de México, México

*Address all correspondence to: jose.ibarra@anahuac.mx

References

[1] Ahuja CS, Wilson JR, Nori S, Kotter MRN, Druschel C, Curt A, et al. Traumatic spinal cord injury. Nature Reviews. Disease Primers. 2017;**3**:17018

[2] Rowland JW, Hawryluk GW, Kwon B, Fehlings MG. Current status of acute spinal cord injury pathophysiology and emerging therapies: Promise on the horizon. Neurosurgical Focus. 2008;**25**(5):E2

[3] Zhou Y, Wang Z, Li J, Li X, Xiao J. Fibroblast growth factors in the management of spinal cord injury. Journal of Cellular and Molecular Medicine. 2018;**22**(1):25-37

[4] Lenehan B, Street J, Kwon BK, Noonan V, Zhang H, Fisher CG, et al. The epidemiology of traumatic spinal cord injury in British Columbia, Canada. Spine (Phila Pa 1976). 2012;**37**(4):321-329

[5] Chen Y, He Y, DeVivo MJ. Changing demographics and injury profile of new traumatic spinal cord injuries in the United States, 1972-2014. Archives of Physical Medicine and Rehabilitation. 2016;**97**(10):1610-1619

[6] van den Berg ME, Castellote JM, Mahillo-Fernandez I, de Pedro-Cuesta J. Incidence of spinal cord injury worldwide: A systematic review. Neuroepidemiology. 2010;**34**(3):184-192; discussion 92

[7] Estrada-Mondaca S, Carreon-Rodriguez A, Parra-Cid del C, Leon CI, Velasquillo-Martinez C, Vacanti CA, et al. Spinal cord injury and regenerative medicine. Salud Pública de México. 2007;**49**(6):437-444

[8] Rouanet C, Reges D, Rocha E, Gagliardi V, Silva GS. Traumatic spinal cord injury: Current concepts and treatment update. Arquivos de Neuro-Psiquiatria. 2017;**75**(6):387-393

[9] Kim YH, Ha KY, Kim SI. Spinal cord injury and related clinical trials. Clinics in Orthopedic Surgery. 2017;**9**(1):1-9

[10] Dalbayrak S, Yaman O, Yilmaz T. Current and future surgery strategies for spinal cord injuries. World Journal of Orthopedics. 2015;**6**(1):34-41

[11] Dumont RJ, Okonkwo DO, Verma S, Hurlbert RJ, Boulos PT, Ellegala DB, et al. Acute spinal cord injury, part I: Pathophysiologic mechanisms. Clinical Neuropharmacology. 2001;**24**(5):254-264

[12] Mautes AE, Weinzierl MR, Donovan F, Noble LJ. Vascular events after spinal cord injury: Contribution to secondary pathogenesis. Physical Therapy. 2000;**80**(7):673-687

[13] Hilton BJ, Moulson AJ, Tetzlaff W. Neuroprotection and secondary damage following spinal cord injury: Concepts and methods. Neuroscience Letters. 2017;**652**:3-10

[14] Oyinbo CA. Secondary injury mechanisms in traumatic spinal cord injury: A nugget of this multiply cascade. Acta Neurobiologiae Experimentalis (Wars). 2011;**71**(2):281-299

[15] Hulsebosch CE. Recent advances in pathophysiology and treatment of spinal cord injury. Advances in Physiology Education. 2002;**26**(1-4):238-255

[16] von Euler M, Li-Li M, Whittemore S, Seiger A, Sundstrom E. No protective effect of the NMDA antagonist memantine in experimental spinal cord injuries. Journal of Neurotrauma. 1997;**14**(1):53-61

[17] Melnikova DI, Khotimchenko YS, Magarlamov TY. Addressing the issue of tetrodotoxin targeting. Marine Drugs. 2018;**16**(10):352

[18] Liu WM, Wu JY, Li FC, Chen QX. Ion channel blockers and spinal cord injury. Journal of Neuroscience Research. 2011;**89**(6):791-801

[19] Rosenberg LJ, Teng YD, Wrathall JR. Effects of the sodium channel blocker tetrodotoxin on acute white matter pathology after experimental contusive spinal cord injury. The Journal of Neuroscience. 1999;**19**(14):6122-6133

[20] Rosenberg LJ, Wrathall JR. Time course studies on the effectiveness of tetrodotoxin in reducing consequences of spinal cord contusion. Journal of Neuroscience Research. 2001;**66**(2):191-202

[21] Teng YD, Wrathall JR. Local blockade of sodium channels by tetrodotoxin ameliorates tissue loss and long-term functional deficits resulting from experimental spinal cord injury. The Journal of Neuroscience. 1997;**17**(11):4359-4366

[22] Wilson JR, Fehlings MG. Riluzole for acute traumatic spinal cord injury: A promising neuroprotective treatment strategy. World Neurosurgery. 2014;**81**(5-6):825-829

[23] Wang SJ, Wang KY, Wang WC. Mechanisms underlying the riluzole inhibition of glutamate release from rat cerebral cortex nerve terminals (synaptosomes). Neuroscience. 2004;**125**(1):191-201

[24] Mu X, Azbill RD, Springer JE. Riluzole improves measures of oxidative stress following traumatic spinal cord injury. Brain Research. 2000;**870**(1-2):66-72

[25] Grossman RG, Fehlings MG, Frankowski RF, Burau KD, Chow DS, Tator C, et al. A prospective, multicenter, phase I matched-comparison group trial of safety, pharmacokinetics, and preliminary efficacy of riluzole in patients with traumatic spinal cord injury. Journal of Neurotrauma. 2014;**31**(3):239-255

[26] Jia YF, Gao HL, Ma LJ, Li J. Effect of nimodipine on rat spinal cord injury. Genetics and Molecular Research. 2015;**14**(1):1269-1276

[27] Cai Y, Fan R, Hua T, Liu H, Li J. Nimodipine alleviates apoptosis-mediated impairments through the mitochondrial pathway after spinal cord injury. Current Zoology. 2015;**57**(3):340-349

[28] Aydoseli A, Can H, Aras Y, Sabanci PA, Akcakaya MO, Unal OF. Memantine and Q-VD-OPh treatments in experimental spinal cord injury: Combined inhibition of necrosis and apoptosis. Turkish Neurosurgery. 2016;**26**(5):783-789

[29] Ehrlich M, Knolle E, Ciovica R, Bock P, Turkof E, Grabenwoger M, et al. Memantine for prevention of spinal cord injury in a rabbit model. The Journal of Thoracic and Cardiovascular Surgery. 1999;**117**(2):285-291

[30] Gaviria M, Privat A, d'Arbigny P, Kamenka J, Haton H, Ohanna F. Neuroprotective effects of a novel NMDA antagonist, gacyclidine, after experimental contusive spinal cord injury in adult rats. Brain Research. 2000;**874**(2):200-209

[31] Gaviria M, Privat A, d'Arbigny P, Kamenka JM, Haton H, Ohanna F. Neuroprotective effects of gacyclidine after experimental photochemical spinal cord lesion in adult rats: Dose-window and time-window effects. Journal of Neurotrauma. 2000;**17**(1):19-30

[32] Liu S, Ruenes GL, Yezierski RP. NMDA and non-NMDA receptor antagonists protect against excitotoxic

injury in the rat spinal cord. Brain Research. 1997;**756**(1):160-167

[33] Mu X, Azbill RD, Springer JE. NBQX treatment improves mitochondrial function and reduces oxidative events after spinal cord injury. Journal of Neurotrauma. 2002;**19**(8):917-927

[34] King VR, Huang WL, Dyall SC, Curran OE, Priestley JV, Michael-Titus AT. Omega-3 fatty acids improve recovery, whereas omega-6 fatty acids worsen outcome, after spinal cord injury in the adult rat. The Journal of Neuroscience. 2006;**26**(17):4672-4680

[35] Zendedel A, Habib P, Dang J, Lammerding L, Hoffmann S, Beyer C, et al. Omega-3 polyunsaturated fatty acids ameliorate neuroinflammation and mitigate ischemic stroke damage through interactions with astrocytes and microglia. Journal of Neuroimmunology. 2015;**278**:200-211

[36] Ward RE, Huang W, Curran OE, Priestley JV, Michael-Titus AT. Docosahexaenoic acid prevents white matter damage after spinal cord injury. Journal of Neurotrauma. 2010;**27**(10):1769-1780

[37] Figueroa JD, Cordero K, Llán MS, De Leon M. Dietary omega-3 polyunsaturated fatty acids improve the neurolipidome and restore the DHA status while promoting functional recovery after experimental spinal cord injury. Journal of Neurotrauma. 2013;**30**(10):853-868

[38] Lim SN, Huang W, Hall JC, Michael-Titus AT, Priestley JV. Improved outcome after spinal cord compression injury in mice treated with docosahexaenoic acid. Experimental Neurology. 2013;**239**:13-27

[39] Lang-Lazdunski L, Blondeau N, Jarretou G, Lazdunski M, Heurteaux C. Linolenic acid prevents neuronal cell death and paraplegia after transient spinal cord ischemia in rats. Journal of Vascular Surgery. 2003;**38**(3):564-575

[40] Hall JC, Priestley JV, Perry VH, Michael-Titus AT. Docosahexaenoic acid, but not eicosapentaenoic acid, reduces the early inflammatory response following compression spinal cord injury in the rat. Journal of Neurochemistry. 2012;**121**(5):738-750

[41] Figueroa JD, Cordero K, Serrano-Illan M, Almeyda A, Baldeosingh K, Almaguel FG, et al. Metabolomics uncovers dietary omega-3 fatty acid-derived metabolites implicated in anti-nociceptive responses after experimental spinal cord injury. Neuroscience. 2013;**255**:1-18

[42] Liu ZH, Yip PK, Priestley JV, Michael-Titus AT. A single dose of docosahexaenoic acid increases the functional recovery promoted by rehabilitation after cervical spinal cord injury in the rat. Journal of Neurotrauma. 2017;**34**(9):1766-1777

[43] Dringen R, Gutterer JM, Hirrlinger J. Glutathione metabolism in brain metabolic interaction between astrocytes and neurons in the defense against reactive oxygen species. European Journal of Biochemistry. 2000;**267**(16):4912-4916

[44] Guizar-Sahagun G, Ibarra A, Espitia A, Martinez A, Madrazo I, Franco-BourlandRE.Glutathionemonoethyl ester improves functional recovery, enhances neuron survival, and stabilizes spinal cord blood flow after spinal cord injury in rats. Neuroscience. 2005;**130**(3):639-649

[45] Santoscoy C, Rios C, Franco-Bourland RE, Hong E, Bravo G, Rojas G, et al. Lipid peroxidation by nitric oxide supplements after spinal cord injury: Effect of antioxidants in rats. Neuroscience Letters. 2002;**330**(1):94-98

[46] Martinon S, Garcia E, Flores N, Gonzalez I, Ortega T, Buenrostro M, et al. Vaccination with a neural-derived peptide plus administration of glutathione improves the performance of paraplegic rats. The European Journal of Neuroscience. 2007;**26**(2):403-412

[47] Barut S, Unlu YA, Karaoglan A, Tuncdemir M, Dagistanli FK, Ozturk M, et al. The neuroprotective effects of z-DEVD.fmk, a caspase-3 inhibitor, on traumatic spinal cord injury in rats. Surgical Neurology. 2005;64(3):213-220. discussion 20

[48] Yakovlev AG, Knoblach SM, Fan L, Fox GB, Goodnight R, Faden AI. Activation of CPP32-like caspases contributes to neuronal apoptosis and neurological dysfunction after traumatic brain injury. The Journal of Neuroscience. 1997;**17**(19):7415-7424

[49] Ray SK, Hogan EL, Banik NL Calpain in the pathophysiology of spinal cord injury: Neuroprotection with calpain inhibitors. Brain Research. Brain Research Reviews. 2003;**42**(2):169-185

[50] Colak A, Karaoglan A, Barut S, Kokturk S, Akyildiz AI, Tasyurekli M. Neuroprotection and functional recovery after application of the caspase-9 inhibitor z-LEHD-fmk in a rat model of traumatic spinal cord injury. Journal of Neurosurgery. Spine. 2005;**2**(3):327-334

[51] Ray SK, Matzelle DD, Sribnick EA, Guyton MK, Wingrave JM, Banik NL. Calpain inhibitor prevented apoptosis and maintained transcription of proteolipid protein and myelin basic protein genes in rat spinal cord injury. Journal of Chemical Neuroanatomy. 2003;**26**(2):119-124

[52] Sun JF, Yang HL, Huang YH, Chen Q, Cao XB, Li DP, et al. CaSR and calpain contribute to the ischemia reperfusion injury of spinal cord. Neuroscience Letters. 2017;**646**:49-55

[53] Schumacher PA, Siman RG, Fehlings MG. Pretreatment with calpain inhibitor CEP-4143 inhibits calpain I activation and cytoskeletal degradation, improves neurological function, and enhances axonal survival after traumatic spinal cord injury. Journal of Neurochemistry. 2000;**74**(4):1646-1655

[54] Arataki S, Tomizawa K, Moriwaki A, Nishida K, Matsushita M, Ozaki T, et al. Calpain inhibitors prevent neuronal cell death and ameliorate motor disturbances after compression-induced spinal cord injury in rats. Journal of Neurotrauma. 2005;**22**(3):398-406

[55] Resnick DK, Graham SH, Dixon CE, Marion DW. Role of cyclooxygenase 2 in acute spinal cord injury. Journal of Neurotrauma. 1998;**15**(12):1005-1013

[56] Resnick DK, Nguyen P, Cechvala CF. Selective cyclooxygenase 2 inhibition lowers spinal cord prostaglandin concentrations after injury. The Spine Journal. 2001;**1**(6):437-441

[57] Popovich PG, Tovar CA, Wei P, Fisher L, Jakeman LB, Basso DM. A reassessment of a classic neuroprotective combination therapy for spinal cord injured rats: LPS/pregnenolone/indomethacin. Experimental Neurology. 2012;**233**(2):677-685

[58] Xing B, Li H, Wang HY, Mukhopadhyay D, Fisher D, Gilpin CJ, et al. RhoA-inhibiting NSAIDs promote axonal myelination after spinal cord injury. Experimental Neurology. 2011;**231**(2):247-260

[59] Ogino K, Hatanaka K, Kawamura M, Katori M, Harada Y. Evaluation of pharmacological profile of meloxicam as an anti-inflammatory agent, with particular reference to its relative selectivity for cyclooxygenase-2 over cyclooxygenase-1. Pharmacology. 1997;**55**(1):44-53

[60] Hakan T, Toklu HZ, Biber N, Celik H, Erzik C, Ogunc AV, et al. Meloxicam exerts neuroprotection on spinal cord trauma in rats. The International Journal of Neuroscience. 2011;**121**(3):142-148

[61] Chen ZR, Ma Y, Guo HH, Lu ZD, Jin QH. Therapeutic efficacy of cyclosporin a against spinal cord injury in rats with hyperglycemia. Molecular Medicine Reports. 2018;**17**(3):4369-4375

[62] Attur MG, Patel R, Thakker G, Vyas P, Levartovsky D, Patel P, et al. Differential anti-inflammatory effects of immunosuppressive drugs: Cyclosporin, rapamycin and FK-506 on inducible nitric oxide synthase, nitric oxide, cyclooxygenase-2 and PGE2 production. Inflammation Research. 2000;**49**(1):20-26

[63] Ibarra A, Correa D, Willms K, Merchant MT, Guizar-Sahagun G, Grijalva I, et al. Effects of cyclosporin-a on immune response, tissue protection and motor function of rats subjected to spinal cord injury. Brain Research. 2003;**979**(1-2):165-178

[64] Gold BG, Udina E, Bourdette D, Navarro X. Neuroregenerative and neuroprotective actions of neuroimmunophilin compounds in traumatic and inflammatory neuropathies. Neurological Research. 2004;**26**(4):371-380

[65] Kaymaz M, Emmez H, Bukan N, Dursun A, Kurt G, Paşaoğlu H, et al. Effectiveness of FK506 on lipid peroxidation in the spinal cord following experimental traumatic injury. Spinal Cord. 2005;**43**(1):22-26

[66] Saganova K, Galik J, Blasko J, Korimova A, Racekova E, Vanicky I. Immunosuppressant FK506: Focusing on neuroprotective effects following brain and spinal cord injury. Life Sciences. 2012;**91**(3-4):77-82

[67] Nottingham S, Knapp P, Springer J. FK506 treatment inhibits caspase-3 activation and promotes oligodendroglial survival following traumatic spinal cord injury. Experimental Neurology. 2002;**177**(1):242-251

[68] Karin N, Mitchell DJ, Brocke S, Ling N, Steinman L. Reversal of experimental autoimmune encephalomyelitis by a soluble peptide variant of a myelin basic protein epitope: T cell receptor antagonism and reduction of interferon gamma and tumor necrosis factor alpha production. The Journal of Experimental Medicine. 1994;**180**(6):2227-2237

[69] Martinon S, Garcia E, Gutierrez-Ospina G, Mestre H, Ibarra A. Development of protective autoimmunity by immunization with a neural-derived peptide is ineffective in severe spinal cord injury. PLoS One. 2012;7(2):e32027

[70] Martiñón S, García E, Gutierrez-Ospina G, Mestre H, Ibarra A. Development of protective autoimmunity by immunization with a neural-derived peptide is ineffective in severe spinal cord injury. PloS one. 2012;7(2):e32027-e

[71] Rodriguez-Barrera R, Fernandez-Presas AM, Garcia E, Flores-Romero A, Martinon S, Gonzalez-Puertos VY, et al. Immunization with a neural-derived peptide protects the spinal cord from apoptosis after traumatic injury. BioMed Research International. 2013;**2013**:827517

[72] del Rayo Garrido M, Silva-Garcia R, Garcia E, Martinon S, Morales M, Mestre H, et al. Therapeutic window for combination therapy of A91 peptide and glutathione allows delayed treatment after spinal cord injury. Basic and Clinical Pharmacology and Toxicology. 2013;**112**(5):314-318

[73] Afshari K, Dehdashtian A, Haddadi NS, Haj-Mirzaian A, Iranmehr A,

Ebrahimi MA, et al. Anti-inflammatory effects of metformin improve the neuropathic pain and locomotor activity in spinal cord injured rats: Introduction of an alternative therapy. Spinal Cord. 2018;**56**(11):1032-1041

[74] Wang C, Liu C, Gao K, Zhao H, Zhou Z, Shen Z, et al. Metformin preconditioning provide neuroprotection through enhancement of autophagy and suppression of inflammation and apoptosis after spinal cord injury. Biochemical and Biophysical Research Communications. 2016;**477**(4):534-540

[75] Zhang D, Xuan J, Zheng BB, Zhou YL, Lin Y, Wu YS, et al. Metformin improves functional recovery after spinal cord injury via autophagy flux stimulation. Molecular Neurobiology. 2017;**54**(5):3327-3341

[76] Markowicz-Piasecka M, Sikora J, Szydłowska A, Skupień A, Mikiciuk-Olasik E, Huttunen KM. Metformin—A future therapy for neurodegenerative diseases. In: Brambilla D, editor. Drug Discovery, Development and Delivery in Alzheimer's Disease. Pharmaceutical Research. 2017;34(12):2614-2627

[77] Sengelaub DR, Xu XM. Protective effects of gonadal hormones on spinal motoneurons following spinal cord injury. Neural Regeneration Research. 2018;**13**(6):971-976

[78] Sengelaub DR, Han Q, Liu NK, Maczuga MA, Szalavari V, Valencia SA, et al. Protective effects of estradiol and dihydrotestosterone following spinal cord injury. Journal of Neurotrauma. 2018;**35**(6):825-841

[79] Samantaray S, Das A, Matzelle DC, Yu SP, Wei L, Varma A, et al. Administration of low dose estrogen attenuates gliosis and protects neurons in acute spinal cord injury in rats. Journal of Neurochemistry. 2016;**136**(5):1064-1073

[80] Yune TY, Kim SJ, Lee SM, Lee YK, Oh YJ, Kim YC, et al. Systemic administration of 17beta-estradiol reduces apoptotic cell death and improves functional recovery following traumatic spinal cord injury in rats. Journal of Neurotrauma. 2004;**21**(3):293-306

[81] Byers JS, Huguenard AL, Kuruppu D, Liu NK, Xu XM, Sengelaub DR. Neuroprotective effects of testosterone on motoneuron and muscle morphology following spinal cord injury. The Journal of Comparative Neurology. 2012;**520**(12):2683-2696

[82] Brotfain E, Gruenbaum SE, Boyko M, Kutz R, Zlotnik A, Klein M. Neuroprotection by estrogen and progesterone in traumatic brain injury and spinal cord injury. Current Neuropharmacology. 2016;**14**(6):641-653

[83] Bains M, Hall ED. Antioxidant therapies in traumatic brain and spinal cord injury. Biochimica et Biophysica Acta. 2012;**1822**(5):675-684

[84] Gao W, Chen SR, Wu MY, Gao K, Li YL, Wang HY, et al. Methylprednisolone exerts neuroprotective effects by regulating autophagy and apoptosis. Neural Regeneration Research. 2016;**11**(5):823-828

[85] Evaniew N, Noonan VK, Fallah N, Kwon BK, Rivers CS, Ahn H, et al. Methylprednisolone for the treatment of patients with acute spinal cord injuries: A propensity score-matched cohort study from a Canadian multi-Center spinal cord injury registry. Journal of Neurotrauma. 2015;**32**(21):1674-1683

[86] Bracken MB, Shepard MJ, Collins WF, Holford TR, Baskin DS, Eisenberg HM, et al. Methylprednisolone or naloxone treatment after acute spinal cord injury: 1-year follow-up data. Results of the second National acute

spinal cord injury study. Journal of Neurosurgery. 1992;**76**(1):23-31

[87] Coutinho AE, Chapman KE. The anti-inflammatory and immunosuppressive effects of glucocorticoids, recent developments and mechanistic insights. Molecular and Cellular Endocrinology. 2011;**335**(1):2-13

[88] Ulndreaj A, Badner A, Fehlings MG. Promising neuroprotective strategies for traumatic spinal cord injury with a focus on the differential effects among anatomical levels of injury. F1000Res. 2017;**6**:1907

[89] Bracken MB, Shepard MJ, Hellenbrand KG, Collins WF, Leo LS, Freeman DF, et al. Methylprednisolone and neurological function 1 year after spinal cord injury. Results of the National acute spinal cord injury study. Journal of Neurosurgery. 1985;**63**(5):704-713

[90] Bracken MB, Shepard MJ, Holford TR, Leo-Summers L, Aldrich EF, Fazl M, et al. Administration of methylprednisolone for 24 or 48 hours or tirilazad mesylate for 48 hours in the treatment of acute spinal cord injury. Results of the third National acute spinal cord injury randomized controlled trial. National acute spinal cord injury study. Journal of the American Medical Association. 1997;**277**(20):1597-1604

[91] Mu X, Azbill RD, Springer JE. Riluzole and methylprednisolone combined treatment improves functional recovery in traumatic spinal cord injury. Journal of Neurotrauma. 2000;**17**(9):773-780

[92] Qian T, Guo X, Levi AD, Vanni S, Shebert RT, Sipski ML. High-dose methylprednisolone may cause myopathy in acute spinal cord injury patients. Spinal Cord. 2005;**43**(4):199-203

[93] Hurlbert RJ, Hadley MN, Walters BC, Aarabi B, Dhall SS, Gelb DE, et al. Pharmacological therapy for acute spinal cord injury. Neurosurgery. 2013;**72**(Suppl 2):93-105

[94] Ibarra A, Hauben E, Butovsky O, Schwartz M. The therapeutic window after spinal cord injury can accommodate T cell-based vaccination and methylprednisolone in rats. The European Journal of Neuroscience. 2004;**19**(11):2984-2990

[95] Festoff BW, Ameenuddin S, Arnold PM, Wong A, Santacruz KS, Citron BA. Minocycline neuroprotects, reduces microgliosis, and inhibits caspase protease expression early after spinal cord injury. Journal of Neurochemistry. 2006;**97**(5):1314-1326

[96] Tator CH, Hashimoto R, Raich A, Norvell D, Fehlings MG, Harrop JS, et al. Translational potential of preclinical trials of neuroprotection through pharmacotherapy for spinal cord injury. Journal of Neurosurgery. Spine. 2012;**17**(1 Suppl):157-229

[97] Garrido-Mesa N, Zarzuelo A, Galvez J. Minocycline: Far beyond an antibiotic. British Journal of Pharmacology. 2013;**169**(2):337-352

[98] Lee SM, Yune TY, Kim SJ, Park DW, Lee YK, Kim YC, et al. Minocycline reduces cell death and improves functional recovery after traumatic spinal cord injury in the rat. Journal of Neurotrauma. 2003;**20**(10):1017-1027

[99] Stirling DP, Koochesfahani KM, Steeves JD, Tetzlaff W. Minocycline as a neuroprotective agent. The Neuroscientist. 2005;**11**(4):308-322

[100] Marchand F, Tsantoulas C, Singh D, Grist J, Clark AK, Bradbury EJ, et al. Effects of etanercept and minocycline in a rat model of spinal cord injury. European Journal of Pain. 2009;**13**(7):673-681

[101] Moini-Zanjani T, Ostad SN, Labibi F, Ameli H, Mosaffa N, Sabetkasaei M. Minocycline effects on IL-6 concentration in macrophage and microglial cells in a rat model of neuropathic pain. Iranian Biomedical Journal. 2016;**20**(5):273-279

[102] Tan AM, Zhao P, Waxman SG, Hains BC. Early microglial inhibition preemptively mitigates chronic pain development after experimental spinal cord injury. Journal of Rehabilitation Research and Development. 2009;**46**(1):123-133

[103] Casha S, Zygun D, McGowan MD, Bains I, Yong VW, Hurlbert RJ. Results of a phase II placebo-controlled randomized trial of minocycline in acute spinal cord injury. Brain. 2012;**135**(Pt 4):1224-1236

[104] Geisler FH, Dorsey FC, Coleman WP. Recovery of motor function after spinal-cord injury—A randomized, placebo-controlled trial with GM-1 ganglioside. The New England Journal of Medicine. 1991;**324**(26):1829-1838

[105] Palmano K, Rowan A, Guillermo R, Guan J, McJarrow P. The role of gangliosides in neurodevelopment. Nutrients. 2015;7(5):3891-3913

[106] Popovich PG, Lemeshow S, Gensel JC, Tovar CA. Independent evaluation of the effects of glibenclamide on reducing progressive hemorrhagic necrosis after cervical spinal cord injury. Experimental Neurology. 2012;**233**(2):615-622

[107] Simard JM, Tsymbalyuk O, Ivanov A, Ivanova S, Bhatta S, Geng Z, et al. Endothelial sulfonylurea receptor 1-regulated NC Ca-ATP channels mediate progressive hemorrhagic necrosis following spinal cord injury. The Journal of Clinical Investigation. 2007;**117**(8):2105-2113

[108] Cordero K, Coronel GG, Serrano-Illan M, Cruz-Bracero J, Figueroa JD, De Leon M. Effects of dietary vitamin E supplementation in bladder function and spasticity during spinal cord injury. Brain Sciences. 2018;**8**(3):38

[109] Taoka Y, Ikata T, Fukuzawa K. Influence of dietary vitamin E deficiency on compression injury of rat spinal cord. Journal of Nutritional Science and Vitaminology (Tokyo). 1990;**36**(3):217-226

[110] Iwasa K, Ikata T, Fukuzawa K. Protective effect of vitamin E on spinal cord injury by compression and concurrent lipid peroxidation. Free Radical Biology and Medicine. 1989;**6**(6):599-606

[111] Robert AA, Zamzami M, Sam AE, Al Jadid M, Al Mubarak S. The efficacy of antioxidants in functional recovery of spinal cord injured rats: An experimental study. Neurological Sciences. 2012;**33**(4):785-791

[112] Zadeh-Ardabili PM, Rad SK, Khazaai H, Sanusi J, Zadeh MH. Palm vitamin E reduces locomotor dysfunction and morphological changes induced by spinal cord injury and protects against oxidative damage. Scientific Reports. 2017;7(1):14365

[113] Yan M, Yang M, Shao W, Mao XG, Yuan B, Chen YF, et al. High-dose ascorbic acid administration improves functional recovery in rats with spinal cord contusion injury. Spinal Cord. 2014;**52**(11):803-808

[114] Wang WG, Xiu RJ, Xu ZW, Yin YX, Feng Y, Cao XC, et al. Protective effects of vitamin C against spinal cord injury-induced renal damage through suppression of NF-kappaB and proinflammatory cytokines. Neurological Sciences. 2015;**36**(4):521-526

[115] Lee JY, Choi HY, Yune TY. Fluoxetine and vitamin C synergistically

inhibits blood-spinal cord barrier disruption and improves functional recovery after spinal cord injury. Neuropharmacology. 2016;**109**:78-87

[116] van Neerven S, Mey J, Joosten EA, Steinbusch HW, van Kleef M, Marcus MA, et al. Systemic but not local administration of retinoic acid reduces early transcript levels of pro-inflammatory cytokines after experimental spinal cord injury. Neuroscience Letters. 2010;**485**(1):21-25

[117] Zhou Y, Zheng B, Ye L, Zhang H, Zhu S, Zheng X, et al. Retinoic acid prevents disruption of blood-spinal cord barrier by inducing autophagic flux after spinal cord injury. Neurochemical Research. 2016;**41**(4):813-825

[118] Lin HY, Tang HY, Davis FB, Davis PJ. Resveratrol and apoptosis. Annals of the New York Academy of Sciences. 2011;**1215**:79-88

[119] Denu JM. Fortifying the link between SIRT1, resveratrol, and mitochondrial function. Cell Metabolism. 2012;**15**(5):566-567

[120] Gut P, Verdin E. Rejuvenating SIRT1 activators. Cell Metabolism. 2013;**17**(5):635-637

[121] Zhao H, Chen S, Gao K, Zhou Z, Wang C, Shen Z, et al. Resveratrol protects against spinal cord injury by activating autophagy and inhibiting apoptosis mediated by the SIRT1/AMPK signaling pathway. Neuroscience. 2017;**348**:241-251

[122] Kesherwani V, Atif F, Yousuf S, Agrawal SK. Resveratrol protects spinal cord dorsal column from hypoxic injury by activating Nrf-2. Neuroscience. 2013;**241**:80-88

[123] Liu C, Shi Z, Fan L, Zhang C, Wang K, Wang B. Resveratrol improves neuron protection and functional recovery in rat model of spinal cord injury. Brain Research. 2011;**1374**:100-109

[124] Hodgetts SI, Harvey AR. Neurotrophic factors used to treat spinal cord injury. Vitamins and Hormones. 2017;**104**:405-457

[125] Weishaupt N, Blesch A, Fouad K. BDNF: The career of a multifaceted neurotrophin in spinal cord injury. Experimental Neurology. 2012;**238**(2):254-264

[126] Hernandez-Torres V, Gransee HM, Mantilla CB, Wang Y, Zhan WZ, Sieck GC. BDNF effects on functional recovery across motor behaviors after cervical spinal cord injury. Journal of Neurophysiology. 2017;**117**(2):537-544

[127] Sharma HS. Neuroprotective effects of neurotrophins and melanocortins in spinal cord injury: An experimental study in the rat using pharmacological and morphological approaches. Annals of the New York Academy of Sciences. 2005;**1053**:407-421

[128] Uchida S, Hayakawa K, Ogata T, Tanaka S, Kataoka K, Itaka K. Treatment of spinal cord injury by an advanced cell transplantation technology using brain-derived neurotrophic factor-transfected mesenchymal stem cell spheroids. Biomaterials. 2016;**109**:1-11

[129] Sharma HS. Neurotrophic factors in combination: A possible new therapeutic strategy to influence pathophysiology of spinal cord injury and repair mechanisms. Current Pharmaceutical Design. 2007;**13**(18):1841-1874

[130] Ji XC, Dang YY, Gao HY, Wang ZT, Gao M, Yang Y, et al. Local injection of Lenti-BDNF at the lesion site promotes M2 macrophage polarization and inhibits inflammatory response after spinal cord injury in mice.

Cellular and Molecular Neurobiology. 2015;**35**(6):881-890

[131] Dobolyi A, Vincze C, Pal G, Lovas G. The neuroprotective functions of transforming growth factor beta proteins. International Journal of Molecular Sciences. 2012;**13**(7):8219-8258

[132] Krieglstein K, Strelau J, Schober A, Sullivan A, Unsicker K. TGF-beta and the regulation of neuron survival and death. Journal of Physiology, Paris. 2002;**96**(1-2):25-30

[133] Prewitt CM, Niesman IR, Kane CJ, Houle JD. Activated macrophage/ microglial cells can promote the regeneration of sensory axons into the injured spinal cord. Experimental Neurology. 1997;**148**(2):433-443

[134] Kohta M, Kohmura E, Yamashita T. Inhibition of TGF-beta1 promotes functional recovery after spinal cord injury. Neuroscience Research. 2009;**65**(4):393-401

[135] Laron Z. Insulin-like growth factor 1 (IGF-1): A growth hormone. Molecular Pathology. 2001;**54**(5):311-316

[136] Davila D, Torres-Aleman I. Neuronal death by oxidative stress involves activation of FOXO3 through a two-arm pathway that activates stress kinases and attenuates insulin-like growth factor I signaling. Molecular Biology of the Cell. 2008;**19**(5):2014-2025

[137] Duarte AI, Santos P, Oliveira CR, Santos MS, Rego AC. Insulin neuroprotection against oxidative stress is mediated by Akt and GSK-3beta signaling pathways and changes in protein expression. Biochimica et Biophysica Acta. 2008;**1783**(6):994-1002

[138] Hung KS, Tsai SH, Lee TC, Lin JW, Chang CK, Chiu WT. Gene transfer of insulin-like growth factor-I providing neuroprotection after spinal cord injury in rats. Journal of Neurosurgery. Spine. 2007;**6**(1):35-46

[139] Sharma HS, Nyberg F, Gordh T, Alm P, Westman J. Topical application of insulin like growth factor-1 reduces edema and upregulation of neuronal nitric oxide synthase following trauma to the rat spinal cord. Acta Neurochirurgica. Supplement. 1997;**70**:130-133

[140] Utada K, Ishida K, Tohyama S, Urushima Y, Mizukami Y, Yamashita A, et al. The combination of insulin-like growth factor 1 and erythropoietin protects against ischemic spinal cord injury in rabbits. Journal of Anesthesia. 2015;**29**(5):741-748

[141] Cheng I, Park DY, Mayle RE, Githens M, Smith RL, Park HY, et al. Does timing of transplantation of neural stem cells following spinal cord injury affect outcomes in an animal model? Journal of Spinal Surgery. 2017;**3**(4):567-571

[142] Salewski RP, Mitchell RA, Shen C, Fehlings MG. Transplantation of neural stem cells clonally derived from embryonic stem cells promotes recovery after murine spinal cord injury. Stem Cells and Development. 2015;**24**(1):36-50

[143] Rong Y, Liu W, Wang J, Fan J, Luo Y, Li L, et al. Neural stem cell-derived small extracellular vesicles attenuate apoptosis and neuroinflammation after traumatic spinal cord injury by activating autophagy. Cell Death and Disease. 2019;**10**(5):340

[144] He BL, Ba YC, Wang XY, Liu SJ, Liu GD, Ou S, et al. BDNF expression with functional improvement in transected spinal cord treated with neural stem cells in adult rats. Neuropeptides. 2013;**47**(1):1-7

[145] Ankeny DP, McTigue DM, Jakeman LB. Bone marrow transplants provide tissue protection and directional guidance for axons after contusive spinal cord injury in rats. Experimental Neurology. 2004;**190**(1):17-31

[146] Kim YC, Kim YH, Kim JW, Ha KY. Transplantation of mesenchymal stem cells for acute spinal cord injury in rats: Comparative study between Intralesional injection and scaffold based transplantation. Journal of Korean Medical Science. 2016;**31**(9):1373-1382

[147] Nakajima H, Uchida K, Guerrero AR, Watanabe S, Sugita D, Takeura N, et al. Transplantation of mesenchymal stem cells promotes an alternative pathway of macrophage activation and functional recovery after spinal cord injury. Journal of Neurotrauma. 2012;**29**(8):1614-1625

[148] Okuda A, Horii-Hayashi N, Sasagawa T, Shimizu T, Shigematsu H, Iwata E, et al. Bone marrow stromal cell sheets may promote axonal regeneration and functional recovery with suppression of glial scar formation after spinal cord transection injury in rats. Journal of Neurosurgery. Spine. 2017;**26**(3):388-395

[149] Ban DX, Ning GZ, Feng SQ, Wang Y, Zhou XH, Liu Y, et al. Combination of activated Schwann cells with bone mesenchymal stem cells: The best cell strategy for repair after spinal cord injury in rats. Regenerative Medicine. 2011;**6**(6):707-720

[150] Allahdadi KJ, de Santana TA, Santos GC, Azevedo CM, Mota RA, Nonaka CK, et al. IGF-1 overexpression improves mesenchymal stem cell survival and promotes neurological recovery after spinal cord injury. Stem Cell Research and Therapy. 2019;**10**(1):146

[151] Wu S, Cui G, Shao H, Du Z, Ng JC, Peng C. The cotransplantation of olfactory ensheathing cells with bone marrow mesenchymal stem cells exerts antiapoptotic effects in adult rats after spinal cord injury. Stem Cells International. 2015;**2015**:516215

[152] Lopez-Vales R, Garcia-Alias G, Fores J, Vela JM, Navarro X, Verdu E. Transplanted olfactory ensheathing cells modulate the inflammatory response in the injured spinal cord. Neuron Glia Biology. 2004;**1**(3):201-209

[153] Zhang J, Chen H, Duan Z, Chen K, Liu Z, Zhang L, et al. The effects of co-transplantation of olfactory ensheathing cells and Schwann cells on local inflammation environment in the contused spinal cord of rats. Molecular Neurobiology. 2017;**54**(2):943-953

[154] Pearse DD, Pereira FC, Marcillo AE, Bates ML, Berrocal YA, Filbin MT, et al. cAMP and Schwann cells promote axonal growth and functional recovery after spinal cord injury. Nature Medicine. 2004;**10**(6):610-616

[155] Pearse DD, Bastidas J, Izabel SS, Ghosh M. Schwann cell transplantation subdues the pro-inflammatory innate immune cell response after spinal cord injury. International Journal of Molecular Sciences. 2018;**19**(9):2550

[156] Wang JM, Zeng YS, Wu JL, Li Y, Teng YD. Cograft of neural stem cells and schwann cells overexpressing TrkC and neurotrophin-3 respectively after rat spinal cord transection. Biomaterials. 2011;**32**(30):7454-7468

[157] Shin JC, Kim KN, Yoo J, Kim IS, Yun S, Lee H, et al. Clinical trial of human fetal brain-derived neural stem/progenitor cell transplantation in patients with traumatic cervical spinal cord injury. Neural Plasticity. 2015;**2015**:630932

[158] Sykova E, Homola A, Mazanec R, Lachmann H, Konradova SL,

Kobylka P, et al. Autologous bone marrow transplantation in patients with subacute and chronic spinal cord injury. Cell Transplantation. 2006;**15**(8-9):675-687

[159] Satti HS, Waheed A, Ahmed P, Ahmed K, Akram Z, Aziz T, et al. Autologous mesenchymal stromal cell transplantation for spinal cord injury: A phase I pilot study. Cytotherapy. 2016;**18**(4):518-522

[160] Karamouzian S, Nematollahi-Mahani SN, Nakhaee N, Eskandary H. Clinical safety and primary efficacy of bone marrow mesenchymal cell transplantation in subacute spinal cord injured patients. Clinical Neurology and Neurosurgery. 2012;**114**(7):935-939

[161] Feron F, Perry C, Cochrane J, Licina P, Nowitzke A, Urquhart S, et al. Autologous olfactory ensheathing cell transplantation in human spinal cord injury. Brain. 2005;**128**(Pt 12):2951-2960

[162] Anderson KD, Guest JD, Dietrich WD, Bartlett Bunge M, Curiel R, Dididze M, et al. Safety of autologous human Schwann cell transplantation in subacute thoracic spinal cord injury. Journal of Neurotrauma. 2017;**34**(21):2950-2963

[163] Scivoletto G, Morganti B, Molinari M. Early versus delayed inpatient spinal cord injury rehabilitation: An Italian study. Archives of Physical Medicine and Rehabilitation. 2005;**86**(3):512-516

[164] Sumida M, Fujimoto M, Tokuhiro A, Tominaga T, Magara A, Uchida R. Early rehabilitation effect for traumatic spinal cord injury. Archives of Physical Medicine and Rehabilitation. 2001;**82**(3):391-395

[165] Marques MR, Nicola FC, Sanches EF, Arcego DM, Duran-Carabali LE, Aristimunha D, et al. Locomotor training promotes time-dependent functional recovery after experimental spinal cord contusion. Neuroscience. 2018;**392**:258-269

[166] Dobkin B, Apple D, Barbeau H, Basso M, Behrman A, Deforge D, et al. Weight-supported treadmill vs over-ground training for walking after acute incomplete SCI. Neurology. 2006;**66**(4):484-493

Chapter 10

Neuroprotective Potentials of Natural Vitamin E for Cerebral Small Vessel Disease

Muzaimi Mustapha, Che Mohd Nasril Che Mohd Nassir, Yuen Kah Hay, Fung Wai Yee and Hafizah Abdul Hamid

Abstract

Cerebral small vessel disease (CSVD) refers to a spectrum of clinical and neuroimaging findings resulting from pathological processes of various etiologies affecting cerebral arterioles, perforating arteries, capillaries, and venules. It is the commonest neurological problem that results in significant disability, but awareness of it remains poor. It affects over half of people over 65 years old and inflicts up to third of acute strokes, over 40% of dementia, and a significant decline in physical ability in otherwise asymptomatic, aging individuals. Moreover, the unifying theory for the pathomechanism of the disease remains elusive and hence the apparent ineffective therapeutic approaches. Given the growing literature for natural vitamin E (tocopherols and tocotrienols) as a potent antioxidant, this chapter attempts to consolidate the contemporary evidence to shed plausible insights on the neuroprotective potentials of natural vitamin E in addressing the heterogenous CSVD spectrum, in health and in disease.

Keywords: cerebral small vessel diseases, vitamin E, antioxidants, dementia, aging

1. Introduction

The recognition of vitamin E for its nutritive value was first linked to reproductive health in laboratory rats, then coined as factor X [1]. While alpha-tocopherol was the first vitamin E isomer to be recognized, there are now eight chemically distinct isomers known, consisting of alpha (α), beta (β), gamma (γ), and delta (δ)-isoforms of tocopherols and tocotrienols [2]. Current recommendations for adequate intake values are established based on α-tocopherol alone, whereas other forms of vitamin E need to meet other criteria [3]. Nature affords tocopherols in abundance, particularly in plants such as peanuts, sunflower seeds, and sesame seeds. The major dietary source of tocopherol is largely from corn and soybean oil consumption [4]. In contrast, the less ubiquitous tocotrienols are found in certain cereals and vegetables such as palm oil and annatto. A non-food source of tocotrienols is also recognized, namely, the latex of the rubber plant [2].

The well-established bioactivity of vitamin E is its antioxidant property by means of lipid peroxidation of cellular membranes [2]. As such, this property lends vitamin E the roles in promoting vascular health in arterial compliance studies and endothelial dysfunction biomarker. Pertinent to this, vitamin E involvement is the vascular endothelium, which lines the intraluminal surface of blood vessels and is involved in the regulation of vascular tone, platelet activity, thrombosis, and the overriding pathogenesis of atherosclerosis [5, 6]. Vitamin E engages with the production of nitric oxide (NO) that relaxes the vascular smooth muscle while limiting free radicals to maintain arterial compliance [7]. More recently, vitamin E has been linked with anti-atherogenic effects that decrease low-density lipoprotein (LDL) oxidation and downstream inhibition of protein kinase C (PKC), adhesion molecules, monocyte transmigration, and vascular smooth muscle cell proliferation [8].

Therefore, the foregoing facts on vascular health and vitamin E profiles offer interrelated perspectives for a largely unexplored neurological condition termed cerebral small vessel diseases (CSVD). CSVD variable manifestations inflict small blood vessels or microcirculation at the subcortical and deeper parts of the brain. It has been widely reported to cause cerebral ischemic stroke or lacunar stroke that accounts for nearly a third of all stroke subtypes worldwide [9–12]. The pathological consequences of small vessel disease on the brain parenchyma rather than the underlying diseases of the vessels is frequently viewed as the basis of CSVD [13]. Notably, CSVD lesions can be silent, and the affected individual may not have any apparent clinical symptoms. This silent (subclinical) lesion, with higher numbers (single or multiple), poses as a risk for vascular cognitive impairment, dementia, Alzheimer's disease, and full-blown stroke [14, 15].

Furthermore, aging and chronic hypertension are known to accelerate CSVD, as the two conditions (physiological and pathological, respectively) may result in less efficient ability to self-regulate cerebral blood flow (cBF) from the concurrent varying systemic blood pressure levels and increased arterial stiffness which increases the speed and flow pulsatility in cerebral arterioles [16]. These hemodynamic changes are postulated to cause variable degrees of endothelial damage in the blood-brain barrier (BBB) and alter its permeability through an increase of the shear stress [17]. Hence, the BBB breakdown is an important etiopathogenesis feature of CSVD [17–19].

In addition, there is an elevated production of reactive oxygen species (ROS) in CSVD that ultimately leads to endothelium dysfunctions [20, 21]. This is mainly due to the cumulative reactions and processes (i.e., high blood pressure, very low density of lipoproteins, diabetes mellitus, homocysteinemia, and smoking) that trigger and escalate the inflammatory responses and oxidative stress [20, 21]. This, in turn, heightens the release of adhesion molecules and recruits leukocytes, causing higher leukocyte-endothelial cell (EC) adhesion and reduced cBF. Accordingly, nicotinamide adenine dinucleotide phosphate (NADPH) oxidases intensify the oxidative stress (a major source of ROS in vessel wall) and the consequent destructive impact on EC-dependent NO signaling [22, 23].

Collectively, this chapter focuses on highlighting the contemporary evidence on vitamin E, especially α-tocopherol and α-tocotrienol, their neuroprotective potential in relation to the heterogenous spectrum of CSVD manifestations, in promoting health as we age, and in mitigating disease.

2. Natural sources of vitamin E

2.1 Forms and structure

Vitamin E was first discovered in 1922 by Herbert Evans and Katherine Bishop at the University of California in Berkeley when they studied nutritive dependencies in reproduction [1]. They observed that rats fed with a purified diet of casein 18%, cornstarch 54%, lard 15%, butterfat 9%, and salts 4% and adequate vitamin A (as cod liver oil), vitamin B (as yeast), and vitamin C (as orange juice) did not reproduce. They observed in females defective placental function, whereas the ovaries, ovulation, and implantation were unimpaired; and in males, there was a complete atrophy of the seminiferous epithelium [24, 25]. The addition of lettuce to the diet prevented embryo resorption during rodent gestation, and healthy pups were born again, thus, leading to the discovery of an anti-sterility factor, then termed as factor X. Wheat germ oil was later found to be a rich source of factor X. It was not until some 10 years later that Evans successfully isolated the components of vitamin E family and named them tocopherols (Greek: *toc* (child), *phero* (to bring forth), and *–ol* because it behaves chemically like an alcohol) [25, 26].

Meanwhile, tocotrienol was named by Bunyan and colleagues, when they identified the unsaturated derivatives of tocols, isolated from the latex of the rubber plant (*Hevea brasiliensis*) [27]. The structure of tocotrienols was further described by Pennock and colleagues, who found that palm oil was a rich source of this "new tocopherol" [28]. Palm oil derived from *Elaeis guineensis* (African oil palm) now represents the richest source of the lesser characterized vitamin E, α-tocotrienol.

α-Tocopherol is currently the only form of vitamin E recognized to meet human requirements, and recommended adequate intake values are established based on α-tocopherol alone. Other forms of vitamin E must fulfill the following to be recognized as vitamin E: (1) converted to α-tocopherol in humans and (2) recognized by the α-tocopherol transfer protein. Plasma α-tocopherol concentrations in humans range from 11 to 37 μmol/L, whereas γ-tocopherol concentrations are roughly 2–5 μmol/L, and tocotrienol concentrations are less than 1 μmol/L in non-supplemented humans [3].

Tocopherols are widely found in nature, predominantly in plant seeds such as peanuts, sunflower seeds, almonds, walnuts, and sesame seeds. The major dietary source of tocopherol comes from the widespread use of corn and soybean oil [4]. Tocotrienols, which are less ubiquitous, are found in certain cereals and vegetables such as palm oil, rice bran oil, and annatto. Lower levels of tocotrienols can be found in grapefruit seed oil, oats, hazelnuts, maize, olive oil, buckthorn berry, rye, flaxseed oil, poppy seed oil, and sunflower oil [3]. A non-food source of tocotrienols is the latex of the rubber plant. While it has been shown that the different vitamin E forms are interconvertible by plants, there has been no convincing evidence that the same is true for animals [29].

While alpha-tocopherol was the first vitamin E isomer to be recognized, there are now eight chemically distinct isomers known, consisting of alpha (α), beta (β), gamma (γ), and delta (δ)-isoforms of tocopherols and tocotrienols [2], as shown in **Figure 1**. The molecular structure of vitamin E is based on a chromanol ring with a side chain at the C2 position. While the lipophilic tail of tocopherols is completely saturated, tocotrienols have three double bonds, at the 3′, 7′, and 11′ positions. Plants synthesize eight different forms of vitamin E, tocopherols and tocotrienols, which include α, β, γ, and δ forms that differ in the number of methyl groups on the chromanol ring [29]. The slight difference in structure between isoforms translates into striking variations in activity. Compared with tocopherols, tocotrienols are more efficiently incorporated into membranes and cultured cells [30], thus giving rise to more potent antioxidant activities.

2.2 Mechanism and regulation of metabolism

Upon oral administration, vitamin E, a lipid-soluble vitamin, requires biliary and pancreatic secretions in order to form micelles for the subsequent uptake by intestinal epithelial cells [3]. Therefore, the absorption of vitamin E is enhanced if

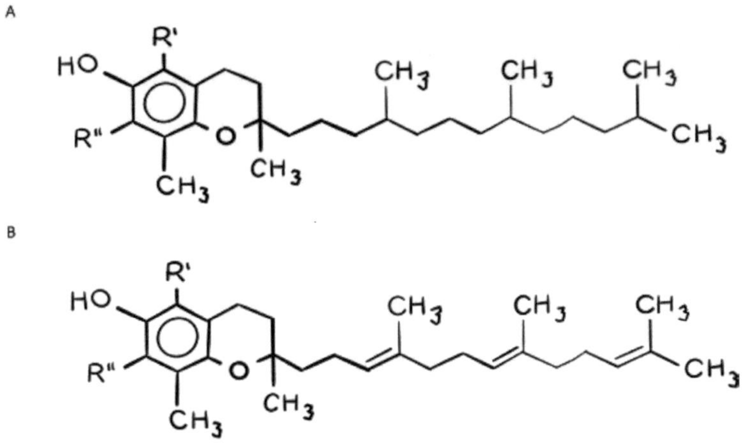

Figure 1.
Chemical structures of (A) tocopherol and (B) tocotrienol. Note the three double bonds in the tocotrienol side chain. Note: Isoforms—α (R' = CH_3, R" = CH_3); β (R' = CH_3, R" = H); γ (R' = H, R" = CH_3); δ (R' = H, R" = H).

taken with food which contributes fat, thereby triggering the secretion of enzymes that facilitate the formation of micelles required for absorption. Despite many years since its discovery, there is still a lack of understanding of the mechanism of absorption, liver trafficking, and disposition of vitamin E isoforms [31].

The general understanding of vitamin E absorption and trafficking is that orally administered vitamin E undergoes intestinal luminal processing, where it accumulates in lipid droplets, which then coalesce with nascent chylomicrons [32]. The vitamin E isoforms are not discriminated during the intestinal absorption or incorporation into chylomicrons. Chylomicrons then transport vitamin E from the intestine through circulation to the liver, which metabolizes or resecretes vitamin E back into the plasma for trafficking to tissues via enriched lipoproteins.

After the liver takes up chylomicron remnants, vitamin E isoforms with greater affinity to α-tocopherol transport protein (αTTP) are preferentially bound for transport to tissues, thereby avoiding catabolism. αTTP expressed in the liver is required to facilitate vitamin E transport from the liver to other tissues and organs. The discrimination of vitamin E isoforms occurs in the liver as a result of differing affinity of isoforms to αTTP. αTTP has the ability to bind to both α-tocotrienol and α-tocopherol, but αTTP binds to α-tocotrienol with approximately 10 fold lower affinity than that for α-tocopherol [33]. All lipoproteins are involved in the trafficking of α-tocopherol to the tissues, although very low-density lipoprotein apparently leaves the liver preferentially enriched in α-tocopherol compared with LDL or high-density lipoprotein (HDL) [29]. Discrimination between dietary forms of vitamin E is dependent upon the hepatic αTTP to maintain circulating α-tocopherol [34]. α-tocopherol is also most retained in tissues due to preferential binding by αTT, facilitating secretion into plasma [2] and trafficking to tissues, whereas large portions of other forms of vitamin E are catabolized through general xenobiotic processes [4].

Interestingly, a study using αTTP knockout mice showed that orally administered α-tocotrienol was absorbed and delivered to vital organs, despite being deficient of αTTP [35]. In organs such as adipose tissue, skin, skeletal muscle, and the heart, α-tocotrienol levels were many folds higher than α-tocopherol in supplemented αTTP knockout mice. Oral supplementation of the female mice with α-tocotrienol also restored fertility, suggesting that it can be successfully delivered to the relevant tissues and that α-tocotrienol supported reproductive function under conditions of α-tocopherol deficiency. These findings suggest TTP-independent mechanisms for the tissue delivery of oral α-tocotrienol. While αTTP may contribute to tocotrienol trafficking, αTTP does not represent a major or sole mechanism of α-tocotrienol transport in the body [35].

Vitamin E is metabolized by ω-hydroxylation by cytochrome P450 (CYP), followed by β-oxidation and conjugation to generate carboxychromanols and conjugated counterparts [2, 29]. The tail of vitamin E isoforms is ω-hydroxylated by CYP 4F2 and subjected to several rounds of β-oxidation, which ultimately results in the formation of carboxyethyl hydroxy chromanol (CEHC) (**Figure 2**). Thus, the tail-shortened, water-soluble metabolite, CEHC, is synthesized and excreted in the urine [36]. Conjugation such as sulfation and glucuronidation of the phenolic on the chromanol may also take place in parallel with β-oxidation when there is a high intake of vitamin E forms [4]. Although α-tocopherol largely escapes catabolism and ends up in the blood circulation, α-CEHC is synthesized endogenously when the quantity of hepatic α-tocopherol exceeds the capacity of αTTP to facilitate α-tocopherol secretion from the liver into the circulation [31].

Traber and colleagues established that urinary α-CEHC might be useful to noninvasively assess α-tocopherol adequacy, especially in populations with metabolic syndrome-associated hepatic dysfunction that likely impairs α-tocopherol trafficking. Their finding also suggests that people with metabolic syndrome may have a higher requirement for vitamin E due to poorer trafficking leading to lower apparent α-tocopherol bioavailability. However, it is still unknown whether urinary α-CEHC excretion reflects α-tocopherol intake from a single meal or whether its changes reflect long-term vitamin E status [31].

Recently, Traber and colleagues, which lead as one of the most prolific research groups in vitamin E tocopherol, suggested novel approaches to assess α-tocopherol absorption and trafficking in order to establish human vitamin E requirements [32]. Their study observed that the absorption of α-tocopherol is not necessarily limited by the absence of fat or fasting and that the absorption is highly dependent on chylomicron assembly processes. The transport of α-tocopherol across the intestines may be prolonged during fasting and

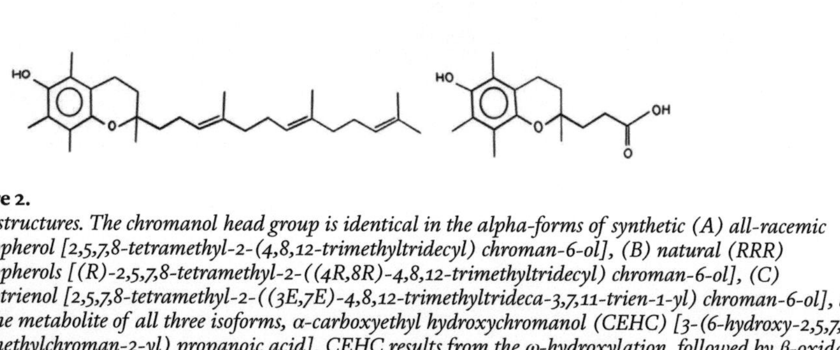

Figure 2.
Tocol structures. The chromanol head group is identical in the alpha-forms of synthetic (A) all-racemic α-tocopherol [2,5,7,8-tetramethyl-2-(4,8,12-trimethyltridecyl) chroman-6-ol], (B) natural (RRR) α-tocopherols [(R)-2,5,7,8-tetramethyl-2-((4R,8R)-4,8,12-trimethyltridecyl) chroman-6-ol], (C) α-tocotrienol [2,5,7,8-tetramethyl-2-((3E,7E)-4,8,12-trimethyltrideca-3,7,11-trien-1-yl) chroman-6-ol], and (D) the metabolite of all three isoforms, α-carboxyethyl hydroxychromanol (CEHC) [3-(6-hydroxy-2,5,7,8-tetramethylchroman-2-yl) propanoic acid]. CEHC results from the ω-hydroxylation, followed by β-oxidation of the side chain (as well as conjugation with glucuronide, sulfate, or other compounds), yielding a water-soluble molecule that is largely excreted in urine [34].

potentiated by eating. However, the authors recognized the conclusion derived from the study has several limitations, including small sample size, lack of randomization or blinding, and compliance issues, leading to an imbalance with attendant potential for baseline and residual confounding. Nevertheless, if proven in a larger trial, this observation changes the conventional thinking that vitamin E needs to be taken with or immediately after meal to enhance absorption and also reflects that there is still much to learn on the absorption and transport of vitamin E in humans.

2.3 Antioxidant activities

The most established bioactivity of vitamin E is its antioxidant property, primarily against lipid peroxidation in biological membranes [2]. By quenching the lipid radicals, vitamin E, as chain-breaking antioxidant, terminates the chain reaction of the oxidation of polyunsaturated fatty acids (PUFAs) [3]. This function is critical to ensure the integrity of cellular membranes and systems which rely on the abundance of PUFAs, such as the nervous system. Hence, neurological symptoms such as progressive ataxia and hyporeflexia are manifestations of vitamin E deficiency as a result of malabsorption.

Tocopherols and tocotrienols are potent antioxidants that scavenge lipid peroxyl radicals by donating hydrogen from the phenolic group on the chromanol ring [4]. A synergistic antioxidant system made up of vitamin C and other hydrogen donors such as thiol antioxidants, namely, glutathione and lipoic acid, reacts with the resulting tocotrienoxyl or tocopheroxyl radicals to regenerate vitamin E [37], returning it to its reduced state for further use (**Figure 3**). There is very little evidence in vivo for more advanced vitamin E oxidation products [34].

Packer and colleagues noted that the substituents on the chromanol nucleus and properties of side chain (saturated vs. unsaturated) were critical to the effectiveness of the different vitamin E homologs [37]. Preferential distribution of α-tocopherol to the tissues in vivo may have contributed to its greater impact compared with other homologs, but the structural differences between α-tocopherol and α-tocotrienol have given rise to differences in reactivity observed in in vitro and in vivo studies.

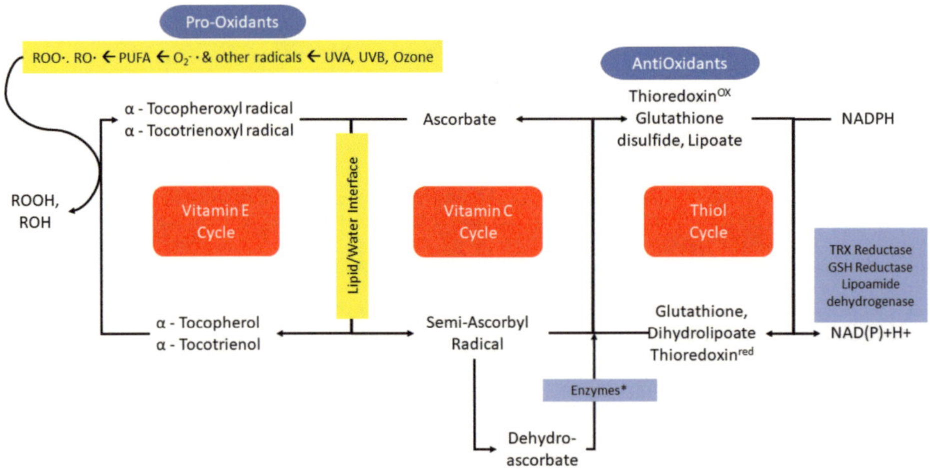

Figure 3.
*The antioxidant network showing the interaction among vitamin E, vitamin C, and thiol redox cycles [37]. Notes: *thiol transferase (glutaredoxin), protein disulfide isomerase, glutathione (GSH)-dependent dehydroascorbate reductase, thioredoxin (TRX) reductase.*

Tocotrienols were suggested to be more effective scavengers of peroxyl radicals due to more even distribution in the phospholipid bilayer, more effective interaction with lipid peroxyl radicals [4], stronger disordering of membrane lipids, and greater recycling of chromanoxyl radical due to closer location to the membrane surface [37]. The chromanoxyl radical of α-tocotrienol was found to be recycled in membranes and lipoproteins more quickly than the corresponding α-tocopheroxyl radical [38].

The antioxidant activity of vitamin E is critical to a healthy nervous system, as evident from the consequences of neurological function under deficient condition. The vitamin E protection of PUFAs leads to neuroprotective effects under pathologic and high oxidative stress conditions. Due to the early discovery of α-tocopherol as an essential vitamer and its ubiquitous nature, most research in vitamin E, concerning the mechanisms of action and physiological implications of deficiency, has centered on tocopherols. Tocotrienols, without having any apparent consequence of deficiency and being not inherently detectable in non-supplemented humans or animals, were not the focus of vitamin E-related research until much later. Since the discovery of rich sources of tocotrienols and subsequent availability as an active ingredient, there is growing evidence that tocotrienols have superior potency in terms of antioxidant activity and modulation of impaired biochemical pathways resulting in physiologically beneficial effects.

Arachidonic acid (AA), one of the most abundant PUFAs of the central nervous system, is highly susceptible to oxidative metabolism under pathologic conditions. [39]. A number of neurodegenerative conditions in the human brain are associated with disturbed PUFA metabolism of AA, including acute ischemic stroke [40]. Cleaved from the membrane phospholipid bilayer by cytosolic phospholipase A_2 ($cPLA_2$), AA is metabolized by both enzymatic and nonenzymatic pathways into neurotoxic metabolites. Palm oil-derived α-tocotrienol at nanomolar concentrations has been shown to attenuate both enzymatic and nonenzymatic mediators of AA metabolism and neurodegeneration [39] (**Figure 4**).

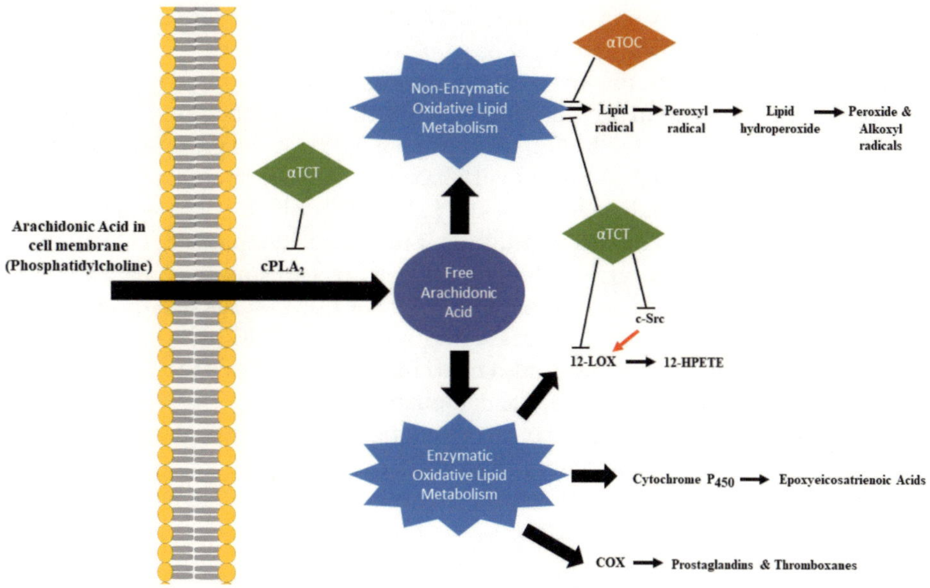

Figure 4.
The arachidonic acid (AA) cascade and potential target sites for α-tocopherols (αTOC) and α-tocotrienols (αTCT) [39]. cPLA2, cytosolic phospholipase A2; 12-LOX, 12-lipoxygenase; c-Src, proto-oncogene tyrosine-protein kinase or simply c-Src (cellular sarcoma); 12-HPETE, 12-hydroperoxyeicosatetraenoic acid; COX, cyclooxygenase.

2.4 Benefits in vascular health

Vitamin E has also been associated with improved vascular health in studies measuring arterial compliance and endothelial dysfunction as biomarkers. Vascular endothelium, which lines the blood luminal surface of vessels, is involved in the regulation of vascular tone, platelet activity, and thrombosis and intimately involved in the pathogenesis of atherosclerosis [5, 6]. The endothelium is an integral part of the vasculature and is involved in promoting an atheroprotective environment via the complementary actions of endothelial cell-derived vasoactive factors [41]. Vasomotor tone is modulated through the release of endothelium-derived relaxing factors (EDRFs) such as NO [6]. Impaired vascular homeostasis can lead to endothelial dysfunction, which contributes to atherosclerosis [41]. Intact endothelium is also needed for normal arterial compliance, a predictor of cardiovascular events. Arterial compliance, which can be assessed by pulse wave velocity (PWV) and augmentation index (AI), can be improved in healthy subjects even with dietary interventions [7].

In a randomized controlled trial, subjects with the following risk factors, hypercholesterolemia (13 subjects), smokers (14 subjects), or both (15 subjects), were supplemented with placebo or vitamin E for 4 months. The authors hypothesized that long-term supplementation with vitamin E would improve endothelium-dependent relaxation in hypercholesterolemic patients and/or chronic smoking, two risk factors that have been associated with increased radical formation, impaired endothelial vasodilator function, and increased plasma levels of autoantibodies against oxidized LDL [6]. The study found the most severe endothelial vasodilator dysfunction in patients with both risk factors present. Vitamin E significantly improved endothelium-dependent relaxation in forearm resistance vessels of hypercholesterolemic smokers. There was a significant relationship between improvement in acetylcholine-induced vasodilation and the change in autoantibody titer against oxidized LDL ($r = -0.59$; $p = 0.002$) [6].

Moreover, in a randomized controlled trial, 36 healthy male volunteers were supplemented with placebo or tocotrienol-rich vitamin (50, 100, 200 mg/day) with self-emulsifying formula for 2 months [7]. Arterial compliance was assessed using carotid-femoral PWV and AI, at baseline and after 2 months of supplementation. Subjects treated with tocotrienols at doses of 100 and 200 mg/day showed significant improvement in arterial compliance with PWV reductions of 0.77 m/s ($p = 0.007$) and 0.65 m/s ($p = 0.002$), respectively. The placebo group did not show a reduction in PWV and AI compared with baseline. The treatment had no effect on blood pressure, serum total cholesterol, and LDL-C [7], which are potential confounding factors to the observed improvement in arterial compliance. The improvement in vascular function can be achieved through mechanisms involving enhanced NO production by the endothelium and inhibition of free radicals that inactivate EDRF. Vitamin E can potentially increase the production of NO, which relaxes the vascular smooth muscle cells, while also neutralizing free radicals which preserve the action of EDRF to maintain arterial compliance [7].

In addition to promoting vascular health, vitamin E is also postulated to exert anti-atherogenic effects via its ability to decrease LDL oxidation, quench free radicals, inhibit protein kinase C (PKC), inhibit expression of adhesion molecules and monocyte transmigration, and impair vascular smooth muscle cell proliferation [8].

3. Cerebral small vessel disease

The general ischemia implicated in CSVD of small blood vessels (i.e., arterial tree occlusion in particular) involving the subcortical and deeper parts of the brain has been widely reported to cause cerebral ischemic stroke or lacunar stroke and accounts for nearly 30% of all stroke subtypes worldwide [9–12].

3.1 Characteristic and classification

The complexity and overlapping pathophysiological mechanism of the disease make the interpretation of CSVD debatable. However, it is a widely accepted view that pathological consequences of small vessel disease (SVD) on the brain parenchyma rather than the underlying diseases of the vessels serve as the basis of CSVD [13]. Hence, the injury in the brain parenchyma that is linked with leptomeningeal and intracerebral vessel pathology that vascularizes with poor collaterals in the deep white matter and subcortical gray matter is the main diagnostic landmark of CSVD. Moreover, CSVD is generally due to several vasculo-pathological processes that affect and cause occlusion to the small perforating cerebral arterioles, capillaries, and venules (of sizes 50–400 mm), which are small arteries (chiefly of middle cerebral artery tributaries) that penetrate and supply the brain subcortical region, resulting in various lesions in the brain [42–46].

Several manifestations of CSVD can be seen through clinical, radiological (i.e., neuroimaging such as CT or MRI), or pathological phenomena with various etiologies [46–49]. Recent advancement in neuroimaging techniques had enabled the imaging-based (such as MRI) identification and characterization of multiple manifestation of CSVD including white matter hyperintensities (WMHs) of presumed vascular origin or leukoaraiosis, lacunes of presumed vascular origin (i.e., small subcortical infarcts and silent brain infarcts, SBI), perivascular spaces, microinfarcts, and cerebral microbleeds (CMBs) [46, 50, 51]. Alarmingly, the aforementioned lesions can be silent, and the affected individual may not have any clinical symptoms. More importantly, this silent lesion with higher number of single or multiple, is associated with higher risk of mild cognitive impairment, dementia, Alzheimer's disease, and full-blown stroke [14, 15].

There are several etiopathogenic classifications of CSVD. However, the most prevalent forms of CSVD are amyloidal CSVD (sporadic and hereditary cerebral amyloid angiopathy [CAA]) and non-amyloidal CSVD (arteriolosclerosis, age-related, vascular risk-factor-related SVD, i.e., microatheroma, lipohyalinosis, fibrinoid necrosis, and segmental arterial disorganization) [42, 52, 53]. Other less common forms of CSVD include inherited or genetic CSVD that is recognizably different from CAA (i.e., Fabry's disease and cerebral autosomal dominant arteriopathy with subcortical ischemic strokes and leukoencephalopathy [CADASIL]), inflammatory and immunologically mediated CSVD (i.e., rheumatoid vasculitis, lupus erythematosus, and CNS vasculitis secondary to infection), venous collagenosis, and other CSVD (i.e., non-amyloid microvessel degeneration in AD and postradiation angiopathy) [42, 52, 53].

3.2 Neuroepidemiology and health burden

Different manifestations of CSVD based on neuroimaging findings result in different and overlapping health burden and epidemiology [54]. Increasing age has been reported to elevate the finding of WMHs, lacunes, perivascular spaces, and CMBs in healthy populations [54–56]. However, increased vascular risk factors are consistent with the prevalence of CMBs but not in other imaging findings [56, 57]. Race, ethnicity, and gender with adjusted age also explain the variability of these imaging findings, whereby some findings had reported that higher WMH grade and volume were found in ethnic or racial minorities than non-Hispanic white [58] and WMHs were much higher in women than men, although no definite mechanism was reported for this gender difference [59]. In addition, previous study had reported stroke-free elderly Hispanic and/or Latino had SBI (16%), especially in subcortical region (82.9%) [60] and perivascular spaces (48%) [61].

In other ethnic groups, previous study had reported that the prevalence of WMHs in South Asians and Europeans is similar, although South Asian elderly individuals with known vascular risk are more likely to be associated with higher WMHs [62]. Meanwhile, data in three Asian countries (Singapore, Hong Kong, and Korea) have shown that elderly Asians with higher SVD burden are associated with cognitive decline [63]. This was further supported by the Taizhou Imaging Study, whereby the authors found increased incidental findings of WMHs (10.68%), lacunes (26.69%), CMBs (18.51%), and perivascular spaces (27.76%) in elderly Chinese with vascular risk [64]. However in the Japanese population, most are having moderate to mild dilated perivascular spaces, especially in the centrum semiovale and basal ganglia [65]. Thus, it is apparent that more data are required to understand the role of racial and/or ethnic contributions for the presence of different CSVD manifestations.

The effects of several manifestations of CSVD on cognition seem to be invariably influenced by the location of the lesion(s). The damaged and reduced white matter integrity in the frontal lobe and its dysfunction are associated with reduced transmission of information to other parts of the brain in the presence of WMHs [54], lacunes (deep nuclear [78.2%], posterior fossa [10.1%]) [66], and perivascular spaces [65, 67]. In contrast, temporal lobe lesion is more associated with the findings of lobar and deep CMBs [68, 69]. Several studies have reported that an increase in WMHs is associated with worse general and specific domain of cognitive performance, especially in executive function, processing speed, and episodic memory [70–73]. Intriguingly, an increase in WMHs with reduced cognitive performance is similar to the individual with amyloid load, mild parkinsonism, and functional impairments [70].

Furthermore, reduced cognitive ability has been reported in elderly and non-demented people with the presence of lacunes of presumed vascular origin [54, 72, 74]. Memory declines have also been associated with thalamic infarcts, whereas decreased psychomotor speed is associated with non-thalamic infarcts [75]. In contrast, the presence of a lesion in the perivascular spaces reduces the individual processing speed [76] and, in others, reported no effect on the cognitive performance [67]. Meanwhile, a decrease in global cognitive performance and domain specific has been linked with the location of CMBs [77].

3.3 Pathomechanism

Despite the growing insights from histopathological, epidemiological, and physiological studies in the past two decades, the underlying pathomechanism of CSVD remains contentious [46, 53]. In general, it is recognized that advanced age and the presence of chronic hypertension may reduce the ability to self-regulate cBF in response to various systemic blood pressure levels and increased arterial stiffness, hence the increased speed and flow pulsatility in cerebral arterioles [16]. These hemodynamic changes are postulated to inflict a certain degree of endothelial damage in the BBB and alter its permeability through an increase of the shear stress [17]. Hence, the BBB breakdown is an important etiopathogenesis feature of CSVD [17–19].

Another key factor thought to contribute to the pathogenesis of CSVD is endothelial dysfunction, with elevated biomarkers as the surrogates [78, 79]. The endothelial dysfunction involvement is also associated with metabolic syndrome [80, 81] and hence a strong link with CSVD. Furthermore, this dysfunction is also implicated for a higher risk of aging-related disease [82, 83]. In addition to the endothelium, cross-talk among cellular components of the BBB, such as pericytes, astrocytes, and oligodendrocyte precursor cells (OPCs), may be involved in the microvascular damage as precursors for the onset and progression of CSVD [84, 85]. In relation to this, reduced white matter integrity due to changes in oligodendrocytes has been shown in CSVD, whereby the EC-OPC signaling became compromised and altered the ECs' ability to secrete the releasing factor crucial for the growth and survival of OPCs to eventually cause oligodendrocytes prone to damage [86]. Therefore, the interaction of multiple BBB components may play a crucial role in the discovery and development of new prevention steps and therapies for CSVD.

In parallel, an increased activity of matrix metalloproteinase-2 (MPP2) from endothelial cell membrane (ECM) also caused tight junctions (TJs) to dissemble. TJ damage eventually leads to basement membrane degradation and endothelial damage and, hence, endothelial dysfunction. This results in BBB damage, making it vulnerable to the infiltration of neutrophils, monocytes, and blood components into the ECM [53]. Activated neutrophils induce the activation of ROS, proteolytic enzymes, and cytokines, thus causing higher leukocyte-EC adhesion and reduced cBF (**Figure 5**). Meanwhile, activated monocytes will be induced by cytokine and neopterin to cause inflammation in the ECs. Cumulatively, the increased shear and oxidative stress from the system also lead to the activation of blood components and increased production of microparticles, reduced tissue factor pathway inhibitor, and increased fibrinogen accumulation that result in lumen narrowing and consequent cBF reduction [53].

Understandably, the role of hypoperfusion or reduced cBF in endothelial dysfunction for CSVD has been hypothesized [87]. Generally, the regulation of cBF is mediated by NO signaling; thus, NO serves as a marker for endothelial dysfunction [88]. Since endothelial dysfunction is associated with increased BBB permeability, this would worsen brain parenchyma and white matter lesions given the reduced integrity of ECs [89]. In addition, the increased expression of the mutated NOTCH3 gene (a genetic determinant of CADASIL) in pericytes was found to contribute to CSVD pathogenesis due to abnormal cross-talk between ECs and pericytes [87]. Therefore, one can posit that increased BBB permeability, reduced cBF, and impaired cerebral autoregulation serve as three main interrelated underlying pathogenesis precursors to the development and progression of CSVD, notwithstanding the role of other potential and novel factors.

3.4 Role of reactive oxygen species

Multiple studies have reported that the early detection of cognitive and motor decline in neurodegenerative disease has been linked with protein, lipids, sugar, and nucleic acid oxidation [90, 91]. Therefore, it can be postulated that changes or damage to the cerebral vasculature, BBB, and cBF is due to localized oxidative stress, hence initiating the neurodegenerative changes in the brain tissue.

Generally, overproduction of oxidants by NADPH oxidases and malfunction or reduced activities of antioxidant enzymes may result in oxidative stress [52]. The imbalance between antioxidants and prooxidants in aging and age-related neurological disease is regarded to be mainly due to ROS [92] which is a large group of oxygen radicals (i.e., superoxide anion radical, hydroxyl radical, peroxyl radical, and alkoxyl radical) and non-radicals (i.e., hydrogen peroxide, organic hydroperoxide, singlet molecular oxygen, electronically excited carbonyls, and ozone) [52, 64]. NADPH oxidase- and superoxide dismutase-mediated enzymatic conversion of molecular oxygen to superoxide initiates the production of ROS; however, the production of ROS can also be mediated by spontaneous transformation of non-radical hydrogen peroxide [93].

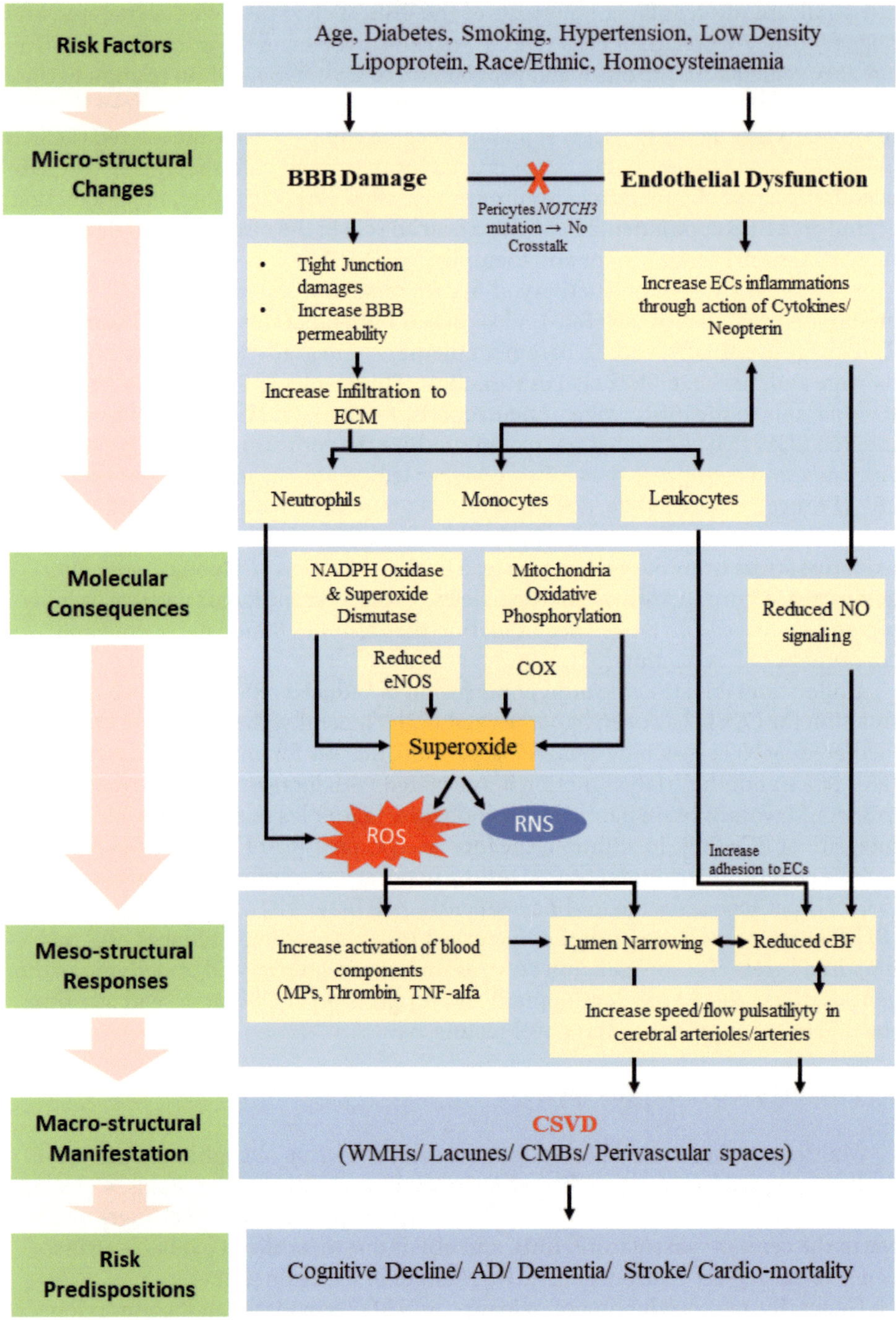

Figure 5.
General pathomechanism and role of ROS in CSVD. ECs, endothelial cells; BBB, blood–brain barrier; ECM, extracellular matrix; cBF, cerebral blood flow; NO, nitric oxide; eNOS, endothelial nitric oxide synthase; ROS, reactive oxygen species; RNS, reactive nitrogen species; COX, cyclooxygenase; NADPH, nicotinamide adenine dinucleotide phosphate; MPs, microparticles; TNF-alpha, tumor necrosis factor-alpha; WMHs, white matter hyperintensities; CMBs, cerebral microbleeds; AD, Alzheimer's disease.

There are multiple oxidative markers used to correlate with neurodegenerative disease including CSVD, for example, thioredoxins (positively correlate with severity of acute ischemic stroke and infarct volume) [94], thioredoxin reductase (reduced thioredoxin reductase attenuates the capacity of endothelium-dependent vasodilatory) [95], and peroxiredoxins (higher during stroke onset and traumatic brain injury) [96]. Moreover, reduced plasma levels of uric acid and vitamins E, A, and C have been used as antioxidant biomarkers for Alzheimer's disease and also Parkinson's disease [97–100]. Similarly, coenzyme Q10 (i.e., ubiquinone Q10) is another antioxidant that has been shown to provide potential protective effects for a spectrum of CSVD and cerebral metabolic syndrome [82].

In CSVD, the elevated production of ROS is mainly due to reactions and process (i.e., high blood pressure, very low density of lipoproteins, diabetes, and homocysteinemia and smoking) that lead to inflammatory mechanism and oxidative stress hence causing endothelium dysfunction [20, 21]. Induction of oxidative stress further enhanced the releasing of adhesion molecules and recruiting of leukocytes causing higher leukocyte-EC adhesion and reduced cBF (**Figure 5**). NADPH oxidases induce oxidative stress (major source of ROS in vessel wall), and its destructive impact on EC-dependent NO signaling has been widely studied [22, 23]. The NADPH oxidases can be stimulated by mechanical forces and vasoactive agonists (i.e., thrombin, platelet-derived growth factor, and tumor necrosis factor-alpha) hence enhancing the production of ROS through superoxide anion radical synthesis [101–103].

Another two key enzymes that facilitate the production of ROS include cyclooxygenase (COX) and enzymatic cascade in mitochondria (i.e., oxidative phosphorylation). COX is an important enzyme that produces superoxide in cerebral blood vessels through prostaglandin H2 synthesis mediated by AA [104, 105]. Superoxide can also be synthesized after endothelial nitric oxide synthase dysfunction that halts the NO production. This eventually reduces the bioavailability of NO and, in turn, facilitates the production of reactive nitrogen species (RNS) to cause reduced anti-inflammatory, reduced vasodilating, increased platelet aggregation, disinhibition of leukocyte adhesion, and reduced antiproliferative effects of NO [52, 106]. Hence, biomarkers of oxidative stress can be used to study the redox imbalance in individuals with WMHs while it draws a plausible therapeutic avenue with targeted dietary supplements to reduced ROS and RNS that would be neuroprotective against CSVD onset and/or manifestations [107].

4. Prospects of vitamin E for CSVD neuroprotection

As remarked in the previous sections, increasing body of evidence indicated that oxidative stress might play a pivotal role in the largely elusive pathomechanism of CSVD and other neurodegenerative disease, including cognitive impairment. Moreover, targeting oxidative stress, as a therapeutic approach of vascular-related disease, has been an area of continuing interest given its significance on the aging world population and the rising trend of noncommunicable disease burden, typically cardio-cerebrovascular disorders which include CSVD. However, informative and converging data on vitamin E and its neuroprotective potential for CSVD are scarce.

Central to this proposition of vitamin E potential in CSVD is the involvement of ROS in the physiological role for normal regulation of cerebral vascular event. Hence, a balance between mitigating oxidative stress and normal physiological role should be considered in this ROS-centric approach for natural vitamin E in CSVD neuroprotective potentials. Nonetheless, the idea of attaining or sustaining certain levels of antioxidants to mitigate vascular oxidative stress remains a contentious issue. For instance, antioxidants such as vitamin E have been proven beneficial for vascular function in small clinical and experimental trials [108], whereby vitamin E supplementation had been shown to reduce the onset of WMHs in small clinical trials [109]. Moreover, natural vitamin E also had been shown favorable to lessen cognitive impairments in CSVD animal models

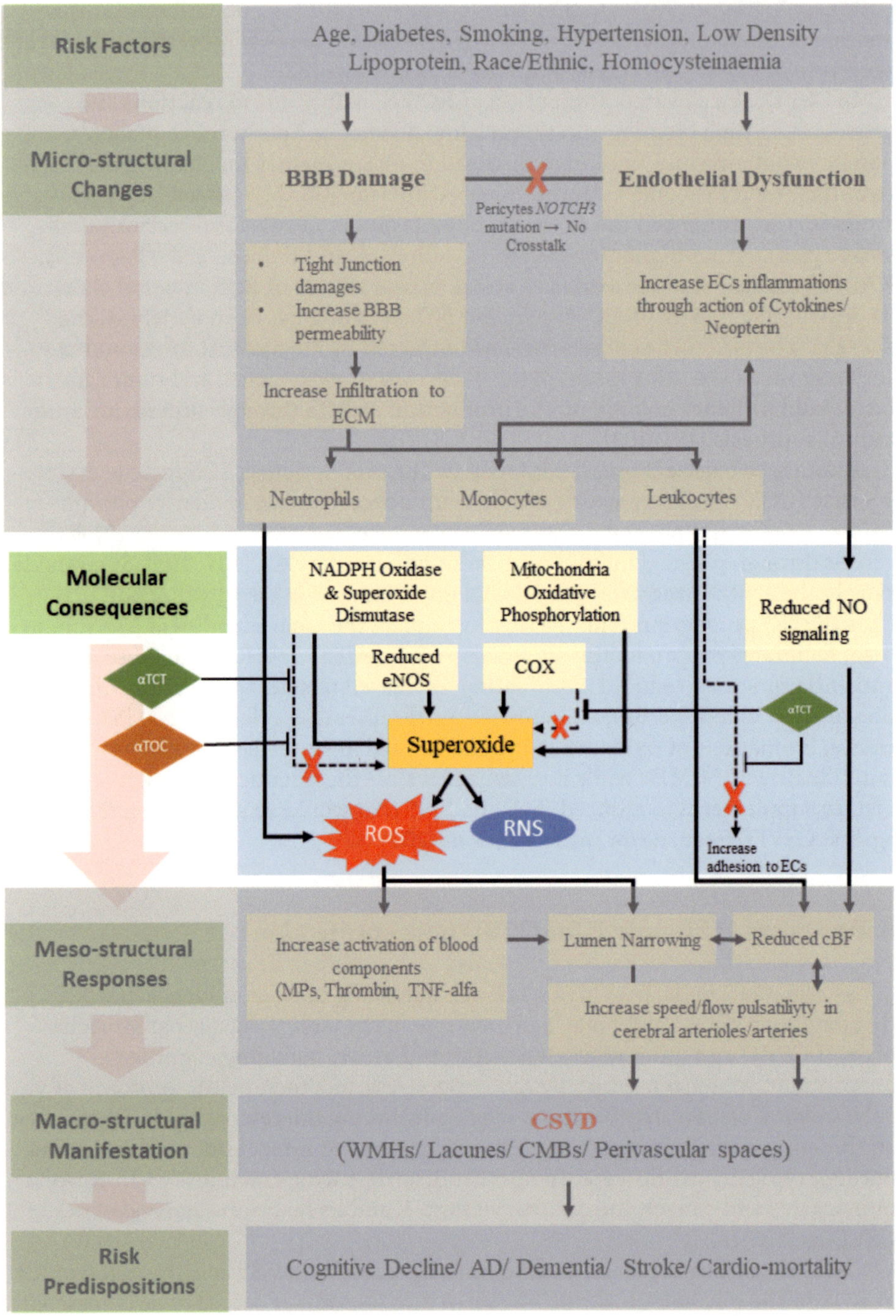

Figure 6.
Putative neuroprotective potentials of natural vitamin E in targeting ROS in CSVD manifestations. αTCT, α-tocotrienols; αTOC, α-tocopherols; ECs, endothelial cells; BBB, blood–brain barrier; ECM, extracellular matrix; cBF, cerebral blood flow; NO, nitric oxide; eNOS, endothelial nitric oxide synthase; ROS, reactive oxygen species; RNS, reactive nitrogen species; COX, cyclooxygenase; NADPH, nicotinamide adenine dinucleotide phosphate; MPs, microparticles; TNF-alpha, tumor necrosis factor-alpha; WMHs, white matter hyperintensities; CMBs, cerebral microbleeds; AD, Alzheimer's disease.

[110, 111]. Notwithstanding, a larger-scale clinical trial had shown less convincing beneficial outcomes on stroke and vascular disease prevention with antioxidant (i.e., vitamin E) supplementation [112].

Moreover, utilizing other antioxidants such as coenzyme Q10 has been reported to have potential neuroprotective effects in treating oxidative stress-induced metabolic syndrome with CSVD-related deterioration with reduced plasma level of coenzyme Q10 in experimental animal model with metabolic syndrome [82]. Nonetheless, recent studies on oxidative stress-induced diet reported weak or no apparent association in modifying the cardiovascular risk in an animal model (normotensive wild-type mice, C57BL/6 J), at least in its impact on systemic blood pressure [113].

The inconsistency in the reports of the potential neuroprotective effects of antioxidant (natural vitamin E) in cerebrovascular disease is partly due to the apparent lack of optimization in terms of concentrations/doses of the vitamin E used. This is despite the supportive data on supra(optimal)-physiological concentration of vitamin E (especially α-tocotrienol) that can interrupt the superoxide and NO reaction [108] to reduce the activation of ROS and endpoint BBB disintegration in CSVD. Hence, we are tempted to posit that appropriate nutritive consumptions of vitamin E could prove advantageous to attenuate BBB damages that underlie CSVD heterogenous manifestations, i.e., by halting the leukocyte-EC adhesion that can further degrade the BBB damages with WMHs. Biomarkers of oxidative stress can serve to monitor the redox imbalance in individuals with WMHs while exploring the putative therapeutic avenue with targeted dietary supplements as neuroprotective potentials against CSVD onset and/or disease manifestations. As such, the vitamin E neuroprotective merits could prevent a comprising reduction of cBF in cerebral ischemia in numerous CSVD manifestations, be it silent or symptomatic, from the ROS-centric targeting (**Figure 6**).

5. Challenge and future direction

Although data on therapeutic regimes had shown promising increased plasma levels of antioxidants, whether this translates to increased levels in the vasculature remains unknown. Even if sufficient levels of antioxidants were achieved in vascular cells, the antioxidants might in fact exert prooxidant effects as a result of their conversion to radical species following their reactions with superoxide [114, 115]. Either way, a single approach of conventional antioxidant supplementation would be suboptimal in combating oxidative stress in CSVD [108].

Corroboratively, with multiple studies having successfully linked the potential therapeutic and neuroprotective potentials of vitamin E in vascular health domains, a multicenter and adequately powered clinical trial is much needed for CSVD. Such data would further strengthen the nutritive value of vitamin E for CSVD neuroprotective supplements. In addition, opportunities exist to examine the connectivity of white matter tracts to exhibit vitamin E role in protection of small vessel collateral circulation as well as an increased expression of proarteriogenic (new blood vessel formation) genes in future research.

6. Conclusion

CSVD, as the commonest neurological condition as we age, could benefit from the potency of vitamin E antioxidant neuroprotective potentials through oxidative stress and BBB integrity modulation. This chapter converges contemporary evidence to shed plausible insights on the neuroprotective potentials of natural vitamin E in addressing the heterogenous CSVD spectrum, in health and disease.

Acknowledgements

Authors thank MIGHT Newton-Ungku Omar Fund, grant number Universiti Sains Malaysia (USM) 304.PPSP.6150151.N118. The authors would like to thank Enago (www.enago.com) for the English language review.

Conflict of interest

The authors acknowledge that there is no conflict of interests in this work.

Author details

Muzaimi Mustapha[1*], Che Mohd Nasril Che Mohd Nassir[1], Yuen Kah Hay[2], Fung Wai Yee[2] and Hafizah Abdul Hamid[3]

1 Department of Neurosciences, School of Medical Sciences, Universiti Sains Malaysia, Kubang Kerian, Kelantan, Malaysia

2 School of Pharmaceutical Sciences, Universiti Sains Malaysia, Minden, Pulau Pinang, Malaysia

3 Department of Human Anatomy, Faculty of Medicine and Health Sciences, Universiti Putra Malaysia (UPM), Serdang, Selangor, Malaysia

*Address all correspondence to: mmuzaimi@usm.my

References

[1] Evans HM, Bishop KS. On the existence of a hitherto unrecognized dietary factor essential for reproduction. Science. 1922;**56**(1458):650-651

[2] Ahsan H, Ahad A, Iqbal J, Siddiqui WA. Pharmacological potential of tocotrienols: A review. Nutrition and Metabolism. 2014;**11**(1):52

[3] Traber MG. Vitamin E regulatory mechanisms. Annual Review of Nutrition. 2007;**27**(1):347-362

[4] Jiang Q. Natural forms of vitamin E: Metabolism, antioxidant, and anti-inflammatory activities and their role in disease prevention and therapy. Free Radical Biology and Medicine. 2014;**72**:76-90

[5] Ross R. The pathogenesis of atherosclerosis: A perspective for the 1990s. Nature. 1993;**362**(6423):801-809

[6] Heitzer T, Herttuala SY, Wild E, Luoma J, Drexler H. Effect of vitamin E on endothelial vasodilator function in patients with hypercholesterolemia, chronic smoking or both. Journal of the American College of Cardiology. 1999;**33**(2):499-505

[7] Rasool AHG, Rahman ARA, Yuen KH, Wong AR. Arterial compliance and vitamin E blood levels with a self-emulsifying preparation of tocotrienol rich vitamin E. Archives of Pharmacal Research. 2008;**31**(9):1212-1217

[8] Mozos I, Stoian D, Luca CT. Crosstalk between vitamins a, B12, D, K, C, and E status and arterial stiffness. Disease Markers. 2017;**2017**:1-14

[9] Rouhl RPW, van Oostenbrugg RJ, Lodder J. White matter lesions: From present to future. In: Westland TB, Calton RN, editors. Handbook on White Matter: Structure, Function and Changes. New York: Nova Science; 2009

[10] Patel B, Markus HS. Magnetic resonance imaging in cerebral small vessel disease and its use as a surrogate disease marker. International Journal of Stroke. 2011;**6**(1):47-59

[11] Heye AK, Thrippleton MJ, Chappell FM, Hernández MDCV, Armitage PA, Makin SD, et al. Blood pressure and sodium: Association with MRI markers in cerebral small vessel disease. Journal of Cerebral Blood Flow & Metabolism. 2015;**36**(1):264-274

[12] Smith EE. Clinical presentations and epidemiology of vascular dementia. Clinical Science. 2017;**131**(11):1059-1068

[13] Wardlaw JM, Smith C, Dichgans M. Mechanisms of sporadic cerebral small vessel disease: Insights from neuroimaging. The Lancet Neurology. 2013;**12**(5):483-497

[14] Debette S, Schilling S, Duperron M-G, Larsson SC, Markus HS. Clinical significance of magnetic resonance imaging markers of vascular brain injury. JAMA Neurology. 2019;**76**(1):81

[15] Georgakis MK, Duering M, Wardlaw JM, Dichgans M. WMH and long-term outcomes in ischemic stroke. Neurology. 2019;**92**(12):e1298-e1308

[16] Cuadrado-Godia E, Dwivedi P, Sharma S, Santiago AO, Gonzalez JR, Balcells M, et al. Cerebral small vessel disease: A review focusing on pathophysiology, biomarkers, and machine learning strategies. Journal of Stroke. 2018;**20**(3):302-320

[17] Zhang CE, Wong SM, Haar HJVD, Staals J, Jansen JF, Jeukens CR, et al. Blood–brain barrier leakage is more widespread in patients with cerebral small vessel disease. Neurology. 2016;**88**(5):426-432

[18] Huisa BN, Caprihan A, Thompson J, Prestopnik J, Qualls CR, Rosenberg GA.

Long-term blood–brain barrier permeability changes in Binswanger disease. Stroke. 2015;**46**(9):2413-2418

[19] Wardlaw JM, Makin SJ, Hernández MCV, Armitage PA, Heye AK, Chappell FM, et al. Blood-brain barrier failure as a core mechanism in cerebral small vessel disease and dementia: Evidence from a cohort study. Alzheimer's & Dementia. 2017;**13**(6):634-643

[20] Blanco M, Rodríguez-Yáñez M, Sobrino T, Leira R, Castillo J. Platelets, inflammation, and atherothrombotic neurovascular disease: The role of endothelial dysfunction. Cerebrovascular Diseases. 2005;**20**(2):32-39

[21] Girouard H, Park L, Anrather J, Zhou P, Iadecola C. Angiotensin II attenuates endothelium-dependent responses in the cerebral microcirculation through Nox-2–derived radicals. Arteriosclerosis, Thrombosis, and Vascular Biology. 2006;**26**(4):826-832

[22] Mayhan WG, Arrick DM, Sharpe GM, Sun H. Age-related alterations in reactivity of cerebral arterioles: Role of oxidative stress. Microcirculation. 2008;**15**(3):225-236

[23] Miller AA, Silva TMD, Judkins CP, Diep H, Drummond GR, Sobey CG. Augmented superoxide production by Nox2-containing NADPH oxidase causes cerebral artery dysfunction during hypercholesterolemia. Stroke. 2010;**41**(4):784-789

[24] Wolf G. The discovery of the antioxidant function of vitamin E: The contribution of Henry A. Mattill. The Journal of Nutrition. 2005;**135**(3):363-366

[25] Evans HM, Emeeson OH, Emerson GA. The isolation from wheat germ oil of an alcohol, α-tocopherol, having the properties of vitamin E. Journal of Biological Chemistry. 1936;**113**:319-332

[26] Evans HM. The Pioneer history of vitamin E. Vitamins and Hormones. 1962;**20**:379-387

[27] Bunyan J, Mchale D, Green J, Marcinkiewicz S. Biological potencies of ε- and ζ1-tocopherol and 5-methyltocol. British Journal of Nutrition. 1961;**15**(2):253-257

[28] Pennock J, Hemming F, Kerr JD. A reassessment of tocopherol chemistry. Biochemical and Biophysical Research Communications. 1964;**17**(5):542-548

[29] Traber MG. Mechanisms for the prevention of vitamin E excess. Journal of Lipid Research. 2013;**54**(9):2295-2306

[30] Saito Y, Nishio K, Akazawa YO, Yamanaka K, Miyama A, Yoshida Y, et al. Cytoprotective effects of vitamin E homologues against glutamate-induced cell death in immature primary cortical neuron cultures: Tocopherols and tocotrienols exert similar effects by antioxidant function. Free Radical Biology and Medicine. 2010;**49**(10):1542-1549

[31] Traber MG, Mah E, Leonard SW, Bobe G, Bruno RS. Metabolic syndrome increases dietary α-tocopherol requirements as assessed using urinary and plasma vitamin E catabolites: A double-blind, crossover clinical trial. The American Journal of Clinical Nutrition. 2017;**105**(3):571-579

[32] Traber MG, Leonard SW, Ebenuwa I, Violet P-C, Wang Y, Niyyati M, et al. Vitamin E absorption and kinetics in healthy women, as modulated by food and by fat, studied using 2 deuterium-labeled α-tocopherols in a 3-phase crossover design. The American Journal of Clinical Nutrition. 2019;**110**(5):1148-1167

[33] Hosomi A, Arita M, Sato Y, Kiyose C, Ueda T, Igarashi O, et al. Affinity for α-tocopherol transfer protein as a determinant of the biological activities of vitamin E analogs. FEBS Letters. 1997;**409**(1):105-108

[34] Niki E, Traber MG. A history of vitamin E. Annals of Nutrition and Metabolism. 2012;**61**(3):207-212

[35] Khanna S, Patel V, Rink C, Roy S, Sen CK. Delivery of orally supplemented αtocotrienol to vital organs of rats and tocopherol-transport protein deficient mice. Free Radical Biology and Medicine. 2005;**39**(10):1310-1319

[36] Schultz M, Leist M, Petrzika M, Gassmann B, Brigelius-Flohé R. Novel urinary metabolite of alpha-tocopherol, 2,5,7,8-tetramethyl-2(2′-carboxyethyl)-6-hydroxychroman, as an indicator of an adequate vitamin E supply? The American Journal of Clinical Nutrition. 1995;**62**(6):1527S-1534S

[37] Packer L, Weber SU, Rimbach G. Molecular aspects of α-tocotrienol antioxidant action and cell signaling. The Journal of Nutrition. 2001;**131**(2):369S-373S

[38] Serbinova E, Kagan V, Han D, Packer L. Free radical recycling and intramembrane mobility in the antioxidant properties of alpha-tocopherol and alpha-tocotrienol. Free Radical Biology and Medicine. 1991;**10**(5):263-275

[39] Sen CK, Rink C, Khanna S. Palm oil–derived natural vitamin E α-tocotrienol in brain health and disease. Journal of the American College of Nutrition. 2010;**29**(Suppl 3):314S-323S

[40] Rink C, Christoforidis G, Khanna S, Peterson L, Patel Y, Khanna S, et al. Tocotrienol vitamin E protects against preclinical canine ischemic stroke by inducing arteriogenesis. Journal of Cerebral Blood Flow and Metabolism. 2011;**31**(11):2218-2230

[41] Sandoo A, van Zanten JJ, Metsios GS, Carroll D, Kitas GD. The endothelium and its role in regulating vascular tone. The Open Cardiovascular Medicine Journal. 2010;**4**:302

[42] Pantoni L. Cerebral small vessel disease: From pathogenesis and clinical characteristics to therapeutic challenges. The Lancet Neurology. 2010;**9**(7):689-701

[43] Novakovic V. Cardiovascular risk factors, white matter abnormalities and diffusion tensor magnetic resonance imaging. Biological Psychiatry and Psychopharmacology. 2010;**12**:103

[44] Hinman JD, Lee MD, Tung S, Vinters HV, Carmichael ST. Molecular disorganization of axons adjacent to human lacunar infarcts. Brain. 2015;**138**(3):736-745

[45] Benjamin P, Zeestraten E, Lambert C, Ster IC, Williams OA, Lawrence AJ, et al. Progression of MRI markers in cerebral small vessel disease: Sample size considerations for clinical trials. Journal of Cerebral Blood Flow & Metabolism. 2015;**36**(1):228-240

[46] Wardlaw JM, Smith C, Dichgans M. Small vessel disease: Mechanisms and clinical implications. The Lancet Neurology. 2019;**18**(7):684-696

[47] Ogata J, Yamanishi H, Ishibashi-Ueda H. Pathology of cerebral small vessel disease. In: Pantoni L, Gorelick P, editors. Cerebral Small Vessel Disease. Cambridge: Cambridge University Press; 2014. pp. 4-15

[48] Sorond FA, Cruz-Almeida Y, Clark DJ, Viswanathan A, Scherzer CR, Jager PD, et al. Aging, the central nervous system, and mobility in older adults: Neural mechanisms of

mobility impairment. The Journals of Gerontology Series A: Biological Sciences and Medical Sciences. 2015;**70**(12):1526-1532

[49] Yakushiji Y, Charidimou A, Noguchi T, Nishihara M, Eriguchi M, Nanri Y, et al. Total small vessel disease score in neurologically healthy Japanese adults in the Kashima scan study. Internal Medicine. 2018;**57**(2):189-196

[50] Wardlaw JM, Smith EE, Biessels GJ, Cordonnier C, Fazekas F, Frayne R, et al. Neuroimaging standards for research into small vessel disease and its contribution to ageing and neurodegeneration. The Lancet Neurology. 2013;**12**(8):822-838

[51] Veluw SJV, Shih AY, Smith EE, Chen C, Schneider JA, Wardlaw JM, et al. Detection, risk factors, and functional consequences of cerebral microinfarcts. The Lancet Neurology. 2017;**16**(9):730-740

[52] Grochowski C, Litak J, Kamieniak P, Maciejewski R. Oxidative stress in cerebral small vessel disease. Role of reactive species. Free Radical Research. 2017Nov;**52**(1):1-13

[53] Mustapha M, Nassir CMNCM, Aminuddin N, Safri AA, Ghazali MM. Cerebral small vessel disease (CSVD)—lessons from the animal models. Frontiers in Physiology. 2019;**10**:1317

[54] Caunca MR, Leon-Benedetti AD, Latour L, Leigh R, Wright CB. Neuroimaging of cerebral small vessel disease and age-related cognitive changes. Frontiers in Aging Neuroscience. 2019;**11**:145

[55] Chowdhury MH, Nagai A, Bokura H, Nakamura E, Kobayashi S, Yamaguchi S. Age-related changes in white matter lesions, hippocampal atrophy, and cerebral microbleeds in healthy subjects without major cerebrovascular risk factors. Journal of Stroke and Cerebrovascular Diseases. 2011;**20**(4):302-309

[56] Akoudad S, Portegies ML, Koudstaal PJ, Hofman A, Lugt AVD, Ikram MA, et al. Cerebral microbleeds are associated with an increased risk of stroke. Circulation. 2015;**132**(6):509-516

[57] Akoudad S, Wolters FJ, Viswanathan A, Bruijn RFD, Lugt AVD, Hofman A, et al. Association of cerebral microbleeds with cognitive decline and dementia. JAMA Neurology. 2016;**73**(8):934

[58] Knopman DS, Penman AD, Catellier DJ, Coker LH, Shibata DK, Sharrett AR, et al. Vascular risk factors and longitudinal changes on brain MRI: The ARIC study. Neurology. 2011;**76**(22):1879-1885

[59] Dijk EJV, Prins ND, Vrooman HA, Hofman A, Koudstaal PJ, Breteler MM. Progression of cerebral small vessel disease in relation to risk factors and cognitive consequences. Stroke. 2008;**39**(10):2712-2719

[60] Wright CB, Dong C, Perez EJ, Rosa JD, Yoshita M, Rundek T, et al. Subclinical cerebrovascular disease increases the risk of incident stroke and mortality: The northern Manhattan study. Journal of the American Heart Association. 2017;**6**(9):e004069

[61] Gutierrez J, Rundek T, Ekind M, Sacco R, Wright C. Perivascular spaces are associated with atherosclerosis: An insight from the northern Manhattan study. American Journal of Neuroradiology. 2013;**34**(9):1711-1716

[62] Sudre CH, Smith L, Atkinson D, Chaturvedi N, Ourselin S, Barkhof F, et al. Cardiovascular risk factors and white matter hyperintensities: Difference in susceptibility in south Asians compared with Europeans. Journal of the American Heart Association. 2018;**7**(21):e010533

[63] Hilal S, Mok V, Youn YC, Wong A, Ikram MK, CL-H C. Prevalence, risk factors and consequences of cerebral small vessel diseases: Data from three Asian countries. Journal of Neurology, Neurosurgery & Psychiatry. 2017;**88**(8):669-674

[64] Li S, Fang F, Cui M, Jiang Y, Wang Y, Kong X, et al. Incidental findings on brain MRI among Chinese at the age of 55-65 years: The Taizhou imaging study. Scientific Reports. 2019;**9**(1):464

[65] Yakushiji Y, Charidimou A, Hara M, Noguchi T, Nishihara M, Eriguchi M, et al. Topography and associations of perivascular spaces in healthy adults: The Kashima scan study. Neurology. 2014;**83**(23):2116-2123

[66] Bryan RN, Wells SW, Miller TJ, Elster AD, Jungreis CA, Poirier VC, et al. Infarctlike lesions in the brain: Prevalence and anatomic characteristics at MR imaging of the elderly—data from the cardiovascular health study. Radiology. 1997;**202**(1):47-54

[67] Yao M, Zhu Y-C, Soumaré A, Dufouil C, Mazoyer B, Tzourio C, et al. Hippocampal perivascular spaces are related to aging and blood pressure but not to cognition. Neurobiology of Aging. 2014;**35**(9):2118-2125

[68] Graff-Radford J, Simino J, Kantarci K, Mosley TH, Griswold ME, Windham BG, et al. Neuroimaging correlates of cerebral microbleeds. Stroke. 2017;**48**(11):2964-2972

[69] Mesker DJ, Poels MMF, Ikram MA, Vernooij MW, Hofman A, Vrooman HA, et al. Lobar distribution of cerebral microbleeds. Archives of Neurology. 2011;**68**(5):656-659

[70] Vemuri P, Lesnick TG, Przybelski SA, Knopman DS, Preboske GM, Kantarci K, et al. Vascular and amyloid pathologies are independent predictors of cognitive decline in normal elderly. Brain. 2015;**138**(3):761-771

[71] Lampe L, Kharabian-Masouleh S, Kynast J, Arelin K, Steele CJ, Löffler M, et al. Lesion location matters: The relationships between white matter hyperintensities on cognition in the healthy elderly. Journal of Cerebral Blood Flow & Metabolism. 2017;**39**(1):36-43

[72] Knopman DS, Griswold ME, Lirette ST, Gottesman RF, Kantarci K, Sharrett AR, et al. Vascular imaging abnormalities and cognition. Stroke. 2015;**46**(2):433-440

[73] Au R, Massaro JM, Wolf PA, Young ME, Beiser A, Seshadri S, et al. Associationofwhitematterhyperintensity volume with decreased cognitive functioning. Archives of Neurology. 2006;**63**(2):246

[74] Koga H, Takashima Y, Murakawa R, Uchino A, Yuzuriha T, Yao H. Cognitive consequences of multiple lacunes and leukoaraiosis as vascular cognitive impairment in community-dwelling elderly individuals. Journal of Stroke and Cerebrovascular Diseases. 2009;**18**(1):32-37

[75] Vermeer SE, Prins ND, Heijer TD, Hofman A, Koudstaal PJ, Breteler MM. Silent brain infarcts and the risk of dementia and cognitive decline. New England Journal of Medicine. 2003;**348**(13):1215-1222

[76] Ding J, Sigurðsson S, Jónsson PV, Eiriksdottir G, Charidimou A, Lopez OL, et al. Large perivascular spaces visible on magnetic resonance imaging, cerebral small vessel disease progression, and risk of dementia. JAMA Neurology. 2017;**74**(9):1105

[77] Ding J, Sigurðsson S, Jónsson PV, Eiriksdottir G, Meirelles O, Kjartansson O, et al. Space and location of cerebral microbleeds, cognitive

decline, and dementia in the community. Neurology. 2017;**88**(22):2089-2097

[78] Farrall AJ, Wardlaw JM. Blood–brain barrier: Ageing and microvascular disease – systematic review and meta-analysis. Neurobiology of Aging. 2009;**30**(3):337-352

[79] Poggesi A, Pasi M, Pescini F, Pantoni L, Inzitari D. Circulating biologic markers of endothelial dysfunction in cerebral small vessel disease: A review. Journal of Cerebral Blood Flow & Metabolism. 2015;**36**(1):72-94

[80] Otero-Losada ME, Loughlin SM, Rodríguez-Granillo G, Müller A, Ottaviano G, Moriondo M, et al. Metabolic disturbances and worsening of atherosclerotic lesions in ApoE−/− mice after cola beverages drinking. Cardiovascular Diabetology. 2013;**12**(1):57

[81] Otero-Losada M, Cao G, Loughlin SM, Rodríguez-Granillo G, Ottaviano G, Milei J. Rate of atherosclerosis progression in ApoE−/− mice long after discontinuation of cola beverage drinking. PLoS One. 2014;**9**(3):e89838

[82] Otero-Losada ME, Grana DR, Müller A, Ottaviano G, Ambrosio G, Milei J. Lipid profile and plasma antioxidant status in sweet carbonated beverage-induced metabolic syndrome in rat. International Journal of Cardiology. 2011;**146**(1):106-109

[83] Otero-Losada M, González J, Müller A, Ottaviano G, Cao G, Azzato F, et al. Exercise ameliorates endocrine pancreas damage induced by chronic cola drinking in rats. PLoS One. 2016;**11**(5):e0155630

[84] Ihara M, Yamamoto Y. Emerging evidence for pathogenesis of sporadic cerebral small vessel disease. Stroke. 2016;**47**(2):554-560

[85] Rajani RM, Williams A. Endothelial cell–oligodendrocyte interactions in small vessel disease and aging. Clinical Science. 2017;**131**(5):369-379

[86] Rajashekhar G, Willuweit A, Patterson CE, Sun P, Hilbig A, Breier G, et al. Continuous endothelial cell activation increases angiogenesis: Evidence for the direct role of endothelium linking angiogenesis and inflammation. Journal of Vascular Research. 2006;**43**(2):193-204

[87] Armulik A, Abramsson A, Betsholtz C. Endothelial/pericyte interactions. Circulation Research. 2005;**97**(6):512-523

[88] Deplanque D, Lavallee PC, Labreuche J, Gongora-Rivera F, Jaramillo A, Brenner D, et al. Cerebral and extracerebral vasoreactivity in symptomatic lacunar stroke patients: A case-control study. International Journal of Stroke. 2012;**8**(6):413-421

[89] Young VG, Halliday GM, Kril JJ. Neuropathologic correlates of white matter hyperintensities. Neurology. 2008;**71**(11):804-811

[90] Halliwell B. Role of free radicals in the neurodegenerative diseases. Drugs & Aging. 2001;**18**(9):685-716

[91] Halliwell B. Antioxidant defence mechanisms: From the beginning to the end (of the beginning). Free Radical Research. 1999;**31**(4):261-272

[92] Mariani E, Polidori M, Cherubini A, Mecocci P. Oxidative stress in brain aging, neurodegenerative and vascular diseases: An overview. Journal of Chromatography B. 2005;**827**(1):65-75

[93] Del Río LA. ROS and RNS in plant physiology: An overview. Journal of Experimental Botany. 2015;**66**:2827-2837

[94] Qi AQ, Li Y, Liu Q, Si J-Z, Tang X-M, Zhang Z-Q, et al. Thioredoxin is a novel diagnostic and prognostic marker in patients with ischemic stroke. Free Radical Biology & Medicine. 2015;**80**:129-135

[95] Choi H, Tostes RC, Webb RC. Thioredoxin reductase inhibition reduces relaxation by increasing oxidative stress and s-nitrosylation in mouse aorta. Journal of Cardiovascular Pharmacology. 2011;**58**:522-527

[96] Richard S, Lapierre V, Girerd N, Bonnerot M, Burkhard PR, Lagerstedt L, et al. Diagnostic performance of peroxiredoxin 1 to determine time-of-onset of acute cerebral infarction. Scientific Reports. 2016;**6**:38300

[97] Kim TS, Pae CU, Yoon SJ, Jang W-Y, Lee NJ, Kim J-J, et al. Decreased plasma antioxidants in patients with Alzheimer's disease. International Journal of Geriatric Psychiatry. 2006;**21**:344-348

[98] Iuliano L, Monticolo R, Straface G, Spoletini I, Gianni W, Caltagirone C, et al. Vitamin E and enzymatic/oxidative stress-driven oxysterols in amnestic mild cognitive impairment subtypes and Alzheimer's disease. Journal of Alzheimer's Disease. 2010;**21**:1383-1392

[99] Cristalli DO, Arnal N, Marra FA, de Alaniz MJT, Marra CA. Peripheral markers in neurodegenerative patients and their first-degree relatives. Journal of the Neurological Sciences. 2012;**314**:48-56

[100] Paganoni S, Schwarzschild MA. Urate as a marker of risk and progression of neurodegenerative disease. Neurotherapeutics. 2017;**14**:148-153

[101] Patterson C, Ruef J, Madamanchi NR, Barry-Lane P, Hu Z, Horaist C, et al. Stimulation of a vascular smooth muscle cell NAD(P)H oxidase by thrombin. Evidence that p47(phox) may participate in forming this oxidase in vitro and in vivo. The Journal of Biological Chemistry. 1999;**274**:19814-19822

[102] Marumo T, Schini-Kerth VB, Fisslthaler B, Busse R. Platelet-derived growth factor-stimulated superoxide anion production modulates activation of transcription factor NF-kappaB and expression of monocyte chemoattractant protein 1 in human aortic smooth muscle cells. Circulation. 1997;**96**:2361-2367

[103] Sundaresan M, Yu ZX, Ferrans VJ, Irani K, Finkel T. Requirement for generation of H2O2 for platelet-derived growth factor signal transduction. Science. 1995;**270**:296-299

[104] Busija DW, Katakam PV. Mitochondrial mechanisms in cerebral vascular control: Shared signaling pathways with preconditioning. Journal of Vascular Research. 2014;**51**:175-189

[105] Santhanam AV, d'Uscio LV, Katusic ZS. Erythropoietin increases bioavailability of tetrahydrobiopterin and protects cerebral microvasculature against oxidative stress induced by eNOS uncoupling. Journal of Neurochemistry. 2014;**131**:521-529

[106] Xie H, Ray PE, Short BL. NF-kappaB activation plays a role in superoxide-mediated cerebral endothelial dysfunction after hypoxia/reoxygenation. Stroke. 2005;**36**:1047-1052

[107] Ulivi L, Maccarrone M, Giannini N, Ferrari E, Caselli M, Montano V, et al. Oxidative stress in cerebral small vessel disease dizziness patients, basally and after polyphenol compound supplementation. Current Molecular Medicine. 2018;**18**(3):160-165

[108] Drummond GR, Selemidis S, Griendling KK, Sobey CG. Combating oxidative stress in vascular disease: NADPH oxidases as therapeutic targets. Nature Reviews Drug Discovery. 2011;**10**(6):453-471

[109] Gopalan Y, Shuaib IL, Magosso E, Ansari MA, Bakar MRA, Wong JW, et al. Clinical investigation of the protective effects of palm vitamin E tocotrienols on brain white matter. Stroke. 2014;**45**(5):1422-1428

[110] Murad LB, Guimarães MRM, Paganelli A, Oliveira CABD, Vianna LM. Alpha-tocopherol in the brain tissue preservation of stroke-prone spontaneously hypertensive rats. Journal of Physiology and Biochemistry. 2013;**70**(1):49-60

[111] Ueno Y, Koike M, Shimada Y, Shimura H, Hira K, Tanaka R, et al. L-Carnitine enhances axonal plasticity and improves white-matter lesions after chronic hypoperfusion in rat brain. Journal of Cerebral Blood Flow & Metabolism. 2015;**35**(3):382-391

[112] Heart Protection Study Collaborative Group. MRC/BHF heart protection study of antioxidant vitamin supplementation in 20 536 high-risk individuals: A randomised placebo-controlled trial. The Lancet. 2002;**360**(9326):23-33

[113] Graneri L, Dalonzo Z, Lam V, Mamo J, Dhaliwal S, Takechi R. Chronic consumption of a commercial energy drink reduces blood pressure in normotensive wild-type mice. Frontiers in Nutrition. 2019;**6**:111

[114] Witting PK, Upston JM, Stocker R. Role of α-tocopheroxyl radical in the initiation of lipid peroxidation in human low-density lipoprotein exposed to horse radish peroxidase. Biochemistry. 1997;**36**(6):1251-1258

[115] Witting PK, Willhite CA, Davies MJ, Stocker R. Lipid oxidation in human low-density lipoprotein induced by metmyoglobin/H2O2: Involvement of α-tocopheroxyl and phosphatidylcholine alkoxyl radicals. Chemical Research in Toxicology. 1999;**12**(12):1173-1181

Chapter 11

Neuroactive Steroids in Hypoxic–Ischemic Brain Injury: Overview and Future Directions

Nicolas Toro-Urrego, Marco Avila-Rodriguez, María Inés Herrera, Andrea Aguilar, Lucas Udovin and Juan P. Luaces

Abstract

Hypoxic–ischemic brain injury is a number one cause of long-term neurologic disability and death worldwide. This public health burden is mainly characterized by a decrease in oxygen concentration and blood flow to the tissues, which lead to an inefficient supply of nutrients to the brain. This condition induces cell death by energy depletion and increases free radical generation and inflammation. Hypoxic–ischemic brain injury may occur in ischemic-stroke and over perinatal asphyxia, being both leading causes of morbidity in adults and children, respectively. Currently, there are no effective pharmaceutical strategies to prevent the triggering of secondary injury cascades, including oxidative stress and metabolic dysfunction. Neuroactive steroids like selective estrogen receptor modulators, SERMs, and selective tissue estrogenic activity regulators, STEARs, exert several neuroprotective effects. These encompass mitochondrial survival, a decrease in reactive oxygen species, and maintenance of cell viability, among others. In this context, these neurosteroids constitute promising molecules, which could modify brain response to injury. Here we show an updated overview of the underlying mechanisms of hypoxic–ischemic brain injury. We also highlight the neuroprotective effects of neurosteroids and their future directions.

Keywords: neuroactive steroids, hypoxia-ischemia, brain injury, oxidative stress, metabolic dysfunction

1. Introduction

Hypoxic–ischemic (HI) brain injury is a major cause of long-term neurologic disability and death worldwide. Brain damage caused by hypoxia-ischemia responds to a wide variety of factors, being the central nervous system (CNS) especially susceptible to changes in energy levels, mainly glucose concentrations and oxygen [1]. The brain has a 25% glucose and 20% oxygen consumption of total body weight [2, 3]. This high energy demand is attributed to the functions performed by brain cells such as synaptic activity, neurotransmitter recycling and ion transport [2]. Thus, ensuring correct brain metabolism results in optimal neuronal functioning. HI brain injury is mainly characterized by a decrease in the concentration of oxygen and blood flow, which causes an insufficient supply of nutrients to the brain. These pathological conditions lead to cell death due to the increase in free radical production and depletion of ATP [4]. This phenomenon is observed both in perinatal asphyxia (PA) and in ischemic stroke (IS) [5–7]. Around 15 to 20% of infants that suffer PA will die in the postnatal period and further 25% will develop severe and long-lasting neurological impairments such as cerebral palsy, epilepsy and neurodevelopmental disorders [8], also representing one of the main causes of morbidity in children and adults in the world [9, 10]. Similarly, at a structural level HI injury mainly affects the layers II, III and VI of the cortex, CA1 and CA3 hippocampal areas, striatum and cerebellum [11]. Therefore, the understanding of the underlying mechanisms of this pathology is essential for the establishment of efficient treatments.

Several neuroprotective strategies have been tested, including Selective Estrogen Receptor Modulators (SERMs) and Selective Tissue Estrogenic Activity Regulators (STEARs), which have shown the same benefits as estrogen, including the decrease of reactive oxygen species (ROS), maintenance of cell viability, mitochondrial survival, among others; without its negative side effects [12–14]. However, there are no effective pharmaceutical strategies to prevent the triggering of secondary injury cascades, including oxidative stress and metabolic dysfunction. In this sense, the present chapter summarizes the underlying mechanisms of HI brain injury and compiles several neuroprotective strategies, including SERMs and STEARs.

2. Mechanisms of brain damage in hypoxia-ischemia

Hypoxia is a condition that affects mainly the brain, and it is characterized by a low concentration of oxygen, affecting the proper functioning of the organs and tissues exposed to it. This insult causes a variety of responses in the brain. An initial response occurs immediately after the insult and is associated with a depletion of ATP, glucose and phosphocreatine inside the brain. This immediate reaction determines the patient's outcome against injury, which in turn triggers a secondary response that occurs several hours later. A temporary energy recovery takes place almost to the initial physiological levels, providing a treatment window between 1 and 6 hours following injury [8, 15, 16]. A third phase of persistent effects lasts for several years [17]. In general terms, global hypoxia affects the cerebral cortex, the sensorimotor cortex, the talamo and the basal ganglia, causing damage in deep gray matter [18].While the complete pathogenic pathways of HI are not fully described, some mechanisms like apoptosis, increased glutamate, calcium overload, mitochondrial dysfunction and oxidative stress have been proposed to contribute to generate neuronal damage [19].

Primary response depends on the energetic failure, which is characterized by the reduction of the energy supply, generating the accumulation of Reactive Oxygen Species (ROS) via lactate production augment, making the cell susceptible to oxidative stress and mitochondrial dysfunction [18]. Besides this, restricted cerebral blood flow causes a switch to anaerobic respiration, reducing ATP and phosphocreatine, and increasing lactic acid production [16]. Low levels of ATP derived from this energetical failure affect the integrity of the cell membrane. Calcium enters easily to the cell causing the membrane depolarization, blocking calcium storage in the cell, which in turn accumulates in the extracellular space. In addition, the ion flux of sodium/potassium is altered by the $Na+/K+$ pump dysfunction [20]. The second phase of injury is related to the recovery of blood flow and the reestablishment of brain metabolism, characterized by an inflammatory response, excitotoxicity and oxidative stress, being the main responsible for the brain cells death after hypoxia [7, 18].

2.1 Second phase of injury

Apoptosis as necrosis are the death pathways of the cell. They are present in brain damage caused by hypoxia, being apoptosis the most common death pathway in the young brain unchained by mitochondrial failure [21]. Apoptosis can follow two pathways, being the extrinsic triggered by external signals like the tumor necrosis factor alpha (TNF-α), Fatty acid synthase (FAS), and the intrinsic path mediated by internal factors such as DNA damage or cell stress [22]. The extrinsic pathway is involved in the action of caspase 8 and 10, which activate caspase effectors directly, interacting with the intrinsic pathway, and triggering a permeabilization of the mitochondrial membrane [23].

The Intrinsic pathway is mediated by the release of apoptotic factors such as cytochrome-c, Serine protease HTRA2, mitochondrial (Omi/HtrA2), apoptosis inducing factor (AIF), endonuclease G (endoG), Second mitochondria-derived activator of caspase/direct inhibitor of apoptosis-binding protein with low pI (Smac / Diablo) after permeabilization of the membrane. These apoptotic factors can trigger cell death processes that can be mediated by caspase-dependent pathways. Each of these factors has a role in programmed death. Cytochrome c interacts with Apoptosis protease-activating factor-1 (Apaf-1), creating the apoptosome. Smac/Diablo interacts with apoptosis inhibitors, AIF and endoG act through a caspase- dependent pathway. These are translocated to the nucleus, causing nuclear fragmentation [24, 25]. Hence, the permeabilization of the mitochondrial membrane has been proposed as a marker of a point of no return in hypoxic injury.

2.2 Excitotoxicity

HI injury triggers responses at both the systemic and cellular levels. When the energy supply is interrupted, excitotoxicity occurs through an uncontrolled release of excitatory neurotransmitters such as glutamate, causing an acute cascade damaging neurons and glial cells at cytoplasmic and mitochondrial levels, and also causing disruption of the BBB [23]. Glutamate activates NMDA receptors, causing the accumulation of Ca ++ and nitric oxide (NO), which in turn cause production of ROS. The increased levels of intracellular calcium in neurons and glial cells in turn results in the activation of calcium-dependent proteases, reactive oxygen species (ROS) production, mitochondrial dysfunction, oxidative stress, cytotoxic edema, lipases and deoxyribonuclease (DNase), and the stimulation of pro-cell death pathways [23, 26, 27].

2.3 Oxidative stress

The balance between the oxidant and the antioxidant levels of the cell is called redox homeostasis. An imbalance in favor of the intracellular level of oxidants results in what is known as oxidative stress. This deregulation occurs mainly in two free radicals, the reactive oxygen species (ROS), and the reactive nitrogen species (RNS) [28, 29]. Oxidative stress plays a major role in the pathophysiology of HI, due to the significant damage to nucleic acids (DNA degeneration), lipids (lipid oxidation), proteins and different organelles such as the mitochondria [7]. There are different sources of free radicals (ROS and RNS) following HI, including mitochondrial electron transport chain (ETC), xanthine oxidase (XO), NADPH oxidases (NOX) and nitric oxide synthase (NOS), and arachidonic acid (12/15 lipoxygenase) [26, 28].

2.4 Mitochondria

Mitochondria plays a vital role in survival of the different cells of the CNS [30]. It is composed of two membranes, one internal and one external, each with different functions. Within these membranes is the matrix. There are enzymes responsible for the main metabolic processes to produce ATP, such as the Krebs cycle, β-oxidation, as well as the metabolism of aminoacids [31]. Additionally, the mitochondria is involved in moderating processes of death (apoptosis) and biogenesis or cell proliferation [31, 32], also in critical processes such the maintenance of neuronal homeostasis, including autophagy, elimination of toxic metabolites like ROS, and calcium homeostasis [26, 30, 31, 33].

Neonatal brain has increased vulnerability to damage by oxidative stress when compared with the adult brain, in part due to lower levels of antioxidants [34]. In adult brain, superoxide dismutase (SOD) 1 can scavenge ROS generating hydrogen peroxide (H2 O2), thus allowing further breakdown by catalases to H2 O. In contrast, neonatal SOD1, although expressed, can exacerbate brain injury caused by HI possibly due to the absence or downregulation of enzymes such as catalase and glutathione peroxidase 1, required downstream of SOD1 [35].

Mitochondria plays a key role in HI injury since the disturbances in energy metabolism trigger a number of pathophysiological responses converging at mitochondrial levels, such as the control of energy metabolism, production of ROS, and the release of apoptotic factors into the cytoplasm [36]. Mitochondria constitutes an important regulator of cell death due to its ability to release proapoptotic proteins following mitochondrial permeabilization. Apoptosis can occur through an intrinsic pathway, where DNA damage or cellular stressors activate apoptosis, or an extrinsic pathway, following activation of death receptors [36].

2.5 Cardiolipin peroxidation

Another consequence of cell death caused by ROS-induced oxidative stress is the peroxidation of a mitochondrial lipid, cardiolipin [37], one of the most critical targets in the components of the evolution of HI injury. This is a unique phospholipid, which is found mostly in the inner mitochondrial membrane, where it has a very close association with the components of oxidative phosphorylation [37, 38]. Cardiolipin plays a crucial role in the insertion into the membrane and the function of cytochrome C, cytochrome C oxidase and other phosphorylation complexes. This is required, therefore, for an optimal functioning of complexes I (NADH: ubiquinone reductase), complex III (NADH: ubiquinone cytochrome C oxidoreductase), complex IV (cytochrome C oxidase) and complex V (ATP synthase) [39].

When HI occurs, enzymatic and non-enzymatic processes induce lipid peroxidation. The non-enzymatic process is triggered by the interaction of ROS with the fatty acyds of the membranes, and the enzymatic process include the activation of lipoxygenases (LOX), cyclooxygenases (COX), phospholipase A2 (PLA2) and Cyt C [40, 41], which leads to an alteration in the structure of this phospholipid responsible for mitochondrial dysfunction. Hence, the release of cytochrome c depends on the integrity of itself. This severe sensitivity to ROS is due to its high content of fatty acids [39].

2.6 Inflammation in HI

Accompanied by the reactions mentioned above, there is a role played by different glial cells in the injury caused by hypoxia, mainly in inflammation. This injury initially triggers an immediate response in neuroglial cells, which contribute to the damage mechanisms mentioned above, due to the secretion of a large amount of proinflammatory cytokines and ROS.

2.7 Astrocytes

In the last 20 years, astrocytes have been granted multiple functions, such as providing support, helping in the maintenance of the cerebral microenvironment for an appropriate function, regulating the blood flow in the brain, which are essential for the adequate functioning of neurons [2, 42]. Another important astrocytic function is the contribution to brain metabolism [43]. Astrocytes takes glucose from blood vessels and provide energy metabolites to neurons [44]. In addition, through the lactate shuttle, astrocytes provide lactate to the neurons as a substrate for the citric acid cycle and can therefore supply their energy requirements [45].

However, the role of astrocytes in injuries such as hypoxia are not fully elucidated. Astrocytes as microglia, when subjected to insults such as hypoxia, may act differently depending on the severity of the injury. Immediately after hypoxia, astrocytes enter in an activated state, which eventually ends in a glial scar [46, 47]. Astrocytes plays important roles in the brain during HI. Because of the tight connection with brain capillaries, astrocytes suffer damage firstly after ischemia, and then, damaged astrocytes kill neighboring neurons. The number of apoptotic astrocytes increases gradually as the extension of ischemic time, which leads to further expand of cerebral infarction area [48].

Astrocytes can exacerbate cytotoxicity death due to secrete inflammatory cytokines such as IL-1, IL-6, interferon-γ, and TNF-α; and can also help the migration of immune cells to the CNS by the secretion of chemokines [49]. Likewise, there is also a protective effect exerted by astrocytes, which play an important role in tolerance to cerebral ischemic injury [50] and inflammation [50, 51].

2.8 Microglia and endothelial cells

Microglia, the immune cells of the CNS, are the first to be activated after hypoxia. They migrate to the place of injury and change their morphology to an amoeboid-lice functional cell, acting in conjunction with monocytes and macrophages [49, 52, 53]. Microglia M1 release proinflammatory agents to the environment such as ROS, cytokines ((IL) -1β, IL-6, tumor necrosis factor-alpha (TNF-α)), glutamate, nitric oxide, creating a cytotoxic environment triggering cell death [49, 52, 53].

The extent of injury noted in HI is not only determined by the biochemical cascades that trigger the apoptosis-necrosis continuum of cell death in the brain parenchyma, but also by the pro-inflammatory factors of the Blood Brain Barrier (BBB), such as the endothelial cells [54]. Endothelial cells can sense variation in the Parcial Oxygen Pressure (PO2) through different mechano-sensors. Then, they can adapt their metabolism to maintain ATP production, switching into an hypoxic metabolism. In this way, endothelial cells augment the production of ROS by making the respiratory chain slower, reduce the cytochrome-c capacity in order to trap O2, and alter the cellular redox potential [54, 55]. In cerebrovascular endothelial cells (cEND) OGD augmented the mRNA expression of IL-1 alpha, IL- 6 glut-1 transporter and total nitric oxide concentration increasing significantly the permeability of the cEND monolayer [56].

2.9 Selective vulnerability of the brain to HI

The pathophysiology of HI is complex. The damage on the developing brain is determined by several factors: timing of asphyxia, intensity, severity of HI and immaturity of the brain. Beside this, different areas of the brain and different cell types present a selective vulnerability to this injury [18].

The immaturity of brain represents a significant factor in the outcome of HI brain injury. Although risk factors of HI in term newborns are similar to those observed in preterm newborns, the immature brain in the last ones, especially those with a very low birth weight, is highly vulnerable to injury [18]. This, due to hypoperfusion caused by the defectively functioning lungs and hearts in preterm newborns, and the poor auto-regulatory capacity the immature brain possess [57].

HI injury induces white matter injury with noticeable oligodendroglia loss, due to the poorly vascularization in white matter compared with cerebral cortex. This injury, known as periventricular leukomalacia (PLV), triggers cognitive, sensory, and motor impairment in preterm infants. Abnormalities of cortical gray matter and hippocampus are also found in the immature brain [18].

In addition, in the developing brain there is a spectrum of lesions caused by HI. Alongside PVL, periventricular hemorrhagic infarction in association with geminal matrix (ganglionic eminence) hemorrhage, with or without intraventricular hemorrhage, or thalamocortical injury (**Table 1**) [58].

The developing brain exhibits selective vulnerability. As it was mentioned above, certain cells and regions appear vulnerable depending on the severity and timing of injury. Projection neurons, especially in the deep gray nuclei, are at greatest risk during ischemic insults in the term brain [18]. Subplate neurons are the earliest and the most transient cell population of the neocortex. The subplate zone peaks at the onset of the developmental window of vulnerability to PVL (GW 24) and undergoes dissolution during the third trimester. Subplate neurons are largely absent at 6 months of postnatal age. HI injury leads to moderate to near-complete subplate neuron cell death, whereas most cortical neurons are intact. This selective vulnerability may be due to early cellular maturation and a developmentally related increase in glutamate receptor expression, including NMDA receptor 1, kainate and AMPA receptors [59]. On the other hand, in the preterm brain, subplate neurons and oligodendrocytes (OL) precursors are most vulnerable. Consequent abnormal thalamocortical connectivity may explain the somatosensory and visual impairment seen in prematurely born infants suffering HI brain injury [60, 61]. OL progenitors appear to be the most vulnerable, showing impaired maturation and development following injury.

Hemorrhagic lesions
Germinal matrix (ganglionic eminence) (frequently associated with PVL)
Limited (grade I[†])
With intraventricular hemorrhage (grade II)
With ventricular expansion (grade III)
With PHI (grade IV)
Subpial
Cerebellar
Subarachnoid space (temporal lobe and cerebellum)
White-matter lesions
Periventricular leukomalacia (PVL)
With focal necrosis
With diffuse white-matter gliosis only
Periventricular hemorrhagic infarction (PHI)
Combined gray- and white-matter lesions
Single cerebral artery–distribution infarcts (porencephaly)
Hydranencephaly (bilateral large hemispheric infarcts)
Multicystic encephalomalacia
Gray-matter lesions
Thalamic and basal ganglionic injury ("status marmoratus")
Neuronal necrosis in basis pontis and subiculum (pontosubicular necrosis)
Mobius syndrome (brainstem neuronal loss and gliosis)
Cerebellar infarct

PHI = periventricular hemorrhagic infarction; PVL = periventricular leukomalacia.
[†]Grade refers to clinical severity assigned based on transfontanelle ultrasonography or other neuroimaging. Adapted from [58].

Table 1.
Lesions caused by HI in the developing brain.

2.10 Oligodendrocytes and astrocytes

Oligodendrocytes, the myelin-forming glia that ensheath axons in the CNS, exhibit four sequential stages of maturation. Oligodendroglial progenitors, the pre-OL (or late oligodendroglial progenitor), the immature OL, and the mature myelin-producing OL [60], are extremely susceptible to HI. The injury involves maturational delays in oligodendrocyte population inducing oxidative stress. Following HI, OLs fail to fully mature, leading to persistent aberrations in myelin ultrastructure, which are associated with permanent disability and neurodevelopmental impairment [62].

Astrocytes are the predominant glial population in the CNS. They play a crucial role in HI as mentioned above. However, sustained HI brain injury can lead to decreased astrocytic function and, thereby, greatly decreased neuronal regeneration [60].

2.11 Blood–brain barrier and vascular fragility

The brain evidences a high requirement of oxygenated blood. This demand has resulted in the development of specific cerebral blood vessel networks with arteriovenous hierarchy. The Blood–Brain Barrier (BBB) is a specific and unique component of the cerebrovascular network. It is a highly specialized biochemical and structural barrier at the interface between blood and brain. BBB is involved in preserving ionic homeostasis within cerebral microenvironment and regulating the entry of molecules into the brain [63].

HI injury in neonatal brain induces an increase in BBB permeability, affecting important cellular and functional components of this vessel network such as pericytes, the tight junctions of endothelial cells and astrocytes [60, 63, 64].

Delicate and thin vessels in the developing brain may not sustain the lack of blood flow to compensate the requirements of oxygen and nutrients that the brain needs, due to the underdeveloped distal arterial network and an immature cerebral auto regulatory capacity. Peripheral arteries in the growing brain lack collateral vessels and exhibit limited vasodilatory function in response to the hypoxic–ischemic event, resulting more susceptible to HI injury [60].

3. Experimental models

In vivo and in vitro models are used for studying hypoxia (**Table 2**). In the most used animal model, a unilateral ligation of the carotid artery (UCCAO) is performed, followed by an exposure to an oxygen atmosphere of 8% for 1–3 hours, mainly developed in rodents [65]. This reproduces the anatomical damage caused by HI in neonates, with gray matter damage in the hippocampus, thalamus and basal ganglia, as well as in white matter [65, 66]. Similarly, it reproduces metabolic damage in parameters such as: cerebral acidosis, decreased cerebral blood flow, and decreased glucose uptake [52] and has the ability to show the neuroprotective effect of different therapeutic approaches like hypothermia [67, 68]. Bilateral ligation of the carotid artery is also used to accentuate white matter damage [69, 70] .

In another animal model, ligation of the common carotid is excluded and hypoxic damage is performed by oxygen deprivation. This experimental paradigm is used to describe milder lesions and to investigate the biochemical alterations of the brain [52]. On the other hand, this model has been used in larger animals such as primates, sheep, pigs and rabbits in order to better replicate the conditions of a human fetus with HI, with the disadvantage of not being able to perform behavioral tests and not having a methodological archetype between experiments [52, 71–73].

3.1 In vitro approaches

The different methodological limitations of in vivo models make in vitro models relevant. In order to replicate the conditions that occur in the presence of a deprivation or decrease in glucose and oxygen levels such as those present in HI, several studies have proposed a model of oxygen and glucose deprivation (OGD) (**Table 2**). This experimental model has the ability to adjust to specific research needs and the versatility of being able to use different cell lines, making possible the study of the bases of the molecular and biochemical mechanisms of HI injury. However, methodological differences have been found in the implementation of this model, especially in the exposure time of hypoxia and reoxygenation. [74–81], making this model dependent on the specific conditions of the tissue or cells used [7].

Another methodological approach used to study the effects of hypoxia in vitro include chemical hypoxia-mimetic agents (HMAs) (**Table 2**). These are based on producing at molecular level the effects caused by low concentration of oxygen, mainly those involved in the expression of Hypoxia-inducible factor-1 (HIF-1) [82, 83]. The activation of this factor depends on oxygen concentration, and HIF-1 is involved in several cellular processes that trigger hypoxia [84–89].

Reference	Species	Animal model	Outcomes
Large animal models			
[73]	*Macaca nemestrina*, near term	UCO	Poor weight gain and cerebellar growth, abnormal brain DTI, behavioral impairment, 43% develop CP.
[90, 91]	Fetal sheep, near term	Bilateral CCAO	Shorter HI (<30 min): selective neuronal loss. Longer HI: cortical necrosis. Post-HI EEG suppression related to insult severity and pathology; prevented by hypothermia.
[92]	Fetal sheep, midgestation	Bilateral CCAO	Necrosis of subcortical white matter, neuronal loss in thalamus and striatum similar to near term fetus. Little loss of final EEG amplitude.
[93]	Fetal sheep, midgestation and near Term	UCO	Hippocampal neuronal loss only in near term group. Degree of injury associated with the severity of hypotension during UCO.
[94]	Pigs, <24 h old	CCAO + hypoxia	Secondary energy failure. Energy metabolism ameliorated by hypothermia (35°C for 12 h) at 24 h–48 h.
[95]	Pigs, P9	Hypotension + hypoxia	~60% fall in CBF, reduced cerebral O2 uptake, phosphorylated metabolites and pH and increased inorganic phosphate.
[71]	Rabbits, 21–22d gestation	Uterine ischemia	P1 pups: overt posture and tone after ischemia >37 min, correlates with microgliosis in basal ganglia and thalamus. MRI: WMI in IC.
Rodent models with global hypoxic or excitotoxic component			
[96]	Mice at E8, P0 or P5	Ibotenate, i.c.v.	Laminar neuronal depopulation of layer V–VIa. P5: neuronal loss in all cortical layers, formation of porencephalic cysts.

Reference	Species	Animal model	Outcomes
[97]	Pregnant Sprague–Dawley rats, embryonic	Hypoxia E5-E20	White matter cysts in offspring P0–P7, increased lipid peroxidation, WMI and macrophages.
Rodent models with hypoxia-ischemia			
[98, 99]	Sprague Dawley rats, P1–P3	CCAL + hypoxia	Selective vulnerability of late OL progenitors, independent of age. Death of sub-plate neurons, motor deficits, altered thalamocortical connections to somatosensory and visual cortex normal.
[65]	Sprague–Dawley rats, P7	CCAL + hypoxia	Unilateral ischemic injury in the cortex, hippocampus, basal ganglia in >90% of survivors.
[100]	Wistar rat, P7	LPS, 4 h prior to CCAL + hypoxia	Blocking lymphocyte trafficking reduced brain inflammation, BBB damage, and improved LPS-induced HI brain injury. No effect with pure HI.
[101]	C57Bl/6 WT, Tg SOD1, GPx1 over-expressing P7 mice	CCAL + hypoxia	Reduced injury in GPx1-Tg mice but not in SOD1-Tg or GPx1/SOD1. NOS inhibition did not improve outcome in SOD-Tg.
[102, 103]	C57BL/6 WT and Gal-3 KO, P9	CCAL + hypoxia	Increased BBB permeability 2–24 h, reduced BBB protein expression. Infarct volume reduction in Gal-3 KO mice.
[104]	C57BL/6 J and TRIF KO mice, P8–9	Poly I:C, 14 h prior to CCAL + hypoxia	Increased infarct volume and WMI, prevented in TRIF KO. Injury linked to inflammatory response & decrease in M2-like microglia.
Focal ischemia rodent models			
[105]	Wistar rat, P7	Permanent MCAO +1 h CCAO	Infarcts in frontoparietal cortex at 3-month recovery. DNA fragmentation from 6 to 96 h.
[106–108]	Sprague Dawley rats, P7	Transient MCAO, 3 h	Severe unilateral perfusion deficits, restoration of CBF upon suture removal. Decreased ADC associated with brain injury at 24 h reperfusion. Demonstrated endogenous neuroprotective role of microglial cells after acute injury.
[109]	Sprague Dawley rats, P10	Transient MCAO, 1.5 h	Time resolved cell-type specific increase in HIF-1a and VEGF expression, gliosis.
[110]	C57/Bl6 mice, CD36 KO and WT, P9	Transient MCAO, 1.5 h and 3 h	Focal ischemia–reperfusion, increased injury and caspase-3 cleavage associated with apoptotic neuronal debris in CD36 KO. Effects independent of NFκB activation.
In vitro models			
Reference	Cell line	Experimental model	Outcomes
[74]	PC12 cells	48 h OGD/ 2 h reperfusion	Significant morphological cell changes
[75]	Primary cortical astrocyte	6 h OGD/ 0, 12, 24, 48 h reperfusion	Significantly increased 2- NBDG uptake by about 1.2 to 2.5 times in cells compared to control

Reference	Species	Animal model	Outcomes
[76]	Primary cerebral cortex neurons	3 h OGD/ 48 h Reperfusion	Damage to neuronal viability, dendrite branch number in neurons deceased significantly
[79]	Primary astrocyte	3, 5, 7 h OGD/ 24 h Reoxygenation	Increases in HMGB1 and TNF-a, induced phosphorylation of PI3K, promoted nuclear translocation of NF-kB
[111]	Primary cortical neurons	2 h OGD	Suppressed significantly cortical neurons proliferation
[112]	SH-SY-5Y cells	6 h OGD/ 1 h reoxygenation	Caused significant mitochondrial fragmentation, excessive mitochondrial fission
[77]	Primary Cortical Neuron	OGD	Decrease in neurite outgrowth
[78]	Neural progenitor cell	6 h OGD	Increased apoptosis
[113]	Mouse hippocampal neurons HT22	4 h OGD/ 24 h Reoxygenation	miR-144-3p expression was significantly downregulated in neurons following OGD/R treatment
[81]	Neuro 2a cells	4 h OGD/ 12 h Reoxygenation	Inhibited cell viability and cell proliferation, reduced phosphorylation levels of p38 MAPK and ERK1/2
[114]	SH-SY5Y cells and primary murine cortical neurons,	4 h OGD	OGDR-induced mitochondrial depolarization, reactive oxygen species production, lipid peroxidation and DNA damages
[115]	Primary astrocytes and microglial cells	2 h OGD/ 48 h Reoxygenation	Induced abnormally opened hemichannels with increased ATP release and EtBr uptake but reduced GJIC permeability. Astrocytic Cx43, hemichannels, and GJIC play critical roles in OGD/R injury-induced neuroinflammatory responses.
[116]	Primary astrocytes	4 h OGD/ 3 h, 6 h, 12 h, 24 h reoxygenation	Expression of Ski was proved to be up-regulated
[117]	Primary hippocampal neurons	2 h OGD/ 24 h reperfusion	Caspase-3 activity and expression increased in the first 24 h,
HMAs models			
Reference	Cell line/species	Experimental model	Outcomes
[82]	Multiple myeloma cell line U266	CoCl2	CoCl2-mediated hypoxia affects the expression profiles of genes that are functionally related to apoptosis and angiogenesis
[83]	Myeloid leukemic cell lines NB4 and U937	CoCl2 and DFO	Apoptosis with a loss of mitochondrial transmembrane potentials, activation of caspase-3/8 and cleavage of anti-apoptotic protein Mcl-1
[118]	U251 human glioblastoma cell line	CoCl2	Increases HIF-1a gene expression
[119]	Glioblastoma cell lines U373MG and DBTRG05MG	DFO	Activation of factors associated with ECM degradation and invasion of glioma cells

Reference	Species	Animal model	Outcomes
[120]	C57BL/6 mice	DFO	DFO up-regulated the expression of vascular endothelial growth factor (VEGF), HIF-1α protein and growth associated protein 43 (GAP43) and down-regulated the expression of divalent metal transporter with iron-responsive element (DMT1 + IRE), α-synuclein, and transferrin receptor (TFR)
[121]	Hippocampal neurons	DFO pretreatment/3 h OGD	45% reduction in cell death
[122]	Sprague–Dawley rats	Subarachnoid hemorrhage/DFO treatment	DFO-induced increase in HIF-1 protein level and activity exerts significant attenuation of BA vasospasm
[123]	Hippocampal cultures	Ppreconditioning CoCl2, DFO or dimethyloxylalyglycine (DMOG), 3 h OGD	Cobalt induced the transcription of the cytokine erythropoietin. Cobalt and DFO, enhanced survival of neurons. DMOG exacerbates OGD-induced neuronal death
[124]	Sprague–Dawley rats	CCA/DFO treatment	Neural-protective and angiogenesis effects through regulating the levels of HIF-1α
[125]	Adipose-derived stem cells	DFO preconditioning	Restored neovascularization potential of ADSCs
[126]	Sprague – Dawley rats	MCA/DFO treatment	Preserved brain volumes, upregulation of HIF1a
[127]	Wistar rats	MCAO/ DFO + Erythropoietin treatment	Reduced the number of cleaved caspase 3-positive cells in the ipsilateral cerebral cortex.

Modified from [7].

Table 2.
Experimental models for HI.

4. Neuroactive steroids

Neuroactive Steroids were defined by Baulieu [128] as steroids synthesized in the nervous system capable of inducing neuronal excitability [129]. Compounds as dehydroepiandrosterone, androstenedione, and deoxycorticosterone meet the requirements to be categorized as neuroactive steroids. Interestingly, neuroactive steroids induce responses on GABA receptors and modulate the activity of 5α and 3α reductases affecting steroid synthesis [130–132]. In this regard, neuroactive steroids can be exogenously synthesized and produce similar effects on the CNS. In the current definition neuroactive steroids are molecules capable of inducing several effects on CNS including ion channel modulation, voltage-dependent calcium channels activation and AMPA-NMDA receptors activation [133–135]. Besides the neuroactive properties of steroids, there are a plethora of protective functions characterized on neurons, astrocyte and microglia [136–139]. The effects of neuroactive steroids on neurons include the increase of dendritic spines, viability, antioxidant capacity [140, 141]. On astrocytes, neuroactive steroids improve the mitochondrial function, modulate the synthesis of antioxidant molecules and growth factors and pro-survival factors as Bcl-2 [142–145]. Finally, on microglia, the effects include the modulation of immune response via regulation of the synthesis and secretion of cytokines and inflammatory mediators [139].

Neuroactive steroids may induce both genomic and non-genomic mechanisms associated with its protective effects [146]. The genomic mechanisms involve the modulation of pro-survival genes, anti-inflammatory [147] and anti-apoptotic functions [148]. For example, the activation of signaling pathways like Akt-PI3K and MAPK, and the upregulation of the anti-apoptotic mediators like Bcl-2 and antioxidant enzymes like SOD and GPx [149] are under control of Neuroactive steroids. Other mechanisms include the downregulation of pro-inflammatory cytokines such as IL-1β, IL-6 and TNF-α [150]. The non-genomic effects include the antioxidant properties of some neurosteroids, especially the ones that include an A-phenolic ring in their chemical structure [151]. Interestingly, some neuroactive steroids are capable of exerting its effects through G-protein coupled receptors, for example via GPR30 receptor [152]. Until now, there is a large body of evidence demonstrating the beneficial effects of neuroactive steroids following ischemia/reperfusion and traumatic brain injury (TBI) in animal models (Liu et al., 2005; O'Connor et al., 2005) as well as steroid-demonstrated effectiveness in glucose deprivation and oxygen–glucose deprivation in in vitro models [148]. Despite this evidence, the direct use of estrogens is not fully recommended and still represents a potential risk for human health [153, 154] (For further evidence, see **Table 3**). In fact, it has been documented that the use of estrogen and progesterone increases the risk to develop breast and uterus cancer, as well as, vascular diseases, brain hemorrhage and clotting disorders [155–159]. To circumvent these issues, selective compounds that mimic the protective action of neuroactive steroid without the side effects were developed. These compounds were defined as selective estrogen receptor modulators (SERMs) and selective tissue-specific estrogenic activity regulators (STEARs). SERMs and STEARs exert their actions as estrogenic agonists or antagonists depending on the target organ [146, 160]. Tissue selective properties of SERM and STEAR are currently under investigation (**Figure 1**).

Reference	Type of study	Outcomes
[197]9	Human Psychiatric study	The evidence summarized supports the idea that MDD and PPD are psychiatric disorders involving neurosteroids and GABAergic dysfunction
[198]	Comparative human and animal studies	The study shows potential mechanisms that underlie sex-related differences in behavior and its implications for stress-related illnesses.
[199]	Animal and human studies	The negative cognitive consequences of sleep deprivation may arise from the effort of the brain to counteract the detrimental effect of sleep loss via compensatory mechanisms
[200]	Animal (neonatal foal) study	Progesterone might be a promissory marker for identifying continuous endogenous production of neuroactive steroids in foals with suspected NMS and other diseases
[201]	Human study	Individual domains of cognitive can be considered as an endophenotype of psychosis. It is possible that higher levels of cortisol and testosterone in siblings are consistent with high-risk states for psychosis
[202]	Animal model	Exposure to neuroactive steroids induced a sustained elevation in tonic current in Fmr1 KO mice. Neuroactive steroids may act to reverse the deficits of tonic inhibition seen in FXS, and thereby reduce aberrant neuronal hyperexcitability associated to this disorder
[203]	Peripartum depressed women	Cortical GABA+/Cr concentrations are associated with postpartum RSFC. It is possible that allopregnanolone may be associated with postpartum intra-DMPFC connectivity.

Reference	Type of study	Outcomes
[204]	Animal and human studies	Nervous diabetic complications show sex dimorphic features. In this regard, sex-oriented therapies with neuroactive steroids might be aimed to counteract nervous damage observed in diabetic pathology.
[205]	Animal and human studies	Neuroactive steroids under pathological conditions may alter their levels involving sex differencies in the outcome. Neuroactive steroid may be considered as neuroprotective factors to be deeply investigated.
[206]	Animal and human studies	Some studies point to a lag between neuroactive steroid dysregulation and subsequent symptoms. The study also consider key interactions with other aspects of neuroactive steroid physiology, such as synthetic enzymes or receptor plasticity.
[207]	Animal and human studies	There is a very close link among neuroactive steroids and the control of metabolic axis to understand the biological basis of many pathologies based on metabolic alterations, for example the metabolic syndrome, obesity or diabetes.
[208]	Women study	Women at both extremes of the weight spectrum have low mean serum allopregnanolone. Neuroactive steroids such as allopregnanolone may be potential therapeutic targets for depression and anxiety in traditionally treatment-resistant groups.
[209]	Animal and human studies	Low levels of neuroactive steroids could have a part in development of depression, neuro-inflammation, multiple sclerosis, experimental autoimmune encephalitis, epilepsy, and schizophrenia. On the other hand, stress and attention deficit disorder could occur during high levels.
[210]	Animal and human studies	Several Compounds have completed a phase 1 single ascending dose (SAD) and multiple ascending dose (MAD) clinical trial and is currently being studied in parallel phase 2 clinical trials for the treatment of postpartum depression (PPD), major depressive disorder (MDD), and essential tremor (ET).
[211]	Animal model	DHEAS and progesterone were good predictors of HPA Axis dysfunction and outcome in hospitalized foals.
[212]	Clinical study	The first-episode antipsychotic-naive schizophrenic patients showed a significantly higher blood level of DHEA-S compared with healthy controls. On the other hand, serum DHEA-S level has an inverse relationship with aggression and may serve as a biological adaptive mechanism to antagonize the neuronal damage caused by cortisol.
[213]	Animal and human studies	Clinical trials designed to test neuroactive steroid therapeutics in PTSD may benefit from such considerations. However it is needed to validate clinically accessible methods for identifying specific neuroactive steroid system abnormalities at the individual level.
[214]	Animal and human studies	Strain variation in neuroactive steroid levels correlated with numerous behavioral phenotypes of anxiety sensitivity accessed in GeneNetwork, consistent with evidence that neuroactive steroids modulate anxiety-like behavior.
[215]	Aged human study	We observed a significant difference in plasma concentration of cortisol and estradiol between experimental groups. In the AIS group, higher levels of these neuroactive steroids were associated with more pronounced neurological, cognitive and functional deficits in women compared to men.

Table 3.
Neuroactive steroids used in experimental models and clinical studies.

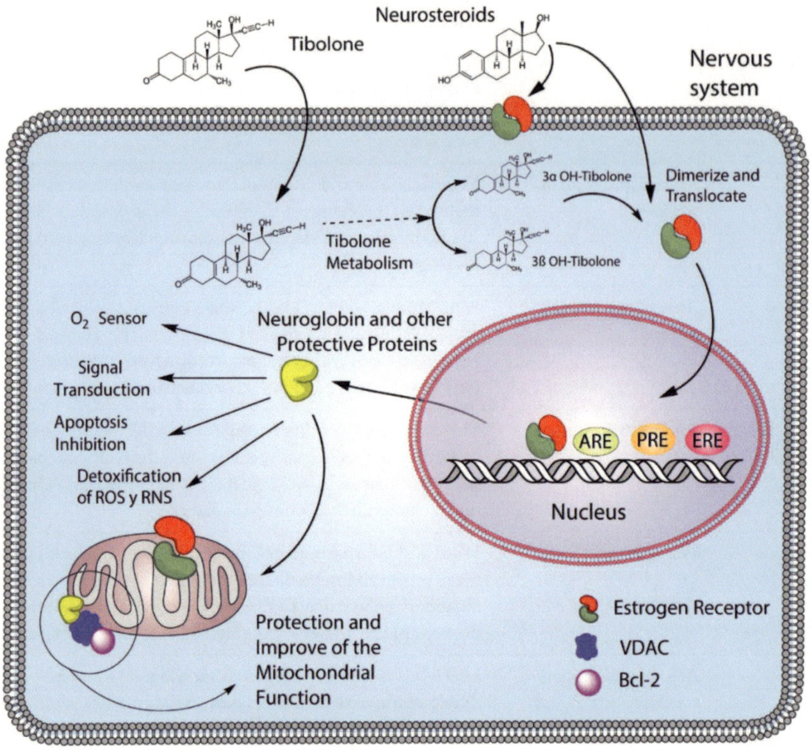

Figure 1.
Potential Neurosteroids action mechanism. The effects of neurosteroids on neurons include the increase of dendritic spines, viability, and antioxidant capacity. The action mechanism is associated to classical (canonical) transduction pathway that includes the transactivation of estrogen receptor to dimerize and promote the transcription of estrogen response elements ERE. For tibolone, it is described the classical transduction pathway but also the transactivation of androgen response elements ARE and progesterone response elements PRE. It is possible that all together response elements explain the beneficial and protective properties of tibolone. Interestingly, the protective properties also has been observed on astrocytes and microglia.

4.1 Selective estrogen receptor modulators

The activation or partial activation of Estrogen receptors (ER) trigger critical signal pathways due to complex molecular mechanisms. ER interact with several endogens and exogenous ligands promoting structural changes with the subsequent transactivation of estrogen response elements (ERE) in the DNA. ER interact also with co-activators, co-repressors and chaperones, affecting the way that the tissues exert their estrogenic response [161, 162]. ER show structural components that may be involved in their particular action mechanism. One of the most striking domain is the ligand binding domain (LBD) that interacts with specific ligands [163] (Cano et al., 2006). It is believed that the high or low affinity of the ligand with LBD plays a central role in the function of ER. Ligand interaction with LBD induces conformational changes that lead to specific bind to activators with co-activators and co-repressors modulating the estrogenic response [161, 164]. In this context, the conformational change is predetermined in part by the chemical nature of the ligand and its interaction with ER [165]. SERMs are capable of exploiting this advantage. A clear example is tamoxifen, a selective compound with estrogenic activity in the liver, but anti-estrogenic activity in breast tissue [166]. These compounds have been widely used in clinics for the treatment of breast cancer and as hormonal replacement therapy (HRT) strategies [167]. SERMs are defined as compounds that are capable of binding ER and produce several responses, ranging from a pure estrogenic agonism to an anti-estrogen activity [146]. SERMs may protect nervous tissue following spinal cord and traumatic brain injuries [168, 169]. Gonzales-Burgos et al. (2012) demonstrated that SERMs increase the number of dendritic spines in hippocampal neurons [170]. Raloxifene, a second-generation SERM, demonstrated to improve sensory motor and working memory deficits following TBI [168], suggesting that SERMs may act as potential therapeutic compounds after CNS injury.

SERMs action mechanisms include the activation of transcription factors such as NF-κB through the PI3K-P38-ERK1/2 pathway [146]. SERMs also induce the production of antioxidant enzymes such as manganese superoxide dismutase (MnSOD) [171] and the endothelial nitric oxide synthase (eNOS) [172]. Interestingly, SERMs may induce the upregulation of anti-apoptotic proteins such as Bcl-2 [173]. Altogether, the activation of these multifactorial protective signaling cascades may improve the outcome of highly heterogeneous pathologies like TBI and HI Brain Injury (HIBI). Currently, SERM are used as primary treatments to counter osteoporosis and some kind of cancer. Compounds like raloxifen (Evista ®) and tamoxifen (Nolvadex®) are routinely prescribed for thousand women [174, 175]. Several reports have described the protective effects of SERMs on the CNS [176–178]. It is well known that tamoxifen is capable of preserving pyramidal neurons following penetrant lesion [179]. Furthermore, raloxifen exerts protective functions by increasing glutamate reuptake via induction of GLT-1 expression on primary astrocytes [180]. However, the complete action mechanism of several SERMs needs to be fully elucidated, due in part, to the complex agonist–antagonist action [181].

4.2 Selective tissue estrogenic activity regulators

The pharmacologic necessity to develop estrogenic safe compounds against climacteric symptoms in post-menopause women lead to synthesize a distinctive compound with selective estrogenic properties. As a result, STEARs are compounds capable of inducing an estrogenic, progestogenic and androgenic response. The most used STEAR compound is tibolone [160]- Tibolone has become a well-known treatment for climacteric symptoms than other HRT compounds, especially in women suffering low libido, persistent fatigue and blunted motivation [172, 182]. Tibolone has been used in the prevention of cardiovascular diseases and osteoporosis [183, 184] Tibolone exhibits weak estrogenic, progestogenic and androgenic properties [160, 183, 185].

The selective action mechanism of tibolone and STEARs is currently under investigation. However, it is well known that tibolone acts as a pro-drug that has complex effects due to its particular mode of action on different steroid receptors. It has been demonstrated that the body metabolized tibolone via two-phase reacts to produce three different metabolites [186]: two hydroxyl-metabolites (3-alpha-hydroxy- and 3-beta-hydroxy tibolone) as a result of 3-alpha and 3-beta hydroxysteroid dehydrogenase enzymes (3α-HSD and 3ß-HSD), and one isomer (delta-4 tibolone) synthesized by 3-beta-hydroxysteroid dehydrogenase [160, 183, 185].

Interestingly, 3α-HSD is predominantly expressed in the liver, whereas 3ß-HSD is expressed in adrenal glands, ovary and placental tissue [160, 183, 185]. Tibolone metabolism is under liver control by α-ketoreductases including hepatic AKR1C1 and AKR1C2 [186]. STEARs like tibolone might be metabolized by the brain, due to brain cells, for example, astrocytes fully expressing all the needed enzymes to carry out the biochemical steps. Kloobsterboer et al. 2017 demonstrated in primates (cynomolgus) the occurrence of 3α OH tibolone and 3β OH tibolone metabolites in the brain. They also detected sulfated tibolone metabolites (inactive chemical compounds) in the brain and plasma. Each metabolite has different features. For example, tibolone perse and delta-4 tibolone are agonists for progesterone receptor PR and androgen receptor AR [185], while 3-alpha and 3-beta hydroxy metabolites are agonists for ER, but antagonists for PR and AR [185, 187]. This tibolone-steroid receptor interaction and other regulatory mechanisms might explain the tissue-selective effects of tibolone [160, 186]. Belenichev et al. (2012) used cortical neurons from neonatal rats to evaluate the neuroprotective activity of tibolone in a model of glutathione depletion that produces oxidative stress and mitochondrial dysfunction. These authors found that tibolone prevented mitochondrial dysfunction and neuronal cell death. Additional studies account for the protective effects of tibolone in an ovariectomized rat model following cerebral ischemia injury [188]. Tibolone has also shown anti-inflammatory effects tested in cardiovascular animal models [184].

Kloosterboer et al. 2007 propose an additional action mechanism of tibolone and STEARs that involves the control of sulfatase and sulfotransferase tissue-specific activity [189]. Since sulfatase and sulfotransferase activity is tissue-specific, it is possible that tibolone exerts its function according to cell type specificity and modulating nuclear receptors activity in the tissues [190]. For instance, it is needed to further investigate the tissue-specific role of tibolone in CNS, for example, in neurons, astrocytes, and microglia. Interestingly, tibolone protects the mitochondrial activity by the preservation of the mitochondrial membrane potential and by increasing the levels of proteins that control the opening of the mitochondrial permeability transition pore (mPTP), such as Bcl-2. Avila-Rodriguez et al. (2014) demonstrated that tibolone protects the mitochondria of T98G glial cells from glucose deprivation [141].

De Marinis' research group recently described and characterized a particular globin belonging to CNS called neuroglobin (Ngb1). Neuroglobin is under control of estrogenic response. In fact, the use of estradiol in several cellular models demonstrated the increase of neuroglobin levels [191–193]. Currently, it is known that neuroglobin is an 18 kDa protein that binds molecular oxygen with more affinity than hemoglobin, probably, increasing the availability of oxygen in the neural tissue [194]. Neuroglobin is expressed in neurons under basal conditions and is also expressed in astrocytes and microglia after brain injury [194]. Avila-Rodriguez et al. 2016 demonstrated that tibolone is capable of increasing the expression of neuroglobin producing a protective effect in a glucose deprivation astrocyte-like model. The action mechanism of tibolone may be associated with ERß receptor as demonstrated by several studies [191, 193].

Other studies demonstrated the protective effect of tibolone against lipid peroxidation and protein oxidation [195]. Tibolone is capable of increasing the density of dendritic spines in hippocampal neurons, indicating a potential role in synaptic plasticity and memory [196]. Guzmán et al. (2007), also showed that tibolone metabolites exert estrogenic activity on human astrocytes and oligodendrocytes-like cell lines [187]. Tibolone may become a promissory option to counter the detrimental effects of TBI and hypoxic injury due to its pleiotropic beneficial properties.

4.3 Selective tissue-specific estrogenic activity regulators and neuroglobin

Pathologic conditions like hypoxia and glucose deprivation, which may lead to neuroinflammation, reduce the expression of ER-α and increase the expression of ER-ß [216]. In this regard, De Marinis et al. (2013) showed that hypoxia may induce the production of pro-inflammatory mediators like IL-6, and INF-γ [193]. Interestingly, estrogen is capable of diminishing the secretion of those pro-inflammatory mediators. It was demonstrated in a pro-oxidant model induced by H2O2 and stimulated via lipopolysaccharide (LPS). Later, it was demonstrated that the anti-inflammatory effect was mediated by NF-κB modulation and ER-ß activation [191, 193]. Therefore, it is reasonable to assume that the activation of ER-ß in hypoxic and glucose deprivation models may be considered as beneficial for brain tissues. Tibolone is capable of inducing the activation of ERß and increasing neuroglobin expression. Avila-Rodriguez et al. (2016) demonstrated that neuroglobin expression depends on ER-ß activation and tibolone favors both mechanisms [217]. Originally, neuroglobin was reported in neurons but later it was detected in other cell types such as astrocytes [218]. Interestingly, neuroglobin has been associated with neuroprotective effects on several injury models including middle cerebral artery occlusion (MCAO), focal cerebral ischemia, ß-amyloid induced toxicity, oxygen and glucose deprivation [217, 219–221].

Neuroglobin may mediate the response against hypoxia by inducing signal pathways. It has also been documented as a reactive oxygen radical scavenger with NADH oxidase activity to favor anaerobic glycolytic metabolism [217]. Controversial studies based on low levels of neuroglobin and low relative oxygen affinity propose that neuroglobin may exert or participate in collateral roles other than solely oxygen store [217, 222] (See **Figure 2** for further illustration). Additionally, photoactivation (NADH/FMN) experiments demonstrated that neuroglobin participates in the ROS and RNS elimination, suggesting a critical role in removing dangerous highly reactive species [223]. The change in the hexacoordinated state of neuroglobin according to normoxic or hypoxic conditions also suggests oxygen sensor capabilities [222]. Proper neuroglobin activity protects neurons and astrocytes against cell death [191]. In this regard, overexpression or induction of neuroglobin may be considered as potential neuroprotective therapies. Interestingly, STEARs such as tibolone are capable of increasing and inducing neuroglobin activity, which have been proposed as potential action mechanisms in

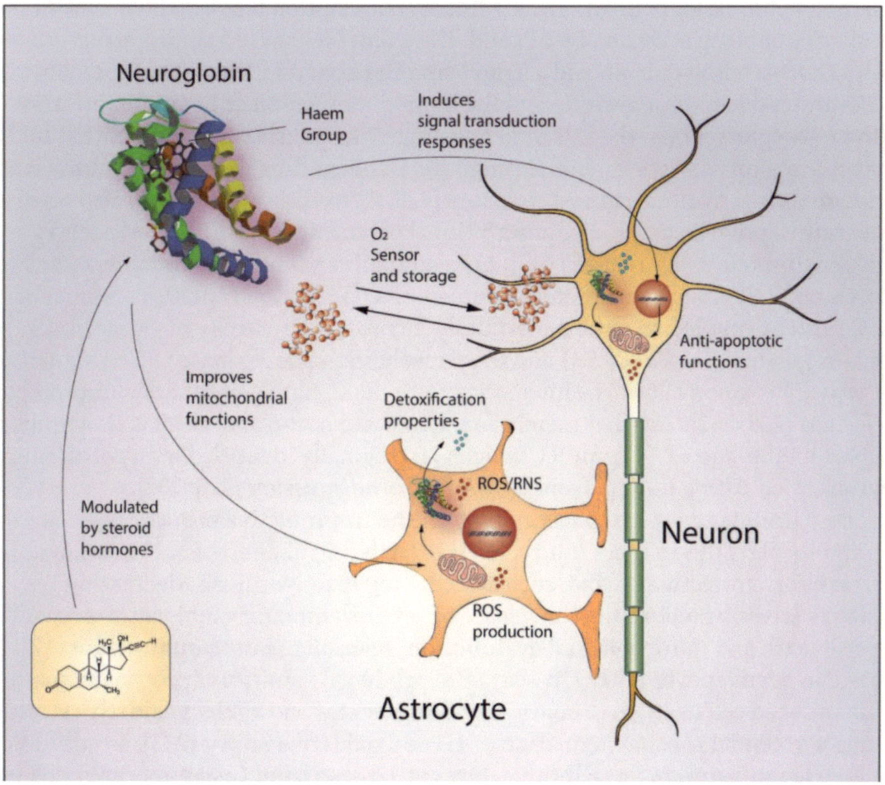

Figure 2.
Neuroglobin exerts interesting beneficial properties. Neuroglobin includes in its protein structure a particular prosthetic haem group to store oxygen. However, it is reported for neuroglobin additional protective functions that include oxygen sensor capabilities and detoxification properties (against reactive oxygen species and reactive nitrogen species). Evidence shows that the protective functions of neuroglobin may be induced via signal transduction mediators including steroid hormones and neurosteroids. For example, some neurosteroids increase neuroglobin production improving mitochondrial functions and inducing anti-apoptotic mechanisms.

brain tissue [191, 217, 222]. According to computations studies and simulations, it has been proposed the neuroglobin may interact with cytochrome c. This apparent interaction may explain the electronic transfer between neuroglobin (ferrous) and cytochrome c (ferric) [191, 224]. Potentially, neuroglobin may modulate cytoplasmic cytochrome c, resulting in diminished apoptotic processes in injured tissues. Surprisingly, De Marinis et al. (2013) showed that neuroglobin hijacks cytochrome c in a neuroblastoma cell model injured via hydrogen peroxide [191]. The estrogenic induction of neuroglobin (and eventually by tibolone) increased neuroglobin expression and diminished the apoptotic cell death mechanism [191].

5. Neuroprotective properties of estrogen and its derivates on brain injury

A derivate of estrogen, 17β-estradiol, is a female sex hormone and neuroactive steroid (NAS) related to the development of secondary sexual characteristics, fat storage and regulation of menstrual cycle [225]. 17β-estradiol, showed beneficial effects in verbal and visual memory performance, which was originally administered as a hormone replacement therapy in order to ameliorate climacteric symptoms [226]. The activity of 17β-estradiol depends on its union with ERs [43, 226, 227]. These receptors are classified in two subtypes: estrogen receptor-beta (ER-β) and estrogen receptor-alpha (ER-α). ERα has its locus in 6 chromosome, while the locus for the Erβ is in the 14 chromosome [226]. These ERs are transcription factors which present the peculiarity of being activated by a ligand. ER-α and ER-β have a similar structure, with a DNA-binding domain and a ligand-binding domain [228]. 17β-estradiol binds to ERs and induces the activation and the homodimerization or heterodimerization of these receptors. Then, the ERs bind to estrogen-responsive elements (EREs) in the promoter region of specific genes through the DNA-binding domain, recruiting transcriptional co-activators and co-repressors [228, 229]. Classical ERs may also regulate gene transcription by acting as transcriptional partners at non-ERE sites, such as activating protein 1 (AP1) sites [230]. 17β-estradiol can bind to membrane-associated non-classical ERs, such as G protein-coupled ERs (GPERs). GPER30, a member of the G protein-coupled receptor superfamily, regulates the activity of extracellular signal-regulated kinases (ERKs) and the phosphoinositide 3-kinase (PI3K) signaling pathway. This union allows the interaction with the signaling of other neuroprotective molecules [228, 231]. Another membrane-associated non-classical ER is Gαq protein-coupled membrane ER (Gq-mER), which was originally identified in hypothalamic neurons, modulating μ-opioid and GABA neurotransmission [228, 232].

These findings have led to research on the neuroprotective properties of estrogen and its derivates in brain injury. In HI brain injury 17β- estradiol has shown several neuroprotective effects, such as: reducing reactive gliosis, decreasing oxidative stress, ameliorating the release of pro inflammatory molecules, preventing cell death and mitochondrial dysfunction, releasing neurotrophic factors [7]. It has also been reported that 17β- estradiol produced significant protection against OGD-induced cell death in primary oligodendrocytes and against oxidative stress, having a potential role in attenuation of HI and oxidative injury [233]. In addition, in neonate rats subjected to HI, three doses of 17β-estradiol (using repeated dosing paradigm) provided approximately 70% protection of the hippocampus, basal ganglia, and amygdala. These results suggest 17β-estradiol acts as a potent neuroprotective agent against HI-induced damage to the developing brain, and that pretreating infants at risk for hypoxic ischemic injury may be advisable [234]. Moreover, treatment with estradiol after PA augmented the expression of IGF-1 and its receptor (IGF-IR). The PI3K/Akt/GSK3 signaling pathway was activated as an increase in Akt and GSK3 phosphorylation [235]. However, it has been found that male sex is a well-established epidemiological risk factor for poor neurodevelopmental outcome after PA. While the mechanisms responsible for this gender difference are unknown, growing evidence has identified neuro-inflammation, oxidative stress and cell death pathways as key players in these differences [236].

Using a mice model of MCAO with a mutant form of ER-α, neuroprotection was absent, showing that protective properties depend on Er-α [237]. Similarly, after emulating hypoxia in the neuroblastoma cell line SH-SY5Y by using CoCl2 (250 μg/mL), an hypoxic mimetic agent, treatment with 17β-estradiol (250 nM) exerted neuroprotection.

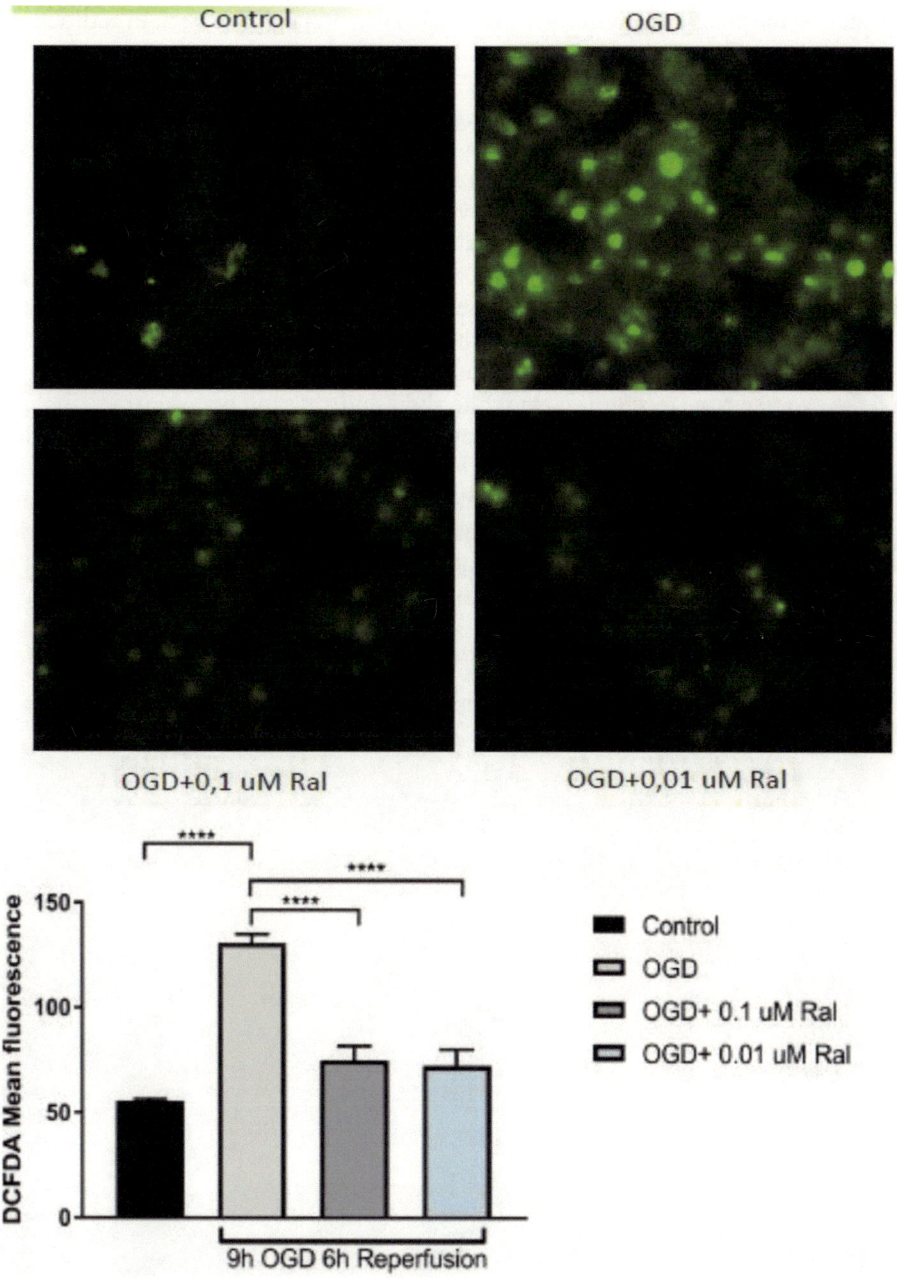

Figure 3.
Ros production.

Afterwards, using ER-α and ER-β agonist (PPT and DPN, respectively) without 17β-estradiol treatment, results showed neuroprotection was mimicked by PPT and suggested that ER-α regulates this protective effect [235]. Likewise, in a model of astrocytic cells it was found that estradiol improved in one of the HI conditions, parameters such as cell viability, mitochondrial membrane potential, reduced ROS production and prevented the loss of mitochondrial mass [38]. Nevertheless, estrogen use can have detrimental effects like the augment in the incidence of breast and uterus cancer [12–14]. In order to maintain the benefits and avoid these side effects, other drugs have been developed, mainly SERMs and STEARs [12–14]. The mechanism of regulation of the SERMs that determines either if they act as agonist or antagonist in an specific cell type depends on the predominant subtype of estrogen receptor alpha or beta. In addition, the co-activators, co- factors and helper proteins of each cell will determine the kind of the response of the tissue exposed to SERMs [238, 239].

In a MCAO rat model, neurogenesis in the ipsilateral subventricular zone (SVZ) after ischemia was significantly higher in estrogen and raloxifene-treated animals compared to rats treated with placebo. Otherwhise, tamoxifen did not show this enhancing effect on neurogenesis. However, both SERMs tamoxifen and raloxifene as well as estrogen, significantly reversed the spine density loss observed in the ischemic cortex at day-5 post ischemia [240]. On the other hand, tibolone action is given by the metabolization of the tibolone to three different metabolites (delta-4 tibolone; alpha-hydroxy tibolone and 3- beta-hydroxy tibolone). Each of them produces different responses. Delta-4 tibolone is an agonist to the androgen receptor and the progesterone receptor, meanwhile alpha-hidroxy and beta-hidroxy tibolone are antagonists of those receptors but agonists of the ER [241]. Keeping this in mind, Avila-Rodriguez et al. (2014) found out that tibolone ameliorates the effects of the GD on an in vitro model of astrocytes, making this molecules interesting for further research in a OGD model [12]. For this reason, in recent years we have been working on the implementation of these neuroprotection strategies in an astrocyte model using Raloxifene as a neuroprotector in the OGD model. **Figures 3** and **4** show the

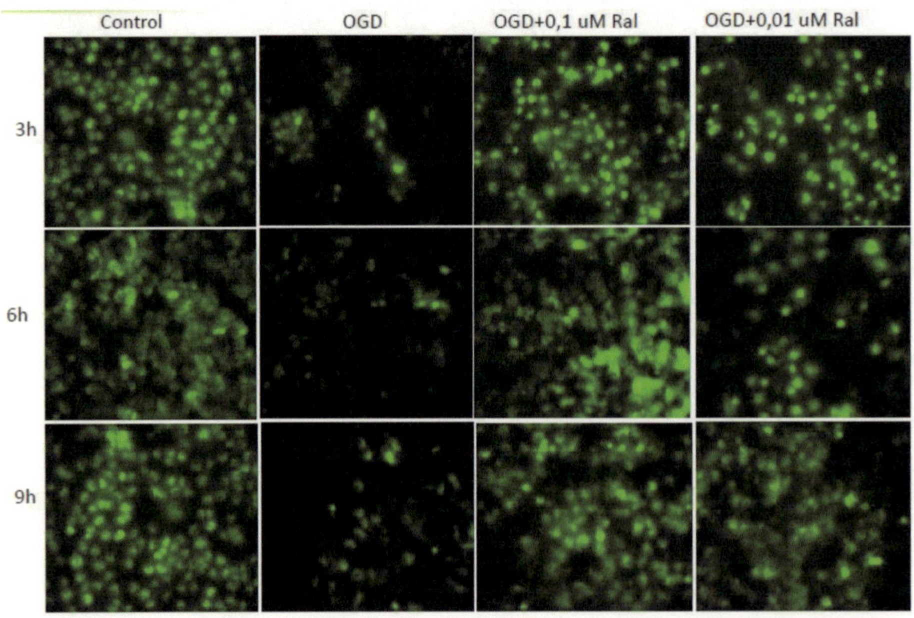

Figure 4.
Mitochondrial mass.

deleterious effect caused by glucose and oxygen deprivation, both in the production of ROS and in the loss of mitochondrial mass, respectively, and how this neuroactive steorid may decrease damage in different concentrations (unpublished data).

6. Conclusion

The different pathologies in which the HI events and with these, the oxygen and glucose deprivation are present, have been shown to exert a high impact on society. Over the years, a multitude of efforts have been directed towards the search for effective treatments that counteract the damage caused by these conditions. The different neuroprotection targets try to combat specific points of damage caused by hypoxia, including oxidative stress, dysregulation of the cell cycle and energy homeostasis [242]. Both in the initial damage phase and in the final one, the different neuroprotective agents may have anti-inflammatory, antioxidant, anti-excitotoxicity or anti-apoptotic capacities [243]. However, due to the complex network of factors that influence these pathologies, such as the cellular interactions (molecular, biochemical, protein, etc.) inherent to the CNS, as well as the gender-dependent response [236] to the use of these neuroprotective agents, the success in the treatments has not been optimal [7]. Estradiol treatment not only prevents neuronal damage, but may also limit the neurodegenerative modifications induced by HI in the early stage of development. The development of SERMs and STEARs brings with it a range of possibilities for the treatment of HI, due to its advantages, focused on the nervous system without having side effects. However, it is necessary to develop new generations of these compounds to improve their neuroprotective effects. Further research is necessary to provide new alternatives in the implementation of new therapeutic strategies and novel approaches.

Author details

Nicolas Toro-Urrego[1*], Marco Avila-Rodriguez[2], María Inés Herrera[1,3], Andrea Aguilar[1], Lucas Udovin[1] and Juan P. Luaces[1]

1 Instituto de Investigaciones Cardiológicas, Universidad de Buenos Aires, Consejo Nacional de Investigaciones Científicas y Técnicas, ININCA, UBA-CONICET, Buenos Aires, Argentina

2 Facultad de Ciencias de la Salud, Departamento de Ciencias Clínicas, Universidad del Tolima, Tolima, Colombia

3 Facultad de Psicología y Psicopedagogía, Centro de Investigaciones en Psicología y Psicopedagogía, Universidad Católica Argentina, Buenos Aires, Argentina

*Address all correspondence to: nicolas.toro3@gmail.com

*Share authorship.

References

[1] Bélanger M, Allaman I, Magistretti PJ. Brain energy metabolism: Focus on astrocyte-neuron metabolic cooperation. Cell Metabolism. 2011 Dec 7;**14**(6):724-738 Available from: https://www.sciencedirect.com/science/article/pii/S1550413111004207

[2] Allaman I, Bélanger M, Magistretti PJ, et al. Trends in Neurosciences. 2011 Feb;**34**(2):76-87. Available from http://www.ncbi.nlm.nih.gov/pubmed/21236501

[3] Dwyer DS, Vannucci SJ, Simpson IA. Expression, regulation, and functional role of glucose transporters (GLUTs) in brain. International Review of Neurobiology. 2002;**51**:159-188. Available from: http://www.ncbi.nlm.nih.gov/pubmed/12420359

[4] Vavilis T, Delivanoglou N, Aggelidou E, Stamoula E, Mellidis K, Kaidoglou A, et al. Oxygen–glucose deprivation (OGD) modulates the unfolded protein response (UPR) and inflicts autophagy in a PC12 hypoxia cell line model. Cellular and Molecular Neurobiology. 2016;**36**(5):701-712 Available from: https://doi.org/10.1007/s10571-015-0250-2

[5] Tian T, Zeng J, Zhao G, Zhao W, Gao S, Liu L. Neuroprotective effects of orientin on oxygen-glucose deprivation/reperfusion-induced cell injury in primary culture of rat cortical neurons. Experimental Biology and Medicine. 2017;**153537021773798** Available from: http://journals.sagepub.com/doi/10.1177/1535370217737983

[6] Yang X, Zheng T, Hong H, Cai N, Zhou X, Sun C, et al. Neuroprotective effects of Ginkgo biloba extract and Ginkgolide B against oxygen–glucose deprivation/reoxygenation and glucose injury in a new in vitro multicellular network model. Frontiers in Medicine. 2017:1-12

[7] Toro-Urrego N, Vesga-Jiménez DJ, Herrera MI, Luaces JP, Capani F. Neuroprotective role of hypothermia in hypoxic-ischemic brain injury: Combined therapies using estrogen. Current Neuropharmacology. 2018 Dec;**6**:17 Available from: http://www.ncbi.nlm.nih.gov/pubmed/30520375

[8] Baburamani AA, Hurling C, Stolp H, Sobotka K, Gressens P, Hagberg H, et al. Mitochondrial optic atrophy (OPA) 1 processing is altered in response to neonatal hypoxic-ischemic brain injury. OPEN ACCESS Int J Mol Sci. 2015;**16**:16 Available from: www.mdpi.com/journal/ijmsArticle

[9] Mozaffarian D, Benjamin EJ, Go AS, Arnett DK, Blaha MJ, Cushman M, et al. Heart disease and stroke statistics—2015 update. Circulation. 2015 Jan 27;**131**(4):e29LP-ee322 Available from: http://circ.ahajournals.org/content/131/4/e29.abstract

[10] Northington FJ, Chavez-Valdez R, Martin LJ. Neuronal cell death in neonatal hypoxia-ischemia. Annals of Neurology. 2011 May;**69**(5):743-758 Available from: http://www.ncbi.nlm.nih.gov/pmc/articles/PMC4000313/

[11] Petito CK, Pulsinelli WA. Delayed neuronal recovery and neuronal death in rat Hippocampus following severe cerebral ischemia: Possible relationship to abnormalities in neuronal processes. Journal of Cerebral Blood Flow and Metabolism. 1984 Jun 28;**4**(2):194-205 Available from: http://journals.sagepub.com/doi/10.1038/jcbfm.1984.28

[12] Ávila Rodriguez M, Garcia-Segura LM, Cabezas R, Torrente D, Capani F, Gonzalez J, et al. Tibolone protects T98G cells from glucose deprivation. The Journal of Steroid Biochemistry and Molecular Biology. 2014;**144**(PART B):294-303

[13] Arevalo MA, Santos-Galindo M, Lagunas N, Azcoitia I, Garcia-Segura LM. Selective estrogen receptor modulators as brain therapeutic agents. Journal of Molecular Endocrinology. 2011;**46**(1)

[14] Garzón D, Cabezas R, Vega N, Ávila-Rodriguez M, Gonzalez J. et al., Novel approaches in astrocyte protection: From experimental methods to computational approaches. Journal of Molecular Neuroscience. 2016;**58**(4):483-492

[15] Blumberg RM, Cady EB, Wigglesworth JS, McKenzie JE, Edwards AD. Relation between delayed impairment of cerebral energy metabolism and infarction following transient focal hypoxia-ischaemia in the developing brain. Experimental Brain Research. 1997 Jan;**113**(1):130-137 Available from: http://www.ncbi.nlm.nih.gov/pubmed/9028781

[16] Thornton C, Jones A, Nair S, Aabdien A, Mallard C, Hagberg H. Mitochondrial dynamics, mitophagy and biogenesis in neonatal hypoxic-ischaemic brain injury. FEBS Letters. Wiley Blackwell. 2018;**592**:812-830

[17] Fleiss B, Gressens P. Tertiary mechanisms of brain damage: A new hope for treatment of cerebral palsy? The Lancet Neurology. 2012;**11**:556-566 Available from: http://www.ncbi.nlm.nih.gov/pubmed/22608669

[18] Li B, Concepcion K, Meng X, Zhang L. Brain-immune interactions in perinatal hypoxic-ischemic brain injury. Progress in Neurobiology. 2017 Dec 1;**159**:50-68 Available from: https://pubmed.ncbi.nlm.nih.gov/29111451/

[19] Noraberg J, Poulsen FR, Blaabjerg M, Kristensen BW, Bonde C, Montero M, et al. Organotypic Hippocampal Slice Cultures for Studies of Brain Damage, Neuroprotection and Neurorepair. Vol. 4. Current Drug Targets: CNS and Neurological Disorders; 2005. pp. 435-452

[20] Berger HR, Brekke E, Widerøe M, Morken TS, Sund Morken T, Morken TS, et al. Neuroprotective treatments after perinatal hypoxic-ischemic brain injury evaluated with magnetic resonance spectroscopy. Developmental Neuroscience. 2017;**39**(1-4):36-48 Available from: http://www.ncbi.nlm.nih.gov/pubmed/28448965

[21] Wu Q, Chen W, Sinha B, Tu Y, Manning S, Thomas N, et al. Neuroprotective agents for neonatal hypoxic–ischemic brain injury. Drug Discovery Today. 2015 Nov;**20**(11):1372-1381 Available from: http://www.ncbi.nlm.nih.gov/pubmed/26360053

[22] Thornton C, Leaw B, Mallard C, Nair S, Jinnai M, Hagberg H. Cell death in the developing brain after hypoxia-ischemia. Frontiers in Cellular Neuroscience. 2017;**11**(August):1-19 Available from: http://journal.frontiersin.org/article/10.3389/fncel.2017.00248/full

[23] Edwards AB, Anderton RS, Knuckey NW, Meloni BP. Perinatal Hypoxic-Ischemic Encephalopathy and Neuroprotective Peptide Therapies: A Case for Cationic Arginine-Rich Peptides (CARPs). Vol. 8. MDPI AG: Brain Sciences; 2018

[24] Descloux C, Ginet V, Clarke PGH, Puyal J, Truttmann AC. Neuronal death after perinatal cerebral hypoxia-ischemia: Focus on autophagy-mediated cell death. International Journal of Developmental Neuroscience. 2015 Oct;**45**:75-85 Available from: http://linkinghub.elsevier.com/retrieve/pii/S0736574815300125

[25] Leaw B, Nair S, Lim R, Thornton C, Mallard C, Hagberg H. Mitochondria. Bioenergetics and Excitotoxicity: New Therapeutic Targets in Perinatal Brain Injury. Front Cell Neurosci. 2017

Jul 12;**11**:199 Available from: http://journal.frontiersin.org/article/10.3389/fncel.2017.00199/full

[26] Cornelius C, Crupi R, Calabrese V, Graziano A, Milone P, Pennisi G, et al. Traumatic brain injury: Oxidative stress and Neuroprotection. Antioxidants & Redox Signaling. 2013 Sep 10;**19**(8):836-853 Available from: http://www.ncbi.nlm.nih.gov/pubmed/23547621

[27] Mehta A, Prabhakar M, Kumar P, Deshmukh R, Sharma PL. Excitotoxicity: Bridge to various triggers in neurodegenerative disorders. European Journal of Pharmacology. 2013 Jan 5;**698**(1-3):6-18 Available from: http://www.ncbi.nlm.nih.gov/pubmed/23123057

[28] Dasuri K, Zhang L, Keller JN. Oxidative stress, neurodegeneration, and the balance of protein degradation and protein synthesis. Free Radical Biology & Medicine. 2013 Sep;**62**:170-185 Available from: http://www.ncbi.nlm.nih.gov/pubmed/23000246

[29] Schimmel S, Acosta S, Lozano D. Neuroinflammation in traumatic brain injury: A chronic response to an acute injury. Brain Circ. 2017;**3**(3):135 Available from: http://www.ncbi.nlm.nih.gov/pubmed/30276315

[30] Venegoni W, Shen Q, Thimmesch AR, Bell M, Hiebert JB, Pierce JD. The use of antioxidants in the treatment of traumatic brain injury. Journal of Advanced Nursing. 2017 Jun;**73**(6):1331-1338 Available from: http://www.ncbi.nlm.nih.gov/pubmed/28103389

[31] Hiebert JB, Shen Q, Thimmesch AR, Pierce JD. Traumatic brain injury and mitochondrial dysfunction. The American Journal of the Medical Sciences. 2015 Aug;**350**(2):132-138 Available from: http://www.ncbi.nlm.nih.gov/pubmed/26083647

[32] Whelan SP, Zuckerbraun BS. Mitochondrial Signaling: Forwards, backwards, and In between. Oxidative Medicine and Cellular Longevity. 2013;**2013**:1-10 Available from: http://www.ncbi.nlm.nih.gov/pubmed/23819011

[33] Zhang L, Wang H, Zhou X, Mao L, Ding K, Hu Z. Role of mitochondrial calcium uniporter-mediated Ca 2+ and iron accumulation in traumatic brain injury. Journal of Cellular and Molecular Medicine. 2019 Feb 12 Available from: http://www.ncbi.nlm.nih.gov/pubmed/30756474

[34] Weidinger A, Kozlov A, Weidinger A, Kozlov AV. Biological activities of reactive oxygen and nitrogen species: Oxidative stress versus signal transduction. Biomolecules. 2015 Apr 15;**5**(2):472-484 Available from: http://www.mdpi.com/2218-273X/5/2/472

[35] Rodríguez-Rodríguez A, Egea-Guerrero JJ, Murillo-Cabezas F, Carrillo-Vico A. Oxidative stress in traumatic brain injury. Current Medicinal Chemistry. 2014 Apr;**21**(10):1201-1211 Available from: http://www.ncbi.nlm.nih.gov/pubmed/24350853

[36] Rousset CI, Baburamani AA, Thornton C, Hagberg H. Mitochondria and perinatal brain injury. In: Journal of Maternal-Fetal and Neonatal Medicine. 2012. pp. 35-38

[37] Kagan VE, Chu CT, Tyurina YY, Cheikhi A, Bayir H. Cardiolipin asymmetry, oxidation and signaling. Chemistry and Physics of Lipids. 2014 Apr;**179**:64-69. Available from http://www.ncbi.nlm.nih.gov/pubmed/24300280

[38] Toro-Urrego N, Garcia-Segura LM, Echeverria V, Barreto GE. Testosterone protects mitochondrial function and regulates Neuroglobin expression in

Astrocytic cells exposed to glucose deprivation. Frontiers in Aging Neuroscience. 2016 Jun;**27**(8):152 Available from: http://www.ncbi.nlm.nih.gov/pubmed/27445795

[39] Paradies G, Petrosillo G, Paradies V, Ruggiero FM. Role of cardiolipin peroxidation and Ca2+in mitochondrial dysfunction and disease. Cell Calcium. 2009;**45**:643-650

[40] Anthonymuthu TS, Kenny EM, Bayır H. Therapies targeting lipid peroxidation in traumatic brain injury. Brain Research. 2016 Jun 1;**1640**(Pt A):57-76 Available from: http://www.ncbi.nlm.nih.gov/pubmed/26872597

[41] Cristofori L, Tavazzi B, Gambin R, Vagnozzi R, Vivenza C, Amorini AM, et al. Early onset of lipid peroxidation after human traumatic brain injury: A fatal limitation for the free radical scavenger pharmacological therapy? Journal of Investigative Medicine. 2001;**49**(5):450-458

[42] Bélanger M, Magistretti PJ. The role of astroglia in neuroprotection. Dialogues in Clinical Neuroscience. 2009;**11**(3):281-295 Available from: http://www.ncbi.nlm.nih.gov/pubmed/19877496

[43] Karki P, Webb A, Zerguine A, Choi J, Son DS, Lee E. Mechanism of raloxifene-induced upregulation of glutamate transporters in rat primary astrocytes. Glia. 2014;**62**(8):1270-1283

[44] Guillamón-Vivancos T, Gómez-PinedoU,Matías-GuiuJ.Astrocitos en las enfermedades neurodegenerativas (I): función y caracterización molecular. Neurología. 2015 Mar;**30**(2):119-129 Available from: http://www.ncbi.nlm.nih.gov/pubmed/23465689

[45] Fuller S, Steele M, Münch G. Activated astroglia during chronic inflammation in Alzheimer's disease—Do they neglect their neurosupportive roles? Mutat Res Mol Mech Mutagen. 2010 Aug 7;**690**(1-2):40-49 Available from: http://www.ncbi.nlm.nih.gov/pubmed/19748514

[46] Lee KM, AG ML. New advances on glial activation in health and disease. World J Virol. 2015 May 12;**4**(2):42-55 Available from: http://www.ncbi.nlm.nih.gov/pubmed/25964871

[47] Sullivan SM, Björkman ST, Miller SM, Colditz PB, Pow DV. Morphological changes in white matter astrocytes in response to hypoxia/ischemia in the neonatal pig. Brain Research. 2010 Mar;**1319**:164-174 Available from: http://linkinghub.elsevier.com/retrieve/pii/S0006899310000491

[48] Wei S, Tong J, Xue Q, Liu Y, Xu X. Effect of puerarin on transcriptome of astrocyte during oxygen-glucose deprivation/reoxygenation injury. Molecular and Cellular Biochemistry. 2017 Jan 1;**425**(1-2):113-123

[49] Rocha-Ferreira E, Hristova M. Antimicrobial peptides and complement in neonatal hypoxia-ischemia induced brain damage. Frontiers in Immunology. 2015;6:56. Available from: http://www.ncbi.nlm.nih.gov/pubmed/25729383 [cited 12 March 2018]

[50] Hirayama Y, Koizumi S. Astrocytes and ischemic tolerance. Neuroscience Research. 2018;**126**:53-59. Available from: http://linkinghub.elsevier.com/retrieve/pii/S0168010217306946 [cited 12 March 2018]

[51] Sofroniew M V. Astrocyte barriers to neurotoxic inflammation. Vol. 16, Nature Reviews Neuroscience. NIH Public Access; 2015. p. 249-263. Available from: http://www.ncbi.nlm.nih.gov/pubmed/25891508 [cited 12 March 2018]

[52] Millar LJ, Shi L, Hoerder-Suabedissen A, Molnár Z. Neonatal

hypoxia Ischaemia: Mechanisms, models, and therapeutic challenges. Frontiers in Cellular Neuroscience. 2017;11:78. Available from: http://www.ncbi.nlm.nih.gov/pubmed/28533743 [cited 12 March 2018]

[53] Ziemka-Nalecz M, Jaworska J, Zalewska T. Insights into the Neuroinflammatory responses after neonatal hypoxia-ischemia. Journal of Neuropathology and Experimental Neurology. 2017 Aug;**76**(8):644-654. Available from: https://academic.oup.com/jnen/article-lookup/doi/10.1093/jnen/nlx046 [cited 12 March 2018]

[54] Lee WLA, Michael-Titus AT, Shah DK. Hypoxic-ischaemic encephalopathy and the blood-brain barrier in neonates. Developmental Neuroscience. 2017;**39**(1-4):49-58

[55] Paternotte E, Gaucher C, Labrude P, Stoltz JF, Menu P. Review: Behaviour of endothelial cells faced with hypoxia. Bio-medical Materials and Engineering. 2008;**18**(4-5):295-299

[56] Salvador E, Burek M, Förster CY. Stretch and/or oxygen glucose deprivation (OGD) in an in vitro traumatic brain injury (TBI) model induces calcium alteration and inflammatory cascade. Frontiers in Cellular Neuroscience. 2015 Aug 21;**9**:323 Available from: http://www.ncbi.nlm.nih.gov/pmc/articles/PMC4543908/

[57] Huang BY, Castillo M. Hypoxic-ischemic brain injury: Imaging findings from birth to adulthood. Radiographics. 2008 Mar;28(2):417-439. Available from: https://pubmed.ncbi.nlm.nih.gov/18349449/ [cited 19 July 2020]

[58] Folkerth RD. Neuropathologic substrate of cerebral palsy. Journal of Child Neurology. 2005 Dec 2;20(12):940-949. Available from: http://journals.sagepub.com/doi/10.1177/08830738050200120301 [cited 19 July 2020]

[59] McQuillen PS, Sheldon RA, Shatz CJ, Ferriero DM. Selective vulnerability of subplate neurons after early neonatal hypoxia-ischemia. The Journal of Neuroscience. 2003 Apr 15;23(8):3308-3315. Available from: /pmc/articles/PMC6742293/?report=abstract [cited 19 July 2020]

[60] Gopagondanahalli KR, Li J, Fahey MC, Hunt RW, Jenkin G, Miller SL, et al. Preterm hypoxic-ischemic encephalopathy. Vol. 4, Frontiers in Pediatrics. Frontiers Media S.A.; 2016. p. 1. Available from: /pmc/articles/PMC5071348/?report=abstract [cited 19 July 2020]

[61] Hoon AH, Stashinko EE, Nagae LM, Lin DDM, Keller J, Bastian A, et al. Sensory and motor deficits in children with cerebral palsy born preterm correlate with diffusion tensor imaging abnormalities in thalamocortical pathways. Developmental Medicine and Child Neurology. 2009;51(9):697-704. Available from: /pmc/articles/PMC2908264/?report=abstract [cited 19 July 2020]

[62] Forbes TA, Goldstein EZ, Dupree JL, Jablonska B, Scafidi J, Adams KL, et al. Environmental enrichment ameliorates perinatal brain injury and promotes functional white matter recovery. Nature Communications. 2020 Dec 1;11(1). Available from: /pmc/articles/PMC7031237/?report=abstract [cited 19 July 2020]

[63] Andjelkovic A V., Stamatovic SM, Phillips CM, Martinez-Revollar G, Keep RF. Modeling blood–brain barrier pathology in cerebrovascular disease in vitro: Current and future paradigms. Fluids Barriers CNS. 2020 Dec 16;17(1):44. Available from: https://fluidsbarrierscns.biomedcentral.com/articles/10.1186/s12987-020-00202-7 [cited 19 July 2020]

[64] Disdier C, Stonestreet BS. Hypoxic-ischemic-related cerebrovascular changes and potential therapeutic strategies in the neonatal brain. Journal of Neuroscience Research. 2020 Jul 14;98(7):1468-1484. Available from: https://onlinelibrary.wiley.com/doi/abs/10.1002/jnr.24590 [cited 19 July 2020]

[65] Rice JE, Vannucci RC, Brierley JB. The influence of immaturity on hypoxic-ischemic brain damage in the rat. Annals of Neurology 1981 Feb;9(2):131-141. Available from: http://www.ncbi.nlm.nih.gov/pubmed/7235629 [cited 15 April 2018]

[66] Drobyshevsky A, Derrick M, Wyrwicz AM, Ji X, Englof I, Ullman LM, et al. White matter injury correlates with hypertonia in an animal model of cerebral palsy. Journal of Cerebral Blood Flow and Metabolism. 2007 Feb 17;27(2):270-281. Available from: http://www.ncbi.nlm.nih.gov/pubmed/16736047 [cited 16 April 2018]

[67] Kida H, Nomura S, Shinoyama M, Ideguchi M, Owada Y, Suzuki M. The effect of hypothermia therapy on cortical laminar disruption following ischemic injury in neonatal mice. Borlongan C V., editor. PLoS One. 2013 Jul 23;8(7):e68877. Available from: http://www.ncbi.nlm.nih.gov/pubmed/23894362 [cited 16 April 2018]

[68] Lin EP, Miles L, Hughes EA, McCann JC, Vorhees C V., McAuliffe JJ, et al. A combination of mild hypothermia and Sevoflurane affords long-term protection in a modified neonatal mouse model of cerebral hypoxia-ischemia. Anesthesia and Analgesia. 2014 Nov;119(5):1158-1173. Available from: http://www.ncbi.nlm.nih.gov/pubmed/24878681 [cited 16 April 2018]

[69] Dominguez R, Zitting M, Liu Q, Patel A, Babadjouni R, Hodis DM, et al. Estradiol protects white matter of male C57BL6J mice against experimental chronic cerebral Hypoperfusion. Journal of Stroke and Cerebrovascular Diseases. 2018 Jul;27(7):1743-1751. Available from: http://www.ncbi.nlm.nih.gov/pubmed/29602614 [cited 2019 Jul 9]

[70] Reddy K, Mallard C, Guan J, Marks K, Bennet L, Gunning M, et al. Maturational change in the cortical response to Hypoperfusion injury in the Fetal sheep. Pediatric Research. 1998 May;43(5):674-682. Available from: http://www.ncbi.nlm.nih.gov/pubmed/9585015 [cited 16 April 2018]

[71] Derrick M, Drobyshevsky A, Ji X, Tan S. A model of cerebral palsy from Fetal hypoxia-ischemia. Stroke. 2007 Feb 1;38(2):731-735. Available from: http://www.ncbi.nlm.nih.gov/pubmed/17261727 [cited 4 March 2018]

[72] Derrick M, Drobyshevsky A, Ji X, Chen L, Yang Y, Ji H, et al. Hypoxia–ischemia causes persistent movement deficits in a perinatal rabbit model of cerebral palsy: Assessed by a new swim test. International Journal of Developmental Neuroscience. 2009 Oct 1;27(6):549-557. Available from: https://www.sciencedirect.com/science/article/pii/S0736574809001002 [cited 17 April 2018]

[73] Traudt CM, McPherson RJ, Bauer LA, Richards TL, Burbacher TM, McAdams RM, et al. Concurrent erythropoietin and hypothermia treatment improve outcomes in a term nonhuman primate model of perinatal asphyxia. Developmental Neuroscience 2013;35(6):491-503. Available from: http://www.ncbi.nlm.nih.gov/pubmed/24192275 [cited 17 April 2018]

[74] Alaa E, Mishima E, Niizuma K, Akiyama Y, Fujimura M, Tominaga T, et al. Stress-induced tRNA cleavage and tiRNA generation in rat neuronal PC12 cells. Journal of Neurochemistry. 2018 Feb 12; Available from: http://www.

ncbi.nlm.nih.gov/pubmed/29431851 [cited 18 April 2018]

[75] Chen Y, Zhang J, Zhang X. 2-NBDG as a marker for detecting glucose uptake in reactive astrocytes exposed to oxygen-glucose deprivation In vitro. Journal of Molecular Neuroscience. 2015 Jan 6;55(1):126-130. Available from: http://www.ncbi.nlm.nih.gov/pubmed/25091860 [cited 18 April 2018]

[76] Cui X, Fu Z, Wang M, Nan X, Zhang B. Pitavastatin treatment induces neuroprotection through the BDNF-TrkB signalling pathway in cultured cerebral neurons after oxygen-glucose deprivation. Neurological Research. 2018 Mar 16;1-7. Available from: http://www.ncbi.nlm.nih.gov/pubmed/29544396 [cited 18 April 2018]

[77] He W, Liu Y, Tian X. Rosuvastatin improves Neurite outgrowth of cortical neurons against oxygen-glucose deprivation via Notch1-mediated mitochondrial biogenesis and functional improvement. Frontiers in Cellular Neuroscience. 2018 Jan 17;12:6. Available from: http://www.ncbi.nlm.nih.gov/pubmed/29387001 [cited 18 April 2018]

[78] Kim M, Jung K, Kim I-S, Lee I-S, Ko Y, Shin JE, et al. TNF-α induces human neural progenitor cell survival after oxygen–glucose deprivation by activating the NF-κB pathway. Experimental & Molecular Medicine. 2018 Apr 6;50(4):14. Available from: http://www.ncbi.nlm.nih.gov/pubmed/29622770 [cited 18 April 2018]

[79] Dong Y-F, Guo R-B, Ji J, Cao L-L, Zhang L, Chen Z-Z, et al. S1PR3 is essential for phosphorylated fingolimod to protect astrocytes against oxygen-glucose deprivation-induced neuroinflammation via inhibiting TLR2/4-NFκB signalling. Journal of Cellular and Molecular Medicine. 2018 Mar 13; Available from: http://www.ncbi.nlm.nih.gov/pubmed/29536648 [cited 18 April 2018]

[80] Wang Z, Guo L, Wang Y, Zhou H, Wang S, Chen D, et al. Inhibition of HSP90α protects cultured neurons from oxygen-glucose deprivation induced necroptosis by decreasing RIP3 expression. Journal of Cellular Physiology. 2018 Jun;**233**(6):4864-4884 Available from: http://www.ncbi.nlm.nih.gov/pubmed/29334122

[81] Wang K, Zhu Y. Dexmedetomidine protects against oxygen-glucose deprivation/reoxygenation injury-induced apoptosis via the p38 MAPK/ERK signalling pathway. The Journal of International Medical Research. 2018 Feb 6;**46**(2):675-686 Available from: http://www.ncbi.nlm.nih.gov/pubmed/29210287

[82] BAE S, H-J JEONG, CHA HJ, KIM K, CHOI YM, I-S AN, et al. The hypoxia-mimetic agent cobalt chloride induces cell cycle arrest and alters gene expression in U266 multiple myeloma cells. International Journal of Molecular Medicine. 2012 Nov 1;**30**(5):1180-1186 Available from: https://www.spandidos-publications.com/10.3892/ijmm.2012.1115

[83] Guo M, Song L-P, Jiang Y, Liu W, Yu Y, Chen G-Q. Hypoxia-mimetic agents desferrioxamine and cobalt chloride induce leukemic cell apoptosis through different hypoxia-inducible factor-1α independent mechanisms. Apoptosis. 2006 Jan 13;**11**(1):67-77 Available from: http://link.springer.com/10.1007/s10495-005-3085-3

[84] Bordt EA. The importance of controlling in vitro oxygen tension to accurately model in vivo neurophysiology. Neurotoxicology. 2018 May;**66**:213-220 Available from: https://linkinghub.elsevier.com/retrieve/pii/S0161813X17302127

[85] Khan M, Khan H, Singh I, Singh AK. Hypoxia inducible factor-1 alpha stabilization for regenerative therapy in traumatic brain injury. Neural Regeneration Research. 2017

May;**12**(5):696-701 Available from: http://www.ncbi.nlm.nih.gov/pubmed/28616019

[86] Semenza GL. Hypoxia-inducible factor 1: Master regulator of O2 homeostasis. Current Opinion in Genetics & Development. 1998 Oct;**8**(5):588-594 Available from: http://www.ncbi.nlm.nih.gov/pubmed/9794818

[87] Ke Q, Costa M. Hypoxia-Inducible Factor-1 (HIF-1). 2006; Available from: http://molpharm.aspetjournals.org.

[88] Huang LE, Gu J, Schau M, Bunn HF. Regulation of hypoxia-inducible factor 1alpha is mediated by an O2-dependent degradation domain via the ubiquitin-proteasome pathway. Proceedings of the National Academy of Sciences of the United States of America. 1998 Jul 7;**95**(14):7987-7992 Available from: http://www.ncbi.nlm.nih.gov/pubmed/9653127

[89] Wenger RH, Gassmann M. Oxygen(es) and the hypoxia-inducible factor-1. Biological Chemistry. 1997 Jul;**378**(7):609-616 Available from: http://www.ncbi.nlm.nih.gov/pubmed/9278140

[90] Tan WKM, Williams CE, Gunn AJ, Mallard CE, Gluckman PD. Suppression of postischemic epileptiform activity with MK-801 improves neural outcome in fetal sheep. Annals of Neurology. 1992 Nov 1;**32**(5):677-682 Available from: http://doi.wiley.com/10.1002/ana.410320511

[91] Gunn AJ, Gunn TR, de Haan HH, Williams CE, Gluckman PD. Dramatic neuronal rescue with prolonged selective head cooling after ischemia in fetal lambs. The Journal of Clinical Investigation. 1997 Jan 15;**99**(2):248-256. Available from http://www.ncbi.nlm.nih.gov/pubmed/9005993

[92] Reddy K, Mallard C, Guan J, Marks K, Bennet L, Gunning M, et al. Maturational change in the cortical response to Hypoperfusion injury in the Fetal sheep. Pediatric Research. 1998 May;**43**(5):674-682 Available from: http://www.ncbi.nlm.nih.gov/pubmed/9585015

[93] Mallard EC, Williams CE, Johnston BM, Gluckman PD. Increased vulnerability to neuronal damage after umbilical cord occlusion in fetal sheep with advancing gestation. American Journal of Obstetrics and Gynecology. 1994 Jan;**170**(1 Pt 1):206-214 Available from: http://www.ncbi.nlm.nih.gov/pubmed/8296824

[94] Thoresen M, Penrice J, Lorek A, Cady EB, Wylezinska M, Kirkbride V, et al. Mild hypothermia after severe transient hypoxia-ischemia ameliorates delayed cerebral energy failure in the Newborn piglet. Pediatric Research. 1995 May;**37**(5):667-670 Available from: http://www.ncbi.nlm.nih.gov/pubmed/7603788

[95] Laptook AR, Hassan A, Peterson J, Corbett RJ, Nunnally RL, et al. NMR in Biomedicine. 1988 Apr;**1**(2):74-79 Available from: http://www.ncbi.nlm.nih.gov/pubmed/3275028

[96] Gressens P, Marret S, Evrard P. Developmental spectrum of the excitotoxic cascade induced by ibotenate: A model of hypoxic insults in fetuses and neonates. Neuropathology and Applied Neurobiology. 1996 May 30;**22**(6):498-502 Available from: https://doi.org/10.1111/j.1365-2990.1996.tb01123.x

[97] Baud O, Daire J-L, Dalmaz Y, Fontaine RH, Krueger RC, Sebag G, et al. Gestational hypoxia induces white matter damage in neonatal rats: A new model of periventricular leukomalacia. Brain Pathology. 2004 Jan;**14**(1):1-10 Available from: http://www.ncbi.nlm.nih.gov/pubmed/14997932

[98] Sheldon A, Chuai J, Ferriero DM. A rat model for hypoxic-ischemic brain

damage in very premature infants. Neonatology. 1996;**69**(5):327-341 Available from: http://www.ncbi.nlm.nih.gov/pubmed/8790911

[99] Back SA, Han BH, Luo NL, Chricton CA, Xanthoudakis S, Tam J, et al. Selective vulnerability of late oligodendrocyte progenitors to hypoxia-ischemia. The Journal of Neuroscience. 2002 Jan 15;**22**(2):455-463 Available from: http://www.ncbi.nlm.nih.gov/pubmed/11784790

[100] Yang D, Sun Y-Y, Bhaumik SK, Li Y, Baumann JM, Lin X, et al. Blocking lymphocyte trafficking with FTY720 prevents inflammation-sensitized hypoxic–ischemic brain injury in Newborns. The Journal of Neuroscience. 2014 Dec 3;**34**(49):16467-16481 Available from: http://www.ncbi.nlm.nih.gov/pubmed/25471584

[101] Sheldon RA, Jiang X, Francisco C, Christen S, Vexler ZS, Täuber MG, et al. Manipulation of antioxidant pathways in neonatal murine brain. Pediatric Research. 2004 Oct;**56**(4):656-662 Available from: http://www.ncbi.nlm.nih.gov/pubmed/15295091

[102] Doverhag C, Hedtjärn M, Poirier F, Mallard C, Hagberg H, Karlsson A, et al. Galectin-3 contributes to neonatal hypoxic–ischemic brain injury. Neurobiology of Disease. 2010 Apr;**38**(1):36-46 Available from: http://www.ncbi.nlm.nih.gov/pubmed/20053377

[103] Ek CJ, D'Angelo B, Baburamani AA, Lehner C, Leverin A-L, Smith PL, et al. Brain barrier properties and cerebral blood flow in neonatal mice exposed to cerebral hypoxia-ischemia. Journal of Cerebral Blood Flow and Metabolism. 2015 May 28;**35**(5):818-827 Available from: http://www.ncbi.nlm.nih.gov/pubmed/25627141

[104] Hagberg H, Mallard C, Ferriero DM, Vannucci SJ, Levison SW, Vexler ZS, et al. The role of inflammation in perinatal brain injury. Nature Reviews. Neurology. 2015 Feb 17;**11**(4):192-208 Available from: http://www.ncbi.nlm.nih.gov/pubmed/25686754

[105] Renolleau S, Aggoun-Zouaoui D, Ben-Ari Y, Charriaut-Marlangue C. A model of transient unilateral focal ischemia with reperfusion in the P7 neonatal rat: Morphological changes indicative of apoptosis. Stroke. 1998 Jul;**29**(7):1454-1460 discussion 1461. Available from: http://www.ncbi.nlm.nih.gov/pubmed/9660403

[106] Derugin N, Ferriero DM, Vexler ZS. Neonatal reversible focal cerebral ischemia: A new model. Neuroscience Research. 1998 Dec;**32**(4):349-353 Available from: http://www.ncbi.nlm.nih.gov/pubmed/9950062

[107] Fernandez-Lopez D, Faustino J, Daneman R, Zhou L, Lee SY, Derugin N, et al. Blood-brain barrier permeability is increased after acute adult stroke but not neonatal stroke in the rat. The Journal of Neuroscience. 2012 Jul 11;**32**(28):9588-9600 Available from: http://www.ncbi.nlm.nih.gov/pubmed/22787045

[108] Faustino JV, Wang X, Johnson CE, Klibanov A, Derugin N, Wendland MF, et al. Microglial cells contribute to endogenous brain Defenses after acute neonatal focal stroke. The Journal of Neuroscience. 2011 Sep 7;**31**(36):12992-13001 Available from: http://www.ncbi.nlm.nih.gov/pubmed/21900578

[109] Mu D, Jiang X, Sheldon RA, Fox CK, Hamrick SEG, Vexler ZS, et al. Regulation of hypoxia-inducible factor 1alpha and induction of vascular endothelial growth factor in a rat neonatal stroke model. Neurobiology of Disease. 2003 Dec;**14**(3):524-534 Available from: http://www.ncbi.nlm.nih.gov/pubmed/14678768

[110] Woo M-S, Wang X, Faustino JV, Derugin N, Wendland MF, Zhou P, et al. Genetic deletion of CD36 enhances injury after acute neonatal stroke. Annals of Neurology. 2012 Dec;**72**(6):961-970 Available from: http://www.ncbi.nlm.nih.gov/pubmed/23280844

[111] Feng S-J, Zhang X-Q, Li J-T, Dai X-M, Zhao F. miRNA-223 regulates ischemic neuronal injury by targeting the type 1 insulin-like growth factor receptor (IGF1R). Folia Neuropathologica. 2018;**56**(1):49-57 Available from: http://www.ncbi.nlm.nih.gov/pubmed/29663740

[112] Guo M, Wang X, Zhao Y, Yang Q, Ding H, Dong Q, et al. Ketogenic diet improves brain ischemic tolerance and inhibits NLRP3 Inflammasome activation by preventing Drp1-mediated mitochondrial fission and endoplasmic reticulum stress. Frontiers in Molecular Neuroscience. 2018 Mar 20;**11**:86 Available from: http://www.ncbi.nlm.nih.gov/pubmed/29662437

[113] Li Y, Zhao Y, Cheng M, Qiao Y, Wang Y, Xiong W, et al. Suppression of microRNA-144-3p attenuates oxygen-glucose deprivation/reoxygenation-induced neuronal injury by promoting Brg1/Nrf2/ARE signaling. Journal of Biochemical and Molecular Toxicology. 2018 Feb 19:e22044 Available from: http://www.ncbi.nlm.nih.gov/pubmed/29457851

[114] Weng Y, Lin J, Liu H, Wu H, Yan Z, Zhao J. AMPK activation by Tanshinone IIA protects neuronal cells from oxygen-glucose deprivation. Oncotarget. 2018 Jan 12;**9**(4):4511-4521 Available from: http://www.ncbi.nlm.nih.gov/pubmed/29435120

[115] Yin X, Feng L, Ma D, Yin P, Wang X, Hou S, et al. Roles of astrocytic connexin-43, hemichannels, and gap junctions in oxygen-glucose deprivation/reperfusion injury induced neuroinflammation and the possible regulatory mechanisms of salvianolic acid B and carbenoxolone. Journal of Neuroinflammation. 2018 Dec 27;**15**(1):97 Available from: http://www.ncbi.nlm.nih.gov/pubmed/29587860

[116] Zhao X, Zhou K-S, Li Z-H, Nan W, Wang J, Xia Y-Y, et al. Knockdown of ski decreased the reactive astrocytes proliferation in vitro induced by oxygen-glucose deprivation/reoxygenation. Journal of Cellular Biochemistry. 2018 Mar 1 Available from: http://www.ncbi.nlm.nih.gov/pubmed/29236326

[117] Zhou T, Lin H, Jiang L, Yu T, Zeng C, Liu J, et al. Mild hypothermia protects hippocampal neurons from oxygen-glucose deprivation injury through inhibiting caspase-3 activation. Cryobiology. 2018 Feb;**80**:55-61 Available from: http://www.ncbi.nlm.nih.gov/pubmed/29223591

[118] Al Okail MS. Cobalt chloride, a chemical inducer of hypoxia-inducible factor-1α in U251 human glioblastoma cell line. Journal of Saudi Chemical Society. 2010 Apr 1;**14**(2):197-201 Available from: https://www.sciencedirect.com/science/article/pii/S1319610310000207

[119] Elstner A, Holtkamp N, von Deimling A. Involvement of Hif-1 in desferrioxamine-induced invasion of glioblastoma cells. Clinical & Experimental Metastasis. 2007 Mar 15;**24**(1):57-66 Available from: http://www.ncbi.nlm.nih.gov/pubmed/17357815

[120] Guo C, Hao L-J, Yang Z-H, Chai R, Zhang S, Gu Y, et al. Deferoxamine-mediated up-regulation of HIF-1α prevents dopaminergic neuronal death via the activation of MAPK family proteins in MPTP-treated mice. Experimental Neurology. 2016 Jun;**280**:13-23 Available from: http://www.ncbi.nlm.nih.gov/pubmed/26996132

[121] Hamrick SEG, McQuillen PS, Jiang X, Mu D, Madan A, Ferriero DM. A role for hypoxia-inducible factor-1α in desferoxamine neuroprotection. Neuroscience Letters. 2005 May 6;**379**(2):96-100 Available from: http://www.ncbi.nlm.nih.gov/pubmed/15823423

[122] Hishikawa T, Ono S, Ogawa T, Tokunaga K, Sugiu K, Date I. Effects of DEFEROXAMINE-activated hypoxia-inducible FACTOR-1 on the brainstem after subarachnoid HEMORRHAGE IN rats. Neurosurgery. 2008 Jan 1;**62**(1):232-241 Available from: http://www.ncbi.nlm.nih.gov/pubmed/18300912

[123] Jones SM, Novak AE, Elliott JP. The role of HIF in cobalt-induced ischemic tolerance. Neuroscience. 2013 Nov 12;**252**:420-430 Available from: http://www.ncbi.nlm.nih.gov/pubmed/23916558

[124] Li L, Yin X, Ma N, Lin F, Kong X, Chi J, et al. Desferrioxamine regulates HIF-1 alpha expression in neonatal rat brain after hypoxia-ischemia. American Journal of Translational Research. 2014;**6**(4):377-383 Available from: http://www.ncbi.nlm.nih.gov/pubmed/25075254

[125] Mehrabani M, Najafi M, Kamarul T, Mansouri K, Iranpour M, Nematollahi MH, et al. Deferoxamine preconditioning to restore impaired HIF-1α-mediated angiogenic mechanisms in adipose-derived stem cells from STZ-induced type 1 diabetic rats. Cell Proliferation. 2015 Oct;**48**(5):532-549 Available from: http://www.ncbi.nlm.nih.gov/pubmed/26332145

[126] Mu D, Chang YS, Vexler ZS, Ferriero DM. Hypoxia-inducible factor 1α and erythropoietin upregulation with deferoxamine salvage after neonatal stroke. Experimental Neurology. 2005 Oct;**195**(2):407-415 Available from: http://www.ncbi.nlm.nih.gov/pubmed/16023639

[127] van der Kooij MA, Groenendaal F, Kavelaars A, Heijnen CJ, van Bel F. Combination of deferoxamine and erythropoietin: Therapy for hypoxia–ischemia-induced brain injury in the neonatal rat? Neuroscience Letters. 2009 Feb 20;**451**(2):109-113 Available from: http://www.ncbi.nlm.nih.gov/pubmed/19103262

[128] Baulieu EE, Robel P, Schumacher M. Neurosteroids: Beginning of the story. International Review of Neurobiology. 2001;**46**:1-32 Available from: http://www.ncbi.nlm.nih.gov/pubmed/11599297

[129] Reddy DS, Estes WA. Clinical potential of Neurosteroids for CNS disorders. Vol. 37, trends in pharmacological sciences. Elsevier Ltd. 2016:543-561

[130] Dubrovsky B. Neurosteroids, neuroactive steroids, and symptoms of affective disorders. Pharmacology, Biochemistry, and Behavior. 2006 Aug;**84**(4):644-655

[131] Ferando I, Mody I. GABA a receptor modulation by neurosteroids in models of temporal lobe epilepsies. Epilepsia. 2012 Dec;**53**:89-101

[132] Gavrilova VA, Ivanova SA, Gusev SI, Trofimova MV, Bokhan NA. Neurosteroids dehydroepiandrosterone and its sulfate in individuals with personality disorders convicted of serious violent crimes. Bulletin of Experimental Biology and Medicine. 2012 Nov;**154**(1):89-91

[133] Borovska J, Vyklicky V, Stastna E, Kapras V, Slavikova B, Horak M, et al. Access of inhibitory neurosteroids to the NMDA receptor. British Journal of Pharmacology. 2012 Jun;**166**(3):1069-1083

[134] González-Usano A, Cauli O, Agustí A, Felipo V. Hyperammonemia alters the modulation by different neurosteroids of the glutamate-nitric oxide-cyclic GMP pathway through NMDA- GABAA- or sigma receptors in cerebellum in vivo. Journal of Neurochemistry. 2013 Apr;**125**(1):133-143

[135] Omura Y, Lu D, Jones MK, Nihrane A, Duvvi H, Shimotsuura Y, et al. Early detection of autism (ASD) by a non-invasive quick measurement of markedly reduced acetylcholine & DHEA and increased β-amyloid (1-42), Asbestos (Chrysotile), titanium dioxide, Al, Hg & often coexisting virus infections (CMV, HPV 16 and 18), bacterial infections etc. in the brain and corresponding safe individualized effective treatment. Acupuncture and Electro-Therapeutics Research. Cognizant Communication Corporation. 2015;**40**:157-187

[136] Biagini G, Marinelli C, Panuccio G, Puia G, Avoli M. Glia-neuron interactions: Neurosteroids and Epileptogenesis. Jasper's Basic Mech Epilepsies. 2012:1-16 Available from: http://www.ncbi.nlm.nih.gov/pubmed/22787673%5Cnhttp://www.ncbi.nlm.nih.gov/pubmed/22787594

[137] Brinton RD. Neurosteroids as regenerative agents in the brain: Therapeutic implications. Nature Reviews Endocrinology. 2013;**9**:241-250

[138] King SR. Neurosteroids and the Nervous System2013. pp. 1-122. Available from. DOI: http://link.springer.com/10.1007/978-1-4614-5559-2_1

[139] Hidalgo Lanussa O, Ávila-Rodriguez M, Miguel García-Segura L, González J, Echeverria V, Aliev G, et al. Microglial dependent protective effects of neuroactive steroids. CNS Neurol Disord - Drug Targets. 2016 Feb 9;**15**(2):242-249

[140] Srivastava DP. Two-step wiring plasticity - a mechanism for estrogen-induced rewiring of cortical circuits. Journal of Steroid Biochemistry and Molecular Biology. 2012;**131**:17-23

[141] Ávila Rodriguez M, Garcia-Segura LM, Cabezas R, Torrente D, Capani F, Gonzalez J, et al. Tibolone protects T98G cells from glucose deprivation. The Journal of Steroid Biochemistry and Molecular Biology. 2014;**144**(PART B):294-303

[142] Wang S, Wang B, Feng Y, Mo M, Du F, Li H, et al. 17β-Estradiol ameliorates light-induced retinal damage in Sprague–Dawley rats by reducing oxidative stress. Journal of Molecular Neuroscience. 2014;**55**(1):141-151

[143] Cardona-Gomez GP, Mendez P, Garcia-Segura LM. Synergistic interaction of estradiol and insulin-like growth factor-I in the activation of PI3K/Akt signaling in the adult rat hypothalamus. Brain Research. Molecular Brain Research. 2002 Oct 30;**107**(1):80-88 Available from: http://www.ncbi.nlm.nih.gov/pubmed/12414126

[144] Garcia-Segura LM, Arevalo MA, Azcoitia I. Interactions of estradiol and insulin-like growth factor-I signalling in the nervous system: New advances. Progress in Brain Research. 2010;**181**(C):251-272

[145] Perillo B, Sasso A, Abbondanza C, Palumbo G. 17beta -Estradiol inhibits apoptosis in MCF-7 cells, inducing bcl-2 expression via two Estrogen-responsive elements present in the coding sequence. Molecular and Cellular Biology. 2000 Apr 15;**20**(8):2890-2901

[146] Arevalo MA, Santos-Galindo M, Lagunas N, Azcoitia I,

Garcia-Segura LM. Selective estrogen receptor modulators as brain therapeutic agents. Journal of Molecular Endocrinology. 2011 Feb 1;**46**(1):R1-R9 Available from: http://www.ncbi.nlm.nih.gov/pubmed/21071476

[147] Vegeto E, Benedusi V, Maggi A. Estrogen anti-inflammatory activity in brain: A therapeutic opportunity for menopause and neurodegenerative diseases. Frontiers in Neuroendocrinology. 2008;**29**:507-519

[148] Guo J, Duckles SP, Weiss JH, Li X, Krause DN. 17β-Estradiol prevents cell death and mitochondrial dysfunction by an estrogen receptor-dependent mechanism in astrocytes after oxygen-glucose deprivation/reperfusion. Free Radical Biology & Medicine. 2012 Jun 1;**52**(11-12):2151-2160

[149] Simpkins JW, Dykens JA. Mitochondrial mechanisms of estrogen neuroprotection. Brain Research Reviews. 2008;**57**:421-430

[150] Mendez P, Garcia-Segura LM. Phosphatidylinositol 3-kinase and glycogen synthase kinase 3 regulate Estrogen receptor-mediated transcription in neuronal cells. Endocrinology. 2006 Jun 1;**147**(6):3027-3039 Available from: http://dx.doi.org/10.1210/en.2005-1224

[151] Prokai L, Prokai-Tatrai K, Perjési P, Simpkins JW. Mechanistic insights into the direct antioxidant effects of estrogens. Drug Development Research. 2005 Oct;**66**(2):118-125 Available from: http://doi.wiley.com/10.1002/ddr.20050

[152] Tang S. ERGDB: Estrogen Responsive Genes Database. Nucleic Acids Research. 2004 Jan 1;**32**(90001):533D-5536D

[153] Colditz GA, Hankinson SE, Hunter DJ, Willett WC, Manson JE, Stampfer MJ, et al. The use of estrogens and progestins and the risk of breast cancer in postmenopausal women. The New England Journal of Medicine. 1995 Jun 15;**332**(24):1589-1593

[154] Manolio TA, Furberg CD, Shemanski L, Psaty BM, O'Leary DH, Tracy RP, et al. Associations of postmenopausal estrogen use with cardiovascular disease and its risk factors in older women. The CHS collaborative research group 86. Circulation. 1993 Nov;**88**(0009-7322 (Print):2163-2171

[155] Brynhildsen J, Hammar M. Lipids and clotting factors during low dose transdermal estradiol/norethisterone use. Maturitas. 2005 Apr 11;**50**(4):344-352

[156] Lemini C, Franco Y, Avila ME, Jaimez R. Contrasting effects of estradiol and 17 beta-aminoestrogens on blood clotting time in rats and mice. European Journal of Pharmacology. 2005 Mar 14;**510**(3):229-233 Available from: http://www.ncbi.nlm.nih.gov/pubmed/15763247

[157] Taxel P, Luthra P, Fall PM, Dauser D. The effect of short-term estradiol therapy on clotting and inflammatory markers in older men receiving hormonal suppression therapy for prostate cancer. The Aging Male. 2008 Jun;**11**(2):71-75

[158] Wise PM, Suzuki S, Brown CM. Estradiol: A hormone with diverse and contradictory neuroprotective actions. Dialogues in Clinical Neuroscience. 2009;**11**:297-303

[159] Liu M, Kelley MH, Herson PS, Hurn PD. Neuroprotection of sex steroids. Minerva Endocrinologica. 2010;**35**:127-143

[160] Kloosterboer HJ. Tissue-selectivity: The mechanism of action of tibolone. In: Maturitas. Elsevier Ireland Ltd; 2004. pp. 30-40

[161] Sanchez AC, Alsina JCI, Dueñas-Díez JL. Selective Estrogen Receptor Modulators: A New Brand of Multitarget Drugs. Selective Estrogen Receptor Modulators: A New Brand of Multitarget Drugs. Springer Berlin Heidelberg; 2006. pp. 1-357

[162] Brzozowski AM, Pike ACW, Dauter Z, Hubbard RE, Bonn T, Engström O, et al. Molecular basis of agonism and antagonism in the oestrogen receptor. Nature. 1997;**389**(6652):753-758

[163] Cano A, Morcillo N, Lopez F, Marquina P, Parrilla JJ, Abad L. Cytoplasmicandnuclearestrogenbinding capacity in the rat uterus during treatment with danazol and testosterone. European Journal of Obstetrics, Gynecology, and Reproductive Biology. 1986 Apr;**21**(4):245-252 Available from: http://www.ncbi.nlm.nih.gov/pubmed/3709924

[164] Díaz Chico BN, Bosch DN, Díaz Chico JC, Escriche EE. Molecular mechanisms of estrogen action in target tissues. In: Selective Estrogen Receptor Modulators: A New Brand of Multitarget Drugs. Berlin Heidelberg: Springer; 2006. pp. 2-47

[165] McKenna NJ, Lanz RB, O'Malley BW. Nuclear receptor Coregulators: Cellular and molecular biology*. Endocrine Reviews. 1999 Jun 1;**20**(3):321-344

[166] Shiau AK, Barstad D, Loria PM, Cheng L, Kushner PJ, Agard DA, et al. The structural basis of estrogen receptor/coactivator recognition and the antagonism of this interaction by tamoxifen. Cell. 1998 Dec 23;**95**(7):927-937 Available from: http://www.ncbi.nlm.nih.gov/pubmed/9875847

[167] Vogelvang TE, Van Der Mooren MJ, Mijatovic V. Hormone replacement therapy, selective Estrogen receptor modulators, and tissue-specific compounds: Cardiovascular effects and clinical implications. Treatments in Endocrinology. 2004;**3**:105-115

[168] Kokiko ON, Murashov AK, Hoane MR. Administration of raloxifene reduces sensorimotor and working memory deficits following traumatic brain injury. Behavioural Brain Research. 2006 Jun 30;**170**(2):233-240

[169] Mosquera L, Colón JM, Santiago JM, Torrado AI, Meléndez M, Segarra AC, et al. Tamoxifen and estradiol improved locomotor function and increased spared tissue in rats after spinal cord injury: Their antioxidant effect and role of estrogen receptor alpha. Brain Research. 2014 May 2;**1561**:11-22

[170] González-Burgos I, Rivera-CervantesMC,Velázquez-ZamoraDA, Feria-Velasco A, Garcia-Segura LM. Selective estrogen receptor modulators regulate dendritic spine plasticity in the hippocampus of male rats. Neural Plasticity. 2012;**2012**

[171] Wakade C, Khan MM, De Sevilla LM, Zhang QG, Mahesh VB, Brann DW. Tamoxifen neuroprotection in cerebral ischemia involves attenuation of kinase activation and superoxide production and potentiation of mitochondrial superoxide dismutase. Endocrinology. 2008 Jan;**149**(1):367-379

[172] Simoncini T, Mannella P, Fornari L, Caruso A, Varone G, Genazzani AR. Genomic and non-genomic effects of estrogens on endothelial cells. Steroids. 2004;**69**(8):537-542 Available from: http://www.sciencedirect.com/science/article/pii/S0039128X04000753

[173] Armagan G, Kanit L, Terek CM, Sozmen EY, Yalcin A. The levels of glutathione and nitrite-nitrate and the expression of BCL-2 mRNA in ovariectomized rats treated by raloxifene against kainic acid. The

International Journal of Neuroscience. 2009 Feb;**119**(2):227-239

[174] Martino S, Cauley JA, Barrett-Connor E, Powles TJ, Mershon J, Disch D, et al. Continuing outcomes relevant to Evista: Breast cancer incidence in postmenopausal osteoporotic women in a randomized trial of raloxifene. Journal of the National Cancer Institute. 2004 Dec 1;**96**(23):1751-1761

[175] Ingle JN, Suman VJ, Mailliard JA, Kugler JW, Krook JE, Michalak JC, et al. Randomized trial of tamoxifen alone or combined with fluoxymesterone as adjuvant therapy in postmenopausal women with resected estrogen receptor positive breast cancer. North central Cancer treatment group trial 89-30-52. Breast Cancer Research and Treatment. 2006 Jul;**98**(2):217-222

[176] Arevalo MA, Diz-Chaves Y, Santos-Galindo M, Bellini MJ, Garcia-Segura LM. Selective oestrogen receptor modulators decrease the inflammatory response of glial cells. Journal of Neuroendocrinology. 2012;**24**:183-190

[177] Belenichev IF, Odnokoz OV, Pavlov SV, Belenicheva OI, Polyakova EN. The neuroprotective activity of tamoxifen and tibolone during glutathione depletion in vitro. Neurochemical Journal. 2012 Jul;**6**(3):202-212

[178] Catalano S, Giordano C, Panza S, Chemi F, Bonofiglio D, Lanzino M, et al. Tamoxifen through GPER upregulates aromatase expression: A novel mechanism sustaining tamoxifen-resistant breast cancer cell growth. Breast Cancer Research and Treatment. 2014;**146**(2):273-285

[179] López Ruiz JR, Osuna Carrasco LP, López Valenzuela CL, Franco Rodríguez NE, de la Torre VB, Jiménez Estrada I, et al. The hippocampus participates in the control of locomotion speed. Neuroscience. 2015 Dec 17;**311**:207-215

[180] Karki P, Webb A, Zerguine A, Choi J, Son DS, Lee E. Mechanism of raloxifene-induced upregulation of glutamate transporters in rat primary astrocytes. Glia. 2014;**62**(8):1270-1283

[181] Shang Y, Brown M. Molecular determinants for the tissue specificity of SERMs. Science (80-). 2002 Mar 29;**295**(5564):2465-2468

[182] Gupta B, Mittal P, Khuteta R, Bhargava A. A comparative study of CEE, tibolone, and DHEA as hormone replacement therapy for surgical menopause. J Obstet Gynecol India. 2013 Jun;**63**(3):194-198

[183] Albertazzi P, Di Micco R, Zanardi E. Tibolone: A review. Maturitas. 1998 Nov 16;**30**(3):295-305 Available from: http://www.ncbi.nlm.nih.gov/pubmed/9881330

[184] Campisi R, Marengo FD. Cardiovascular effects of tibolone: A selective tissue estrogenic activity regulator. Cardiovascular Drug Reviews. 2007;**25**:132-145

[185] Escande A, Servant N, Rabenoelina F, Auzou G, Kloosterboer H, Cavaillès V, et al. Regulation of activities of steroid hormone receptors by tibolone and its primary metabolites. The Journal of Steroid Biochemistry and Molecular Biology. 2009 Aug;**116**(1-2):8-14

[186] Vos RME, Krebbers SFM, Verhoeven CHJ, Delbressine LPC. The in vivo human metabolism of tibolone. Drug Metabolism and Disposition. 2002;**30**(2):106-112

[187] Guzmán CB, Zhao C, Deighton-collins S, Kleerekoper M, Benjamins JA, Skafar DF. Agonist activity of the 3-hydroxy metabolites of tibolone through the oestrogen receptor in the

mouse N20.1 oligodendrocyte cell line and normal human astrocytes. Journal of Neuroendocrinology. 2007 Dec;**19**(12):958-965

[188] Tian WY, Zhang HY, Su LK, Shen WZ. Effects of tibolone on apoptosis of neurons after cerebral ischemia-reperfusion injury in rats. Acad J Second Mil Med Univ. 2009 Jul;**30**(7):790-792

[189] Kloosterboer HJ, Löfgren L, Von Schoulz E, Von Schoultz B, Verheul HAM. Estrogen and tibolone metabolite levels in blood and breast tissue of postmenopausal women recently diagnosed with early-stage breast cancer and treated with tibolone or placebo for 14 days. Reproductive Sciences. 2007 Feb;**14**(2):151-159

[190] Falany JL, Falany CN. Interactions of the human cytosolic sulfotransferases and steroid sulfatase in the metabolism of tibolone and raloxifene. The Journal of Steroid Biochemistry and Molecular Biology. 2007 Nov;**107**(3-5):202-210

[191] De Marinis E, Fiocchetti M, Acconcia F, Ascenzi P, Marino M. Neuroglobin upregulation induced by 17β-estradiol sequesters cytocrome c in the mitochondria preventing H2 O2 -induced apoptosis of neuroblastoma cells. Cell Death & Disease. 2013 Feb;**4**:2

[192] De Marinis E, Ascenzi P, Pellegrini M, Galluzzo P, Bulzomi P, Arevalo MA, et al. 17β-Estradiol - a new modulator of neuroglobin levels in neurons: Role in neuroprotection against H 2O 2-induced toxicity. Neuro-Signals. 2011 Mar;**18**(4):223-235

[193] De Marinis E, Acaz-Fonseca E, Arevalo MA, Ascenzi P, Fiocchetti M, Marino M, et al. 17β-Oestradiol anti-inflammatory effects in primary astrocytes require oestrogen receptor β-mediated neuroglobin up-regulation. Journal of Neuroendocrinology. 2013 Mar;**25**(3):260-270

[194] Acaz-Fonseca E, Sanchez-Gonzalez R, Azcoitia I, Arevalo MA, Garcia-Segura LM. Role of astrocytes in the neuroprotective actions of 17β-estradiol and selective estrogen receptor modulators. Molecular and Cellular Endocrinology. 2014;**389**:48-57

[195] Pinto Almazán R, Rivas Arancibia S, Farfán García ED, Rodríguez Martínez E, Guerra AC. Efecto neuroprotector de la tibolona contra el estrés oxidativo inducido por la exposición a ozono. Revista de Neurologia. 2014;**58**(10):441 Available from: https://www.neurologia.com/articulo/2013357

[196] Beltrán-Campos V, Díaz-Ruiz A, Padilla-Gómez E, Aguilar Zavala H, Ríos C, Díaz Cintra S. Effect of tibolone on dendritic spine density in the rat hippocampus. Neurol(English Ed.). 2015 Sep;**30**(7):401-406

[197] Maguire J. Neuroactive steroids and GABaergic involvement in the neuroendocrine dysfunction associated with major depressive disorder and postpartum depression. Frontiers in Cellular Neuroscience, Frontiers Media S.A. 2019;**13**

[198] Hillerer KM, Slattery DA, Pletzer B. Neurobiological mechanisms underlying sex-related differences in stress-related disorders: Effects of neuroactive steroids on the hippocampus. Frontiers in Neuroendocrinology. 2019;**55**

[199] Frau R, Traccis F, Bortolato M. Neurobehavioural complications of sleep deprivation: Shedding light on the emerging role of neuroactive steroids. Journal of Neuroendocrinology. 2019

[200] Aleman M, McCue PM, Chigerwe M, Madigan JE. Plasma concentrations of steroid precursors, steroids, neuroactive steroids, and neurosteroids in healthy neonatal foals from birth to 7 days of age. Journal of

Veterinary Internal Medicine. 2019 Sep 1;**33**(5):2286-2293

[201] Knytl P, VoráCková V, Dorazilová A, Rodriguez M, CvrCková A, Kofronová E, et al. Neuroactive steroids and cognitive functions in first-episode psychosis patients and their healthy siblings. Frontiers in Psychiatry. 2019;**10** (Jun)

[202] Modgil A, Parakala ML, Ackley MA, Doherty JJ, Moss SJ, Davies PA. Endogenous and synthetic neuroactive steroids evoke sustained increases in the efficacy of GABAergic inhibition via a protein kinase C-dependent mechanism. Neuropharmacology. 2017 Feb 1;**113**:314-322

[203] Deligiannidis KM, Fales CL, Kroll-Desrosiers AR, Shaffer SA, Villamarin V, Tan Y, et al. Resting-state functional connectivity, cortical GABA, and neuroactive steroids in peripartum and peripartum depressed women: A functional magnetic resonance imaging and spectroscopy study. Neuropsychopharmacology. 2019 Feb 1;**44**(3):546-554

[204] Giatti S, Diviccaro S, Melcangi RC. Neuroactive steroids and sex-dimorphic nervous damage induced by diabetes mellitus. Cellular and Molecular Neurobiology. 2019;**39**:493-502

[205] Giatti S, Garcia-Segura LM, Barreto GE, Melcangi RC. Neuroactive steroids, neurosteroidogenesis and sex. Progress in Neurobiology. 2019;**176**:1-17

[206] McEvoy K, Payne JL, Osborne LM. Neuroactive steroids and perinatal depression: A review of recent literature. Current Psychiatry Reports. 2018;**20**

[207] Melcangi RC, Panzica GC. Neuroactive steroids and metabolic axis. Frontiers in Neuroendocrinology. 2018;**48**:1-2

[208] Dichtel LE, Lawson EA, Schorr M, Meenaghan E, Paskal ML, Eddy KT, et al. Neuroactive steroids and affective symptoms in women across the weight Spectrum. Neuropsychopharmacology. 2018 May 1;**43**(6):1436-1444

[209] Tuem KB, Atey TM. Neuroactive steroids: Receptor interactions and responses. Frontiers in Neurology. 2017 Aug;**8**(Aug):28

[210] Martinez Botella G, Salituro FG, Harrison BL, Beresis RT, Bai Z, Blanco MJ, et al. Neuroactive steroids. 2. 3α-Hydroxy-3β-methyl-21-(4-cyano-1H-pyrazol-1′-yl)-19-nor-5β-pregnan-20-one (SAGE-217): A clinical next generation Neuroactive steroid positive allosteric modulator of the (γ-Aminobutyric acid) a receptor. Journal of Medicinal Chemistry. 2017;**60**(18):7810-7819

[211] Dembek KA, Timko KJ, Johnson LM, Hart KA, Barr BS, David B, et al. Steroids, steroid precursors, and neuroactive steroids in critically ill equine neonates. Veterinary Journal. 2017 Jul 1;**225**:42-49

[212] Solanki RK, Sharma P, Tyagi A, Singh C. Serum levels of neuroactive steroids in first-episode antipsychotic-na'ive schizophrenic patients and its correlation with aggression: A case-control study. East Asian Archives of Psychiatry. 2017 Jun 1;**27**(2):79-84

[213] Rasmusson AM, Marx CE, Pineles SL, Locci A, Scioli-Salter ER, Nillni YI, et al. Neuroactive steroids and PTSD treatment. Neuroscience Letters. 2017;**649**:156-163

[214] Porcu P, O'Buckley TK, Lopez MF, Becker HC, Miles MF, Williams RW, et al. Initial genetic dissection of serum neuroactive steroids following chronic intermittent ethanol across BXD mouse strains. Alcohol. 2017 Feb 1;**58**:107-125

[215] Casas S, Gonzalez Deniselle MC, Gargiulo-Monachelli GM, Perez AF, Tourreilles M, Mattiazzi M, et al. Neuroactive steroids in acute ischemic stroke: Association with cognitive, functional, and neurological outcomes. Hormone and Metabolic Research. 2017 Jan 1;**49**(1):16-22

[216] Straub RH. The complex role of estrogens in inflammation. Endocrine Reviews. 2007;**28**:521-574

[217] Brunori M, Vallone B. Neuroglobin, seven years after. Cellular and Molecular Life Sciences. 2007 May;**64**(10):1259-1268 Available from: http://www.ncbi.nlm.nih.gov/pubmed/17385072

[218] Xiao QC, Lu YQ, Chen GZ, Li TY, Gao Z, Liu S, et al. Presence of neuroglobin in cultured astrocytes. Glia. 2005 Apr 15;**50**(2):182-186

[219] Venis S. Neuroglobin might protect brain cells during stroke. Lancet. 2001;**358**(9298):2055

[220] Gao XY, Huang JO, Hu YF, Gu Y, Zhu SZ, Bin HK, et al. Combination of mild hypothermia with neuroprotectants has greater neuroprotective effects during oxygen-glucose deprivation and reoxygenation-mediated neuronal injury. Scientific Reports. 2014;**4**

[221] Li Y, Dai Y. Bing, Sun J yun, Xiang Y, Yang J, Dai S yang, et al. Neuroglobin attenuates Beta amyloid-induced apoptosis through inhibiting Caspases activity by activating PI3K/Akt Signaling pathway. Journal of Molecular Neuroscience. 2016 Jan 1;**58**(1):28-38

[222] Trent JT, Watts RA, Hargrove MS. Human Neuroglobin, a Hexacoordinate Hemoglobin that reversibly binds oxygen. The Journal of Biological Chemistry. 2001 Aug 10;**276**(32):30106-30110

[223] Hua S, Antao ST, Corbet A, Witting P. k. Retraction notice: The significance of Neuroglobin in the brain. Current Medicinal Chemistry. 2009 Dec 21;**17**(2):160-172

[224] Brittain T, Skommer J, Raychaudhuri S, Birch N. An Antiapoptotic Neuroprotective Role for Neuroglobin. International Journal of Molecular Sciences. 2010 May 27;**11**(6):2306-2321 Available from: http://www.mdpi.com/1422-0067/11/6/2306

[225] Sadava DE, Hillis DM, Heller CH, Berenbaum M. Libro Life 10th.Pdf2014. pp. 893-894

[226] Zhao L, O'Neill K, Diaz BR. Selective estrogen receptor modulators (SERMs) for the brain: Current status and remaining challenges for developing NeuroSERMs. Brain Research Reviews. 2005;**49**(3):472-493

[227] Paterni I, Granchi C, Katzenellenbogen JA, Minutolo F. Estrogen receptors alpha (ERα) and Beta (ERβ): Subtype-selective ligands and clinical potential. Steroids. 2014 Nov 15:13-29 Available from: http://www.ncbi.nlm.nih.gov/pmc/articles/PMC4192010/

[228] Arevalo MA, Azcoitia I, Garcia-Segura LM. The neuroprotective actions of oestradiol and oestrogen receptors. Nature Reviews. Neuroscience. 2015;**16**(1):17-29 Available from: http://dx.doi.org/10.1038/nrn3856

[229] Shang Y, Hu X, DiRenzo J, Lazar MA, Brown M. Cofactor dynamics and sufficiency in Estrogen receptor–regulated transcription. Cell. 2000 Dec 8;**103**(6):843-852 Available from: https://doi.org/10.1016/S0092-8674(00)00188-4

[230] Safe S, Kim K. NONCLASSICAL GENOMIC ER/Sp AND ER/AP-1 SIGNALING PATHWAYS. Journal of Molecular Endocrinology. 2008 Nov

4;**41**(5):263-275 Available from: http://www.ncbi.nlm.nih.gov/pmc/articles/PMC2582054/

[231] Ruiz-Palmero I, Hernando M, Garcia-Segura LM, Arevalo M-A. G protein-coupled estrogen receptor is required for the neuritogenic mechanism of 17β-estradiol in developing hippocampal neurons. Molecular and Cellular Endocrinology. 2013;**372**(1-2):105-115 Available from: http://europepmc.org/abstract/MED/23545157

[232] Qiu J, Bosch MA, Tobias SC, Grandy DK, Scanlan TS, Ronnekleiv OK, et al. Rapid signaling of estrogen in hypothalamic neurons involves a novel G-protein-coupled estrogen receptor that activates protein kinase C. The Journal of Neuroscience. 2003 Oct 22;**23**(29):9529-9540 Available from: http://www.ncbi.nlm.nih.gov/pubmed/14573532

[233] Gerstner B, Lee J, DeSilva TM, Jensen FE, Volpe JJ, Rosenberg PA. 17β-Estradiol protects against hypoxic/ischemic white matter damage in the neonatal rat brain. Journal of Neuroscience Research. 2009 Jul;**87**(9):2078-2086 Available from: http://www.ncbi.nlm.nih.gov/pmc/articles/PMC2770176/

[234] Nuñez J, Yang Z, Jiang Y, Grandys T, Mark I, Levison SW. 17β-Estradiol protects the neonatal brain from hypoxia-ischemia. Experimental Neurology. 2007 Dec 12;**208**(2):269-276 Available from: http://www.ncbi.nlm.nih.gov/pmc/articles/PMC2194656/

[235] Barreto G, Saraceno E, Gonzalez J, Kolliker R, Castilla R, Capani F. Chapter 8 - Neuroprotection with Estradiol in Experimental Perinatal Asphyxia: A New Approach A2 - Duncan, Kelli a. BT - Estrogen Effects on Traumatic Brain Injury. San Diego: Academic Press; 2015. pp. 113-124 Available from: https://www.sciencedirect.com/science/article/pii/B9780128014790000085

[236] Charriaut-Marlangue C, Besson VC, Baud O. Sexually dimorphic outcomes after neonatal stroke and hypoxia-ischemia. International Journal of Molecular Sciences. 2018;**19**:1

[237] Elzer JG, Muhammad S, Wintermantel TM, Regnier-Vigouroux A, Ludwig J, Schütz G, et al. Neuronal Estrogen receptor-α mediates Neuroprotection by 17β-Estradiol. Journal of Cerebral Blood Flow and Metabolism. 2009 Dec 16;**30**(5):935-942 Available from: https://doi.org/10.1038/jcbfm.2009.258

[238] Nelson ER, Wardell SE, McDonnell DP. The molecular mechanisms underlying the pharmacological actions of estrogens, SERMs and oxysterols: Implications for the treatment and prevention of osteoporosis. Bone. 2013;**53**(1):42-50

[239] Marín F, Barbancho MC. Action of selective Estrogen receptor modulators (SERMs) through the classical mechanism of Estrogen action. In: Selective Estrogen Receptor Modulators. Berlin Heidelberg: Springer; 2006. pp. 71-77. Available from. DOI: http://link.springer.com/10.1007/3-540-34742-9_3

[240] Khan MM, Wakade C, de Sevilla L, Brann DW. Selective estrogen receptor modulators (SERMs) enhance neurogenesis and spine density following focal cerebral ischemia. The Journal of Steroid Biochemistry and Molecular Biology. 2015 Feb;**146**:38-47 Available from: http://www.ncbi.nlm.nih.gov/pubmed/24815952

[241] Lopez-Rodriguez AB, Ávila-Rodriguez M, Vega-vela NE, Capani F, Gonzalez J, Garciá-Segura LM, et al. Estrogen Effects on Traumatic Brain Injury. 2015.

[242] Leaw B, Nair S, Lim R, Thornton C, Mallard C, Hagberg H. Mitochondria, bioenergetics and Excitotoxicity: New therapeutic targets in perinatal

brain injury. Frontiers in Cellular Neuroscience. 2017 Jul 12;**11**:199 Available from: http://journal.frontiersin.org/article/10.3389/fncel.2017.00199/full

[243] Wu Q, Chen W, Sinha B, Tu Y, Manning S, Thomas N, et al. Neuroprotective agents for neonatal hypoxic-ischemic brain injury. Drug Discovery Today. 2015;**20**:1372-1381 Available from: https://www.sciencedirect.com/science/article/pii/S1359644615003414?via%3Dihub

Section 3

Mechanisms of Action of Other Potential Neuroprotective Treatments

Chapter 12

Glyproline Pro-Ampakine with Neuroprotective Activity

Ksenia N. Koliasnikova, Polina Yu. Povarnina, Anna V. Tallerova, Yulia N. Firsova, Sergei V. Nikolaev, Tatiana A. Antipova, Anna V. Nadorova, Larisa G. Kolik, Tatiana A. Gudasheva and Sergei B. Seredenin

Abstract

Previously it was shown that neuropeptide cyclo-L-prolylglycine (CPG) is a positive modulator of AMPA receptors, which increases BDNF level in neuronal cell cultures. The spectrum of CPG's pharmacological effects corresponds to that of BDNF. Dipeptide N-phenylacetyl-glycyl-L-proline ethyl ester (GZK-111) was designed and synthesized as a linear analog of CPG. The aim of the present work was to reveal the pharmacological profile of GZK-111. Dipeptide GZK-111 was shown to metabolize into CPG in vitro and increased cell survival by 28% at concentrations of 10-7–10-6 M in a Parkinson's disease cell model. In a model of cerebral ischemia, GZK-111, at a dose of 0.5 mg/kg, i.p., was found to have neuroprotective effects, reducing the cerebral infarct volume by 1.6 times. Similar to CPG, GZK-111, at the range 0.1–1.0 mg/kg, i.p., possessed a stereospecific antiamnesic activity. A significant anxiolytic effect was observed at a dose of 1.5 mg/kg. GZK-111, at the range 0.5–4.0 mg/kg, i.p., demonstrated analgesic activity. GZK-111, at a dose of 10 mg/kg/7 days, i.p., possessed antidepressant-like activity. So, the neuroprotective, nootropic, antihypoxic, anxiolytic, antidepressant-like, and analgesic effects of GZK-111 were revealed. Thus, GZK-111 can be considered as a pharmacologically active pro-ampakine with a BDNF-ergic mechanism of action.

Keywords: glyproline GZK-111, pro-ampakine, cyclo-prolylglycine, BDNF, neuroprotective activity

1. Introduction

Cyclo-*L*-prolylglycine (CPG) was designed as a potential peptide prototype of piracetam, the classic nootropic drug [1] and was subsequently discovered as endogenous compound in the brain of intact rats in micromolar concentration [2]. CPG is similar to piracetam both in structure and main pharmacological effects; it possesses nootropic [3], anxiolytic [4, 5], antihypoxic [6], neuroprotective [6, 7], analgesic [8], and antidepressant [9, 10] activities at central administration at doses 100–1000 times smaller than those for piracetam. Recently, we have demonstrated CPG to be ampakine, i.e., a positive modulator of AMPA receptors [11]. Like other ampakines, it increases brain-derived neurotrophic factor (BDNF) content in neuronal cell cultures [12]. The range of CPG pharmacological effects corresponds both to that of piracetam and BDNF. In view of this, CPG can be regarded as a basis for creation of new group of drugs with neuroprotective properties.

CPG is a hydrophilic compound. The task to create an amphiphilic CPG prodrug with improved pharmacokinetic properties, converted to active molecule in the brain, was established to increase drug passage through biological membranes, including the blood-brain barrier. Two variants of substituted dipeptides, based on the Pro-Gly or Gly-Pro sequence, could be used for this purpose. We selected the second one (i.e., Gly-Pro), following the known information that an imide bond with proline in Gly-Pro dipeptide sequence increased the proportion of the cisoid peptide bond [13, 14], which, in turn, promoted cyclization of the dipeptide [15, 16].

In this work, we synthesized substituted glyproline *N*-phenylacetyl-glycyl-*L*-proline ethyl ester (GZK-111) to prove the hypothesis, confirmed the CPG formation during GZK-111 metabolism in the presence of blood plasma enzymes, and demonstrated the compound pharmacological effects typical for CPG and BDNF, namely, neuroprotective, nootropic, antihypoxic, anxiolytic, antidepressant, and analgesic activities.

2. Materials and methods

2.1 Chemical experimental part

The chemical reagents used in the synthesis were obtained from commercial suppliers and used without purification. All solvents were dried and purified by standard procedures if required. Melting points were measured in open capillary tubes using OptiMelt melting point apparatus (Stanford Research Systems, USA). The structures of the compounds were confirmed by elemental analysis and ^{1}H NMR spectroscopy. The NMR spectra were obtained on a Bruker Fourier 300 (Bruker, Germany) spectrometer using tetramethylsilane as an internal standard. The NMR peaks were designated as follows: s, singlet; d, doublet; t, triplet; and m, multiplet. Microanalyses for C, H, and N agreed with calculated values within 0.4%. Specific optical rotations were recorded by automatic polarimeter ADP 440 (Bellingham + Stanley Ltd., England). The TLC was carried out on Merck silica gel 60 F 254 plates with spot visualization by iodine vapor or UV light.

***N*-Phenylacetyl-glycine.** 13.24 ml (0.1 mol) of N-phenylacetyl chloride and 25 ml of 4 M NaOH were added dropwise successively to a solution of 7.5 g (0.1 mol) of glycine in 25 ml of 4 M NaOH under stirring at −10°C. The reaction mixture was stirred for 30 min on cooling, extracted by ethyl acetate (3 × 15 ml) to remove impurities and unreacted N-phenylacetyl chloride. Then the solution was acidified by 4 M HCl to pH 2–3; the resulting precipitate was filtered, washed with cooled distilled water, and dried in air. The yield of N-phenylacetyl-glycine was 5.83 g (30%); m.p. 143–144°C; R_f 0.8 (BuOH/AcOH/H_2O, 4:1:1). ^{1}H-NMR spectrum (DMSO-d_6 + CF_3COOD, d, ppm): 3.47 (s, 2H, CH_2Ar), 3.76 (d, *J* 6.0 Hz, 2H, CH_2 Gly), 7.27 (m, 5H, ArH), 8.40 (t, *J* 6.0 Hz, 1H, NH Gly). Lit. data [17]: m.p. 138–143°C.

H-*L*-Pro-OC_2H_5·HCl. 2.54 ml (35 mmol) of thionyl chloride was added dropwise to 60 ml of anhydrous ethanol cooled to −20°C. Then 2.0 g (17.5 mmol) of *L*-proline was added portionwise under vigorous stirring. The resulting mixture was stirred for 2 h at −5°C and then for 2 h at room temperature. The solvent was removed in vacuo. This operation was repeated twice, each time adding 30 ml of anhydrous ethyl alcohol to afford 2.4 g (77%) of *L*-proline ethyl ester hydrochloride as an oil. $[\alpha]^{23}{}_{D}$ −43° (*c* 3, EtOH); R_f 0.75 (i-PrOH/NH_3, 7:3). ^{1}H-NMR spectrum ($DMSO-d_6$, d, ppm): 1.19 (m, 3H, CH_3CH_2O), 1.8–2.1 (m, 4H, $C^{\gamma}H_2$ Pro, $C^{\beta}H_2$ Pro), 3.2 (m, 2H, $C^{\delta}H_2$ Pro), 4.2 (m, 2H, CH_3CH_2O), 4.5 (m, 1H, $C^{\alpha}H$ Pro), 9.9 (br. s, 1H, NH). Lit. data [18]: oil; $[\alpha]^{23}{}_{D}$ −44.8° (*c* 3.03, EtOH).

H-*D*-Pro-OC_2H_5·HCl. Obtained similarly to H-*L*-Pro-OC_2H_5·HCl from *D*-proline. $[\alpha]^{23}{}_{D}$ + 42.0° (*c* 3, EtOH); R_f 0.75 (i-PrOH/NH_3, 7:3). ^{1}H-NMR spectrum ($DMSO-d_6$, d, ppm): 1.18 (m, 3H, CH_3CH_2O), 1.8–2.1 (m, 4H, $C^{\gamma}H_2$ Pro, $C^{\beta}H_2$ Pro), 3.19 (m, 2H, $C^{\delta}H_2$ Pro), 4.2 (m, 2H, CH_3CH_2O), 4.5 (m, 1H, $C^{\alpha}H$ Pro), 9.9 (br. s, 1H, NH). Lit. data [18]: oil; $[\alpha]^{23}{}_{D}$ +44.16° (*c* 3.03, EtOH).

***N*-Phenylacetyl-glycyl-*L*-proline ethyl ester.** 1.1 ml (10.0 mmol) of *N*-methylmorpholine and 1.35 ml (10.0 mmol) of isobutyl chloroformate were added simultaneously at −10°C to a vigorously stirred solution of 1.93 (10.0 mmol) *N*-phenylacetyl-glycine in dimethylformamide (10 mL). After 2 min a mixture of 1.79 g (10.0 mmol) of proline ethyl ester hydrochloride and 1.1 ml (10.0 mmol) of *N*-methylmorpholine in dimethylformamide (20 mL) was added dropwise. The reaction mixture was stirred at −10°C for 30 min and then at room temperature for 1 h. The precipitate was separated by filtration; the solvent was evaporated in vacuo; the residue was dissolved in chloroform (25 ml). The solution was washed with 3% solution of $NaHCO_3$ (3 × 7 ml), water (3 × 7 ml), and 1 N HCl (3 × 7 ml). The organic layer was dried with anhydrous Na_2SO_4, filtered, and evaporated to dryness. The yield of chromatographically homogeneous product was 2.87 g (90%), an orange oil, finally crystallized from ethyl acetate/hexane system. M.p. 111–112°C; $[a]^{23}{}_{D}$ −90.0° (*c* 1, water); R_f = 0.80 (dioxane/H_2O, 9:1). ^{1}H-NMR spectrum ($DMSO-d_6$, d, ppm): 1.2 (m, 3H, CH_3CH_2O), 1.8–2.1 (m, 4H, $C^{\gamma}H_2$ Pro, $C^{\beta}H_2$ Pro), 3.5 (s, 2H, CH_2ArH), 3.6 (m, 2H, $C^{\delta}H_2$ Pro), 3.85 and 4.0 (2 dd, *J* 17.6 Hz, *J* 5.6 Hz, 2H, $C^{\alpha}H_2$ Gly), 4.2 (m, 2H, CH_3CH_2O), 4.5 (dd, *J* 4.0 Hz, *J* 8.5 Hz, 1H, $C^{\alpha}H$ Pro), 6.4 (br. t, *J* 5.6 Hz, 1H, NH), 7.3 (m, 5H, ArH). Calcd. for $C_{17}H_{22}N_2O_4$, %: C, 64.27; H, 7.05; N, 8.63. Found, %: C, 64.13; H, 6.97; N, 8.80.

C_6H_5-CH_2-C(O)-Gly-*D*-Pro-OEt (GZK-121). Obtained similarly to the *L*-enantiomer. Yield 64%. M.p. 112–113°C; $[a]^{23}{}_{D}$ +90.0° (*c* 1, water); R_f = 0.80 (dioxane/H_2O, 9:1). ^{1}H-NMR spectrum ($DMSO-d_6$, d, ppm): 1.2 (m, 3H, CH_3CH_2O), 1.85–2.2 (m, 4H, $C^{\gamma}H_2$ Pro, $C^{\beta}H_2$ Pro), 3.5 (s, 2H, CH_2Ar), 3.6 (m, 2H, $C^{\delta}H_2$ Pro), 3.86 and 4.0 (2 dd, *J* 17.6 Hz, *J* 5.6 Hz, 2H, $C^{\alpha}H_2$ Gly), 4.2 (m, 2H, CH_3CH_2O), 4.5 (dd, *J* 4.0 Hz, *J* 8.5 Hz, 1H, $C^{\alpha}H$ Pro), 6.4 (br. t, *J* 5.6 Hz, 1H, NH), 7.3 (m, 5H, Ar). Calcd. for $C_{17}H_{22}N_2O_4$., %: C, 64.27; H, 7.05; N, 8.63. Found, %: C, 63.91; H, 6.90; N, 8.71.

2.2 Biological experimental

2.2.1 Study of GZK-111 metabolism

Blood plasma preparation. Blood plasma of outbred male rats weighing 250–280 g was used. Animals were decapitated, blood was collected in BD Vacutainer® tubes with EDTA, and plasma was obtained by centrifugation at 3000 rpm for 10 min.

Incubation and extraction. A solution of 3 mg of GZK-111 in 100 μl of saline was added to 900 μl of rat plasma. The mixture was incubated at 37°C in a water bath for 10 h. Then, an equal volume of acetonitrile was added to 100 μl of the incubated mixture, the samples were vigorously shaken for 10 min and centrifuged at 12,000 rpm for 10 min, and the supernatant was collected and then chromatographed.

Reverse-phase high-performance liquid chromatography (*RP HPLC*). HPLC was performed on a Gilson 41 chromatograph (Gilson, USA) with a Gilson 116 UV detector (Gilson, USA). Detection was carried out at 220 nm. A Nucleosil C18 column (4.6 × 150 mm, 5 μm) was used with a flow rate of 0.5 ml/min. The sample volume was 20 μl. The following eluents were used: (solution A) 3.7 mM sodium 1-hexanesulfonate/water (pH 3.5) and (solution B) 3.7 mM sodium 1-hexanesulfonate/40% acetonitrile. The elution was carried out in a gradient according to the following program: (1) 0% B for 3 min, (2) from 0 to 100% B in 20 min, and (3) 100% B for 6 min. The signal was recorded using the Multichrom 1.5 software (Ampersend, RF). Cyclo-*L*-prolylglycine and *N*-phenylacetyl-glycyl-*L*-proline, synthesized in the Medicinal Chemistry Department of the V.V. Zakusov Research Institute of Pharmacology, were used as standards for HPLC.

Calibration curve. Standard solutions of synthetic cyclo-L-prolylglycine were prepared in acetonitrile at the concentrations of 0, 0.1, 0.2, 0.4, 0.8, 1.6, and 3.2 mg/L. The 20 μl aliquot of the solutions were chromatographed under RP HPLC conditions as described above. The calibration curve was calculated based on the peak areas.

2.2.2 *In vitro pharmacological study*

Cell culture. The studies were carried out on SH-SY5Y human neuroblastoma cells received from the cell bank of the N.N. Blokhin National Medical Research Center of Oncology of the Ministry of Health of the Russian Federation. Cells were grown at 37°C and 5% CO_2 in DMEM (HyClone, USA) with 10% FBS (Gibco, USA) and 2 mM L-glutamine (MP Biomedicals, Germany). After the monolayer formation, the cells were counted and placed into 96-well culture plates (Costar-Corning, USA) at a density of 3.5 thousand per well and into 6-well culture plates (Costar-Corning, USA) at a density of 280 thousand per well; both plates were pre-coated with a 0.1 mg/ml solution of poly-D-lysine (BD Bioscience, UK) for 1 h.

Parkinson's disease model in culture of SH-SY5Y human neuroblastoma cells. Neurotoxin 6-hydroxidopamine (6-OHDA) used in an experimental model of in vitro dopaminergic neuron degeneration according to [19] was applied to simulate Parkinson's disease in the culture of SH-SY5Y human neuroblastoma cells. 6-OHDA was added into the cell medium at a final concentration of 100 μM 24 h after cell seeding. Then the cells were incubated for 24 h. The neuroprotective effect was investigated by addition of compounds to the culture medium at final concentrations of 10^{-8}–10^{-5} M 24 h before 6-OHDA. Cell viability was determined after 24 h using the MTT test.

Neuronal viability assessment in culture using the MTT test. MTT (3-[4,5-dimethylthiazol-2-yl]-2,5-diphenyltetrazolium bromide) is a yellow water-soluble tetrazolium salt that easily penetrates into cells. In living cells, MTT transforms into water-insoluble violet formazan crystals, which are dissolved in organic solvents (isopropanol, dimethylformamide, dimethyl sulfoxide) upon completion of the reaction followed by absorption measurements.

At the end of the experiment, the culture medium was replaced with MTT solution (0.5 mg/ml) and incubated for 30 min at 37°C. Then, a MTT solution was removed from the wells, and DMSO was added to dissolve the formazan. Absorbance was measured at 600 nm using a 96-well plate reader Multiscan (Thermo, USA).

2.2.3 *In vivo pharmacological studies*

In vivo studies were performed in outbred male rats weighing 200–270 g (nootropic and a anxiolytic activity), in outbred male mice weighing 25–28 g (antihypoxic and antidepressant-like activity), and in C57Bl/6 male mice weighing

25–29 g (analgesic activity), received from the Stolbovaya Branch of the Scientific Center of Biomedical Technologies of the Federal Medical Biological Agency (FMBA) of Russia, and in Wistar male rats weighing 200–250 g (neuroprotective activity) received from the Andreevka Branch of the Scientific Center of Biomedical Technologies of the FMBA of Russia. The animals were kept in vivarium under natural circadian light/dark cycles with free access to standard granular feed and water. The study complied with the requirements of Order of the Ministry of Health of the Russian Federation No. 199 "On Approval of the Rules of Good Laboratory Practice" and Decision of the Council of the Eurasian Economic Commission No. 81 "On Approval of the Rules of Good Laboratory Practice of the Eurasian Economic Union in the Area of Circulation of Medicines." All manipulations with animals were approved by the Bioethical Commission of the Zakusov Research Institute of Pharmacology. The experiments were carried out from 10 to 16 pm. The test substances were dissolved in saline or in distilled water and administered, i.p. The animals of the control groups were injected with saline or with distilled water, respectively.

2.2.4 Neuroprotective activity

A model of focal cerebral ischemia (ischemic stroke). Focal cerebral ischemia was induced by transient middle cerebral artery occlusion (MCAO) using a modification of the intraluminal filament model originally described in [20]. All surgical procedures were performed using titanium microsurgical instruments.

The rats were anesthetized with an i.p. injection of chloral hydrate (350 mg/kg) as a 5% solution in saline. The right common carotid artery, internal carotid artery, and external carotid artery were surgically exposed. A nylon suture (0.25 mm in diameter) with a silicon-coated tip was inserted from the external carotid artery into the internal carotid artery and then to the circle of Willis to occlude the origin of the middle cerebral artery. After 1 h of MCAO, the suture was carefully removed to induce reperfusion. Sham-operated rats (n = 6) underwent identical surgery except that the suture was not inserted. During the surgery the body temperature was maintained at $37.0 \pm 0.5°C$ using a heating pad. Three rats received MCAO without any neurological deficits observed after awakening was excluded.

Design of the study. The rats with experimental ischemic stroke were randomly divided into two groups: a "stroke" group with water treatment (n = 10) and "stroke + GZK-111" group treated with GZK-111 (n = 7). Solution of GZK-111 in distilled water was administered, i.p., at a dose 0.5 mg/kg 6 h after surgery and then once a day for 6 days. Neurological functions were evaluated 3 and 6 days after surgery using the limb-placing test [21]. The infarct volume was evaluated according to [22] using 2,3,5-triphenyltetrazolium chloride (TTC) staining and computerized image analysis 7 days after surgery.

Limb-placing test. Neurological functions were evaluated using the limb-placing test [21], a modified version of the test described by De Ryck et al. [23]. This test assessed the forelimb and hind limb responses to tactile and proprioceptive stimulation and consisted of seven limb-placing tasks. The following scores were used to detect impairment of the forelimb and hind limb: 2 points, the rat performed normally; 1 point, the rat performed with a delay of more than 2 s and/or incompletely; and 0 point, the rat did not perform the task. The maximum possible score for the sham-operated rats for each side of the body was 14. Rats with experimental stroke exhibited decreased neurological score on the side of the body which is opposite to the ischemic lesion.

Evaluation of cerebral infarct volume. The cerebral infract volumes measured with TTC staining were used to describe the severity of cerebral ischemia. The animals were deeply anesthetized with chloral hydrate (350 mg/kg, i.p.) and then decapitated. The brains were removed rapidly, frozen in −20°C for 10 min and then sectioned coronally into 2-mm-thick slices. The brain slices were incubated with 2% TTC at 37°C for 30 min. Stained slices were fixed in 10% formalin solution. The slices were digitalized on a flatbed scanner at 2400 dpi. The infarct volumes were measured using the ImageJ (National Institutes of Health, Bethesda, MD, USA) image analysis software program. The total infarct volume for each brain was calculated by summation of unstained areas of the subsequent slices and multiplying by the thickness (2 mm).

Nootropic antiamnesic activity. The antiamnesic effect of the substances was evaluated by their ability to prevent impaired reproduction of the conditioned passive avoidance reflex (passive avoidance reaction) caused by electroconvulsive shock (ECS). Compounds GZK-111 and GZK-121 were administered once, i.p., at the doses of 0.1, 0.5, and 1.0 mg/kg 40 min before training. Control animals were injected with the same volume of physiological saline.

Passive avoidance reaction was developed in rats in a certified Lafayette Instrument Co installation (USA) according to the method of [24] using a single training procedure. The illuminated start platform (25 × 7 cm) was connected to a dark 40 × 40 × 40 cm chamber equipped with an electrified floor through a square guillotine door. The animal was placed on the start platform with its tail to a dark chamber. When governed by the hole exploratory behavior, the rat found the entrance and passed into the dark compartment; the hole was closed. In the dark chamber, eight unavoidable electric pain stimuli were applied through the floor to the rat (the training current was 0.45 mA, the duration of each pulse was 1 s, and the interval between consecutive pulses was 2 s). Immediately after this, the rat was removed from the dark chamber and subjected to EKS (250 V, 120–122 mA, 0.1 s) applied transcorneally using a certified Harvard apparatus (Germany). After 24 h, the animal was again placed on the illuminated platform for learning test. The latent period of the first animal entry into the dark chamber was recorded. Antiamnesic activity (AA) was calculated as Eq. (1):

$$AA\% = \frac{LPtest - LPamn}{LPcontrol - LPamn} \times 100\% \qquad (1)$$

where AA% is antiamnesic activity, LPtest is the average latent period of entry into the chamber in the animals administered with the test compound and subjected to amnesia, LPamn is the average period of entry into the chamber in the animals administered with 0.9% NaCl and subjected to amnesia, and LPcontrol is the average latent period of entry into the chamber in animals administered with 0.9% NaCl without amnesia.

Antihypoxic activity was studied in a model of normobaric hypoxia with hypercapnia ("canned" hypoxia), according to [25]. Tests were performed on animals of the same weight (scatter in groups of ≤2 g). Each group consisted of 10 animals. The substances were administered, i.p., in saline 1 h before the start of the experiment. Antihypoxic activity of the compounds was studied at doses of 0.1, 0.5, and 1.0 mg/kg. Control animals received an equivalent volume of saline. Animals were placed singly into 200 cm^3 containers that were hermetically sealed. Deaths of animals were recorded as the final agonal gasp.

Anxiolytic activity was studied in an elevated plus maze test according to Pellow [26]. Compounds were administered once, i.p., 15 min before the experiment. GZK-111 was administered at doses of 0.75, 1.5, and 3.0 mg/kg and GZK-121 at a dose of 1.5 mg/kg. The control animals were administered with the saline. The apparatus consisted of four arms elevated 60 cm above the floor, with each arm positioned at 90° relative to the adjacent arms. Two opposite arms were enclosed with high opaque walls ($50 \times 15 \times 30$ cm), and the other arms were open ($50 \times 15 \times 1$ cm) connected via a central area (14×14 cm) to form a plus sign. At the beginning of the experiment, the rats were placed in the center of the maze, randomly orientated relative to the arm entrance. The behavior of the animals was evaluated within 5 min. The following indicators were recorded: the number of visits to all arms, the number of visits to open arms, the time spent in all arms, and the time spent in open arms. The anxiolytic effect of the compound was estimated by the increase in the number of visits to the light arms and in the time spent in the light arms and on the central platform.

Antidepressant-like activity was assessed in a forced swimming test [27]. Mice were placed into cylinders (30 cm high and 10 cm in diameter), filled in two-thirds with water at a temperature of 22°C for 5 min; the time of preservation of the characteristic immobilization posture (rejection of active defensive and research behavior) was estimated. The behavior of animals was recorded using a video camera. Video recording of the experiment was processed in semiautomatic mode using the RealTimer program (Open Joint-Stock Company Open Science LLC). A decrease in the immobilization duration was regarded as a manifestation of antidepressant activity.

Analgesic activity. The hot plate test was used to evaluate the nociceptive response. Latent reaction period (the time before the hind paw pulling and/or jumping) was recorded with a Ugo Basile analgesimeter (Italy). 1–2 hours before the experiment, animals were selected following the basic response in the experimental model conditions and excluding mice that remained on a plate heated to 55 ± 0.5°C for longer than 10 s. A latent period of 20 s (cutoff value) was regarded as 100% analgesia. Hot plate tests were performed before and 30, 60, 90, and 120 min after i. p. drug injection. If no response occurred within 20 s, the mice were removed from the hot plate to avoid tissue injury. The percentage of the maximum possible effect (% MPE) was calculated as follows: $(\text{postdrug latency} - \text{predrug latency}) \times 100/(\text{cutoff value} - \text{predrug latency})$.

Statistical analysis of the biological results was performed using the standard software package "Statistica 10.0" (StatSoft, Inc., USA). To evaluate statistically significant differences between the experimental and control groups of animals, the following tests were used: nonparametric Mann-Whitney U test for nootropic, anxiolytic, antihypoxic, and neuroprotective effects, the unpaired Student t-test for antidepressant effect, and Duncan criterion for analgesic effect. The means and standard errors of the mean ($m \pm SEM$) were calculated. Kruskal-Wallis ANOVA followed by Dunn's posttest was used to compare three or more samples in in vitro experiments. The means and standard errors of the mean ($m \pm SD$) were calculated. The results were evaluated as significant at $p \leq 0.05$.

3. Results and discussions

3.1 Synthesis of GZK-111

N-Phenylacetyl-glycyl-L-proline ethyl ester was prepared according to **Figure 1** by the mixed anhydride method under Anderson conditions [28] using isobutyl chloroformate. *N*-phenylacetylglycine obtained from glycine and phenylacetic acid chloride according to Schotten-Baumann procedure [29] was used as carboxylic component, and proline ethyl ester obtained with thionyl chloride in absolute ethanol according to Brenner method [30] was used as amine component. The D-enantiomer of GZK-111 (GZK-121) was prepared by the same procedure.

3.2 Biotransformation of GZK-111 to CPG

Synthesized GZK-111 was subjected to biotransformation in the presence of plasma enzymes to show the fundamental possibility of its conversion to CPG. The initial plasma contained endogenous CPG at a concentration of 1 μM, according to RP HPLC. Upon GZK-111 incubation with plasma at 37°C for 10 h, an increase of the CPG peak and appearance of a peak corresponding to the retention time of the compound with an open carboxyl group, N-phenylacetyl-glycyl-L-proline, were observed (see **Figure 2**). Thus, CPG is actually formed from GZK-111 in the presence of blood plasma enzymes. The scheme of GZK-111 metabolism is shown in **Figure 3**.

3.3 Pharmacological effects of GZK-111

Based on the previously established pharmacological effects of CPG, the pharmacological activity of GZK-111 (viz., neuroprotective, antiamnesic, antihypoxic, anxiolytic, antidepressant-like, and analgesic effects) was studied.

The **neuroprotective effect** of GZK-111 was studied **in vitro** in a 6-OHDA toxicity model in SH-SY5Y cells (cellular model of Parkinson's disease) [19, 31], which demonstrated the neuroprotective effect of CPG previously [6]. GZK-111 was introduced 24 h before 6-OHDA, because pharmacological effects of its metabolite (CPG) were probably caused by BDNF synthesis [12], which took no less than 6 h [32]. When introduced 24 h before the injury, GZK-111 was revealed to have neuroprotective activity at concentrations of 10^{-7} and 10^{-6} M (**Figure 4**). The range of active concentrations of CPG was 10^{-8}–10^{-5} M in this model [6].

The **neuroprotective activity** of GZK-111 was studied **in vivo** in a model of ischemic stroke caused by transient occlusion of the middle cerebral artery in rats, according to [20]. This model allows to simulate the most common cerebrovascular accident—an extensive ischemic stroke in the middle cerebral artery basin—and provides a reproducible volume of ischemic injury [33]. The compound was administered, i.p., at a dose of 0.5 mg/kg/day for 7 days; the first injection was given 6 h after surgery. The GZK-111 dose was taken accordingly to the results of other pharmacological studies (see **Tables 1** and **2**). The duration of substance introduction corresponds to the period of poststroke treatment in a hospital with consideration to differences in the metabolic rates of animals and humans [34]. The first administration of the compound 6 h after ischemia is explained by preservation of penumbra zone during this period [35], which makes it possible to decrease the volume of ischemic damage. Neurological functions were evaluated 3 and 6 days after surgery using the limb-placing test [21]. The infarct volume was evaluated 7 days after surgery according to [22] with 2,3,5-triphenyltetrazolium chloride staining and computerized image analysis. GZK-111 was found to have pronounced neuroprotective effects, reducing the volume of the infarct zone by 1.6 times (**Figure 5**) and improving the neurological status of animals by approximately 30% (**Figure 6**).

The neuroprotective activity of CPG (1.0 mg/kg, i.p., subchronic) was revealed previously in a model of incomplete global cerebral ischemia induced by permanent bilateral common carotid arteries occlusion in rats [7].

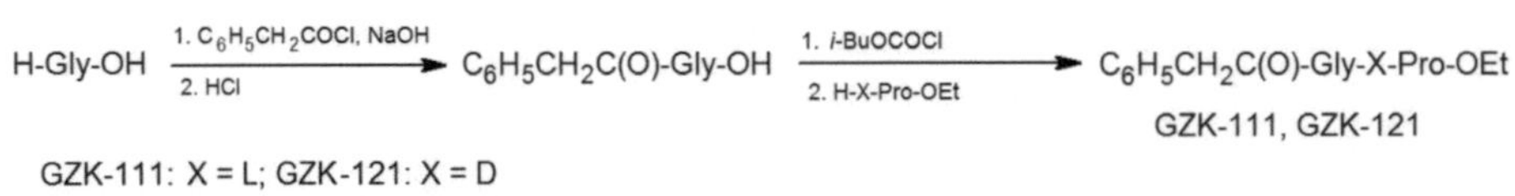

Figure 1.
The scheme of synthesis of N-phenylacetyl-glycyl-L-proline ethyl ester enantiomers.

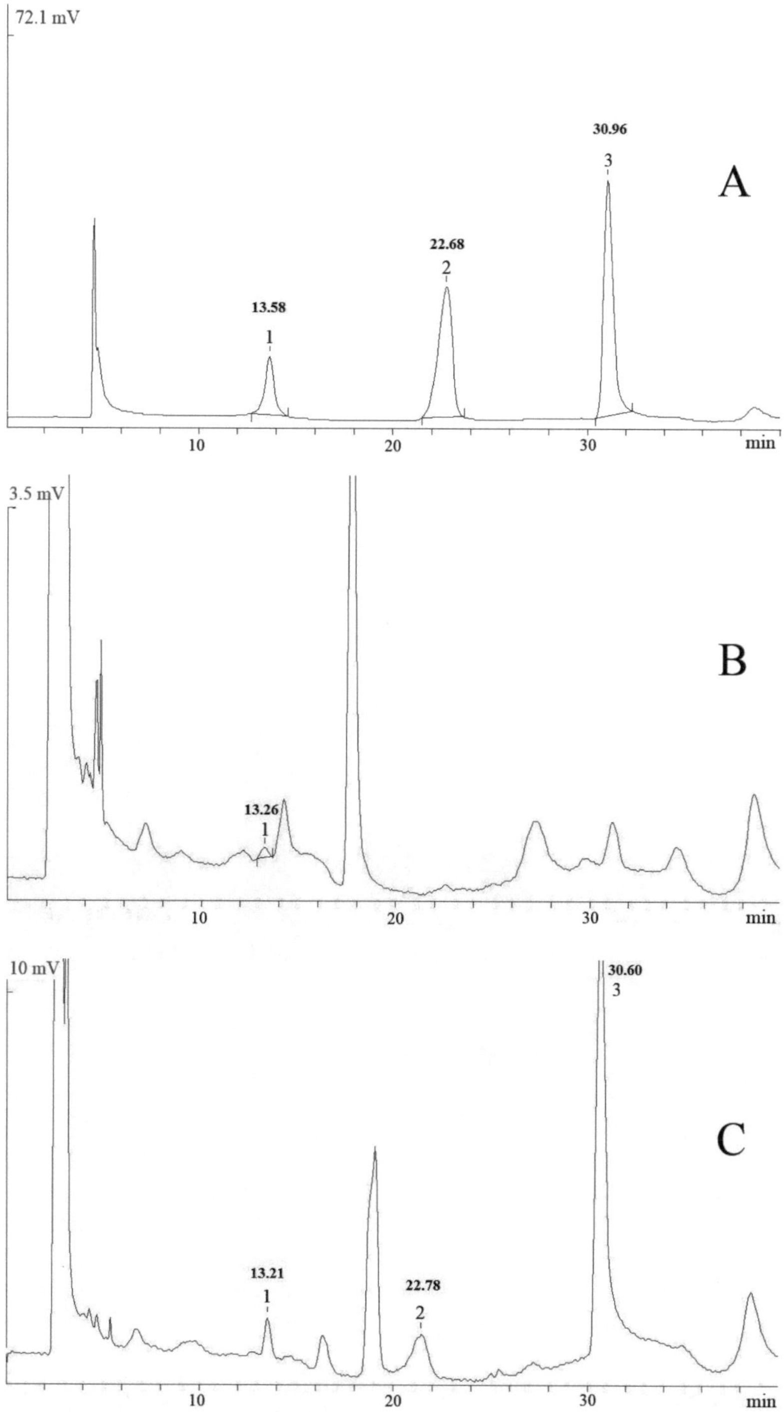

Figure 2.
The investigation of GZK metabolism in blood plasma by HPLC method. (A) Standards: (1) cyclo-L-prolylglycine, (2) N-phenylacetyl-glycyl-L-proline, and (3) N-phenylacetyl-glycyl-L-proline ethyl ester; (B) control blood plasma; (C) blood plasma + GZK-111, 10-h incubation.

The **nootropic antiamnesic effect** of GZK-111 was evaluated by its ability to prevent impaired reproduction of the conditioned passive avoidance reflex (passive avoidance reaction) in rats caused by electroconvulsive shock (ECS) by the Ader method [24]. The test is based on the inborn hole exploratory behavior of rodents.

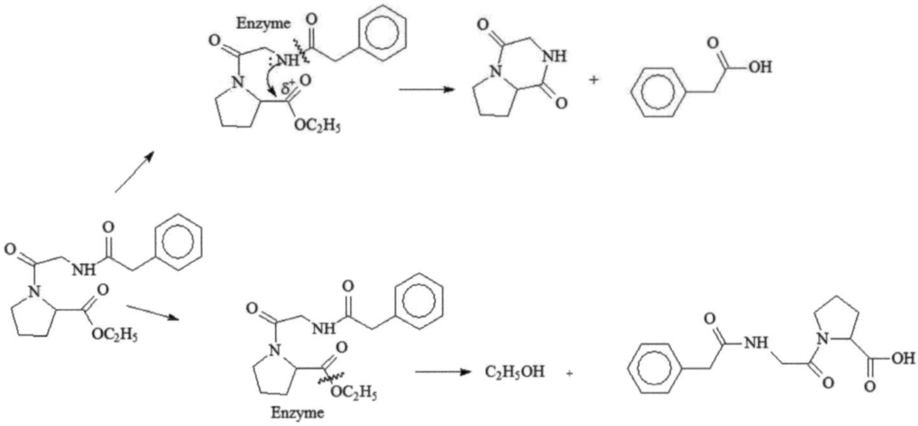

Figure 3.
The scheme of GZK-111 metabolism.

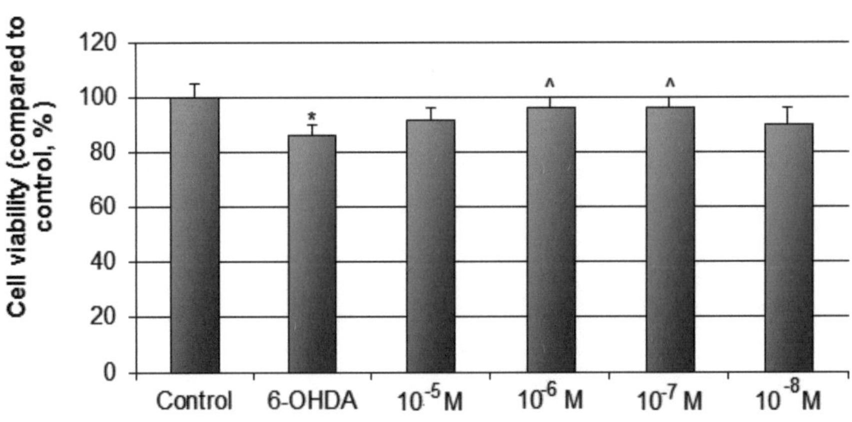

Figure 4.
*The neuroprotective effect of GZK-111 in a 6-OHDA toxicity model, SH-SY5Y cells. Notes: *p < 0.05 comparison with the control, ^p < 0.05 comparison with the damage group (Kruskal-Wallis ANOVA test with Dunn's post hoc).*

An animal learns not to enter the dark compartment using electric pain stimulation. Once the animal is subjected to EKS after training, the memorial trail is erased, and the animal again enters the dark chamber. Nootropic activity is defined as the ability to decrease the amnesic effect of ECS. GZK-111 was demonstrated to have antiamnesic activity at doses of 0.1, 0.5, and 1.0 mg/kg, i.p. (see **Table 1**), i.e., at least in the same dose range as CPG. Unlike the L-isomer, the D-stereoisomer of GZK-111, ethyl ester of *N*-phenylacetyl-glycyl-*D*-proline (GZK-121), had no antiamnesic activity.

Thus, GZK-111 possesses an antiamnesic activity similarly to CPG, and its effect is stereospecific, like that of CPG. However, if the *D*-enantiomer of CPG exhibits a pro-amnesic effect, the *D*-enantiomer of GZK-111 (GZK-121) has no activity. The possible explanation is that *D*-CPG blocks the receptor, while GZK-121 is not metabolized to CPG at all.

The **antihypoxic activity** of GZK-111 was studied in the normobaric hypoxia test with hypercapnia ("canned" hypoxia) in mice, which is the simplest method to assess antihypoxic activity [25]. GZK-111 was administered at doses of 0.1, 0.5, and 1.0 mg/kg, i.p., 60 min before test. Likewise CPG, the compound was found to

Compound	Dose, mg/kg, i.p. (n = 10)	Latent period, s			Effect, %
		Control	Amnesia	Amnesia + compound	
L-CPG [3]	0.05	91 ± 34	19 ± 8°	25 ± 7	+8
	0.1	91 ± 34	19 ± 8°	73 ± 26*	+75*
	1.0	91 ± 34	19 ± 8°	43 ± 19*	+33*
D-CPG [36]	0.1	113 ± 12	48 ± 11°	27 ± 8*	−32*
GZK-111	0.1	180 ± 0	129 ± 28°	169 ± 10*	+76*
	0.5	180 ± 0	100 ± 25	176 ± 6*	+95*
	1.0	180 ± 0	129 ± 28°	179 ± 2*	+98*
GZK-121	0.5	180 ± 0	95 ± 31°	133 ± 23	+44

Notes: n, number of animals;
°p < 0.05 comparison with the control;
**p < 0.05 comparison with the amnesia group (Mann-Whitney U test with a Bonferroni correction).*
Antiamnesic activity (AA) was calculated as follows: $AA\% = \frac{LPtest-LPamn}{LPcontrol-LPamn} \times 100\%$. *where AA% is antiamnesic activity, LPtest is the average latent period of entry into the chamber in the animals administered with the test compound and subjected to amnesia, LPamn is the average period of entry into the chamber in the animals administered with 0.9% NaCl and subjected to amnesia, and LPcontrol is the average latent period of entry into the chamber in animals administered with 0.9% NaCl without amnesia.*

Table 1.
The effects of GZK-111 and GZK-121 in passive avoidance reaction test, compared to CPG.

Compound	Dose, mg/kg, i.p. (n = 10)			
	Control	0.1	0.5	1.0
	Life expectancy, min			
L-CPG [6]	20.9 ± 0.6	20.2 ± 0.8	24.0 ± 0.7*	25.0 ± 1.6**
D-CPG [37]	21.8 ± 1.7	23.3 ± 1.5	22.7 ± 0.5	22.3 ± 1.4
GZK-111	27.1 ± 0.9	25.2 ± 0.5	30.2 ± 0.7*	26.2 ± 0.3
GZK-121	25.8 ± 0.8	23.9 ± 0.7	26.0 ± 0.7	23.5 ± 0.8

Notes: The outbred white male mice were used in the experiments;
n, number of animals;
**p < 0.05;*
***p < 0.01 comparison with the control (Mann-Whitney U test).*

Table 2.
The effects of GZK-111 and GZK-121 in normobaric hypoxia test with hypercapnia in mice, compared to CPG.

exhibit an antihypoxic effect at a dose of 0.5 mg/kg, significantly increasing the life expectancy of animals (see **Table 2**). The stereoisomer GZK-121 at doses of 0.1, 0.5, and 1.0 mg/kg showed no antihypoxic activity in this test.

The **anxiolytic activity** of GZK-111 was studied in rats at doses of 0.75, 1.5, and 3.0 mg/kg, i.p., using the elevated plus maze test (EPM) according to Pellow [26]. This test is the primary model for anxiolytic activity detection; it is based on the conflict between rodents' inherent fear of open spaces and natural exploratory behavior. A significant anxiolytic effect was observed at a dose of 1.5 mg/kg. GZK-111 increased the time rats spent in the open arms by 12 times relative to the control, which is comparable with the effect of CPG. The enantiomer, GZK-121, was inactive at a dose of 1.5 mg/kg (see **Table 3**).

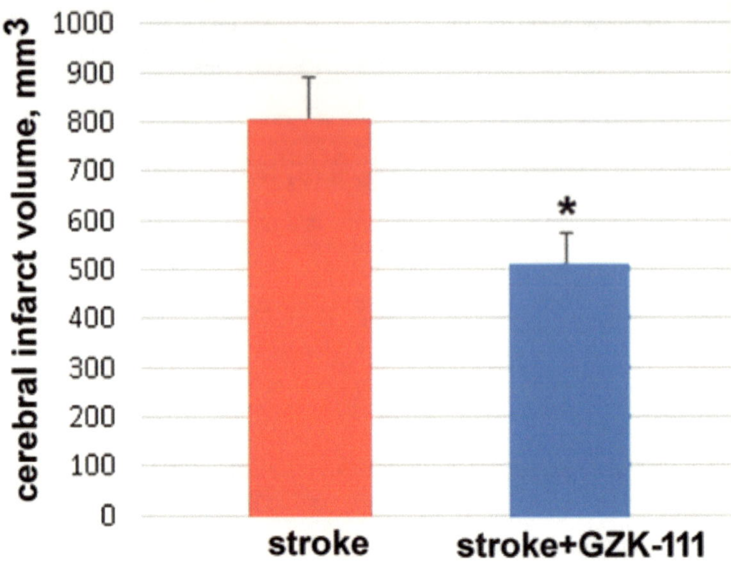

Figure 5.
*GZK-111 reduces the cerebral infarct volumes in rats with experimental stroke. Notes: Morphometric measurements of infarct volume were performed using TTC staining. The data are presented as mean ± SEM. *p = 0.05 compared to the "stroke" group (Mann-Whitney U test).*

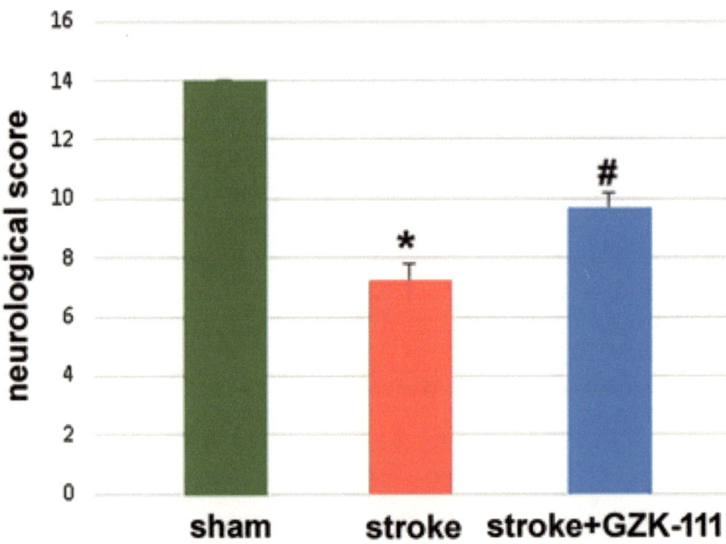

Figure 6.
*GZK-111 improves neurological status in rats with experimental stroke. Notes: Neurological status is given for the injured side of the body (which is the opposite to the ischemic lesion) in the limb-placing test. The data are presented as mean ± SEM. *p = 0.003 compared to the "sham" group, #p = 0.01 compared to the "stroke" group (Mann-Whitney U test).*

The **antidepressant-like effect** of GZK-111 was studied in the forced swimming test [27], one of the most widely used for this purpose [38]. The test is based on the ability of antidepressants to reduce the time of immobility in case of unavoidable swimming of the animal in a cylinder with water. The study was performed in mice at daily i.p. administration at a dose range of 0.01–20.0 mg/kg within 7 or 14 days.

Compound	Dose, mg/kg, i.p. (n = 10)	Number of entries into the open arms		Time spent in the open arms	
		m	%	s	%
L-CPG [4]	Control 1	0.20	100	2.15	100
	0.1	1.79*	895*	13.8*	641*
	1.0	0.25	125	1.46	68
	Control 2	0.58	100	6.38	100
	0.05	1.60**	276**	57.4**	900**
	0.2	1.50	259	19.3	303
D-CPG [4]	Control	0.20	100	2.15	100
	0.05	0.34	170	3.87	180
	0.1	0.26	132	2.58	120
GZK-111	Control	0.9 ± 0.6	100	4.8 ± 2.5	100
	0.75	1.3 ± 0.5	170	14.8 ± 7.0	180
	1.50	3.2 ± 1.1	355	58.2 ± 13.3**	1212**
	3.0	1.0 ± 0.5	132	6.4 ± 2.9	120
GZK-121	Control	0.2 ± 0.2	100	4.1 ± 1.5	100
	1.5	0.2 ± 0.2	100	4.7 ± 1.5	114

Notes: Number of entries into the open arms and time spent in the open arms were taken as 100% for control animals.
n, number of animals; m, number of entries into the open arms of the maze;
$^{*}p < 0.05$;
$^{**}p < 0.001$ comparison with the control (Mann-Whitney U test).

Table 3.
The effects of GZK-111 and GZK-121 in EPM test in rats, compared to CPG.

The tricyclic antidepressant amitriptyline (10.0 mg/kg, i.p.) was used as a comparison drug. GZK-111 administered at a dose of 10 mg/kg for 7 days was established to statistically significantly reduce the immobility time by 11% (**Table 4**), which is comparable to the effect of amitriptyline at a dose of 10 mg/kg.

With a 14-day administration, GZK-111 had a significant antidepressant effect at a dose of 10 mg/kg, i.p., and showed a tendency to decrease immobility time at a dose of 1.0 mg/kg, i.p. ($p = 0.08$) and 10 mg/kg p.o. ($p = 0.06$) (**Table 5**).

Recently, the antidepressant activity of started CPG was also discovered in the forced swimming test in mice (**Table 5**) [9] and in an experimental model of learned helplessness in rats [10] at i.p. administration for 14 days.

The **analgesic properties** of GZK-111 were determined in the hot plate test in inbred male C57Bl/6 mice [39] at acute i.p. administration at doses of 0.5, 1.0, 2.0, and 4.0 mg/kg. This test was widely used to study the pain sensitivity in rodents at supraspinal level, and the effectiveness of analgesics evaluates the pain response on paw pad contact with a hot surface; the time until the hind paw pulling and/or jumping is measured. The average baseline nociceptive response for C67Bl/6 mice was 8.2 ± 0.2 s. GZK-111 showed no analgesic effect ($F(4, 44) = 11{,}163$, $p = 0{,}36{,}098$) 30 min after administration at each of the doses studied. At a dose of 2.0 mg/kg, GZK-111 statistically significantly increased the latent period of the nociceptive reaction ($F(4, 44) = 3.1489$, $p = 0.02319$) 60 min ($p < 0.01$) and 120 min ($p < 0.05$) after administration, compared with the control group. At a

Experimental groups	Dose, mg/kg, i.p. (n = 10)	Immobilization time, s	Immobilization time compared to the control, %
Experiment 1			
Control	0.0	235.8 ± 11.8	100
GZK-111	0.1	240.2 ± 19.8	101
GZK-111	0.5	235.3 ± 17.7	100
GZK-111	1.0	240.0 ± 22.1	101
GZK-111	5.0	253.9 ± 9.2	108
Amitriptyline	10.0	218.5 ± 17.9*	93
Experiment 2			
Control		275.3 ± 8.7	100
GZK-111	0.01	260.1 ± 7.3	94
GZK-111	5.0	268.7 ± 10.2	98
GZK-111	10.0	245.5 ± 9.1*	89
GZK-111	20.0	259.9 ± 9.2	94

Notes: Immobilization time was taken as 100% for control animals.
n, number of animals;
$^*p < 0.05$, the statistical significance of the differences relative to control group by the unpaired t-Student criterion.

Table 4.
The effect of GZK-111 on immobilization time in the Porsolt forced swimming test in mice after 7-day administration.

Compound	Dose, mg/kg, i.p. (n = 10)	Immobilization time, s	Immobilization time compared to the control, %
GZK-111	Control	180.1 ± 10.7	100
	0.1	188.4 ± 9.3	105
	1.0	163.2 ± 11.2 (p = 0.08)	91
	10.0	157.7 ± 9.2*	88
	10.0 (p.o.)	160.3 ± 10.4 (p = 0.06)	89
CPG [9]	Control	139 ± 8	100
	1.0	97 ± 6#	70
	2.0	101 ± 8#	73
Fluoxetine [9]	10.0	87 ± 9#	63

Notes: Immobilization time was taken as 100% for control animals.
n, number of animals;
$^*p < 0.05$, the statistical significance of the differences relative to control group by the unpaired t-Student criterion;
$^\#p < 0.05$;

Table 5.
The effect of GZK-111 on immobilization time in the Porsolt forced swimming test in mice after 14-day administration, compared to CPG.

dose of 4 mg/kg, an increase of the reaction thresholds induced by GZK-111 was observed after 90 min ($F(4, 44) = 3.8743$, $p = 0.00881$) that persisted for up to 2 h ($F(4, 44) = 3.2141$, $p = 0.02124$), compared with the control group ($p < 0.05$ and $p < 0.05$, respectively) (**Figure** 7). The data obtained indicate that GZK-111 exhibits dose-dependent analgesic activity, like CPG in rats [40].

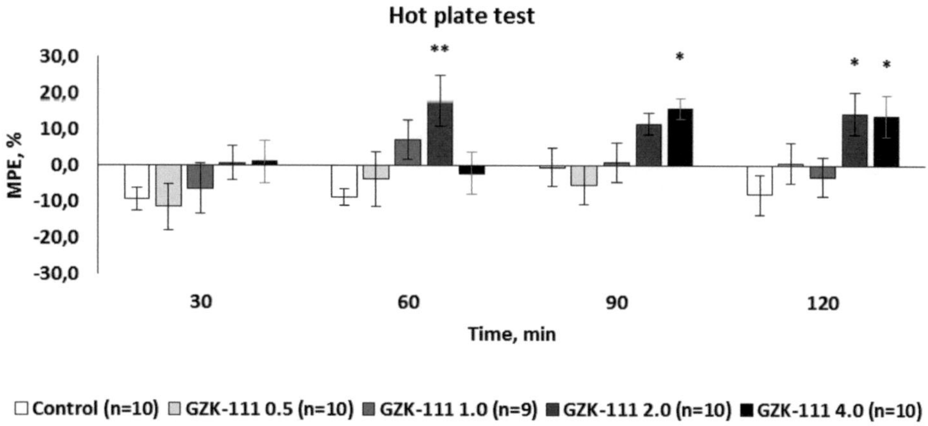

Figure 7.
*GZK-111 influences the pain response threshold during thermal stimulation in C57BL/6 mice. X-axis, time of the effect development after substance administration (min); y-axis, maximum possible effect (MPE), %. *$p < 0.05$; **$p < 0.01$, statistically significant in relation to the corresponding control; according to Duncan criterion, the number of animals in groups $n = 10$; data are presented as mean values.*

4. Conclusions

Thus, GZK-111 exhibits nootropic, anxiolytic, antihypoxic, antidepressant, neuroprotective, and analgesic effects being characteristic to CPG. The compound is similar to CPG both in the spectrum of activities and in the stereospecificity and its nature. The ampakine CPG identical to endogenous one was proven to form during the fermentolysis of GZK-111. Therefore, GZK-111 can be considered as a "prodrug" of CPG and a pharmacologically active pro-ampakine with a BDNF-ergic mechanism of action.

Conflict of interest

The authors declare no conflict of interest, financial or otherwise.

Funding

This work was supported by RFBR (project 20-015-00102).

Author details

Ksenia N. Koliasnikova[1], Polina Yu. Povarnina[1], Anna V. Tallerova[1], Yulia N. Firsova[1], Sergei V. Nikolaev[2], Tatiana A. Antipova[2], Anna V. Nadorova[3], Larisa G. Kolik[3], Tatiana A. Gudasheva[1]* and Sergei B. Seredenin[2]

1 Department of Medicinal Chemistry, V.V. Zakusov Research Institute of Pharmacology, Russia

2 Department of Pharmacogenetics, V.V. Zakusov Research Institute of Pharmacology, Russia

3 Laboratory of Pharmacological Regulation of Alcohol and Drug Dependence, V.V. Zakusov Research Institute of Pharmacology, Russia

*Address all correspondence to: tata-sosnovka@mail.ru

References

[1] Gudasheva TA, Vasilevich NI, Zolotov NN, Lezina VP, Rozenberg SG, Kravchenko EV, et al. Nootropic action of proline-based topological analogs of piracetam. Pharmaceutical Chemistry Journal. 1991;**25**(6):363-367. DOI: 10.1007/BF00772132

[2] Gudasheva TA, Boyko SS, Akparov VK, Ostrovskaya RU, Skoldinov SP, Rozantsev GG, et al. Identification of a novel endogenous memory facilitating cyclic dipeptide cyclo-prolylglycine in rat brain. FEBS Letters. 1996;**391**: 149-152

[3] Gudasheva TA, Ostrovskaya RU, Trofimov SS, Voronina TA, Skoldinov AP, Seredenin SB. New endogenous dipeptide cycloprolylglycine is similar to piracetam by its mnemotropic selectivity. Bulletin of Experimental Biology and Medicine. 1999;**128**(4):1012-1014

[4] Gudasheva TA, Konstantinopol'skii MA, Ostrovskaya RU, Seredenin SB. Anxiolytic activity of endogenous nootropic dipeptide cycloprolylglycine in elevated plus-maze test. Bulletin of Experimental Biology and Medicine. 2001;**131**(5):464-466. DOI: 10.1023/a: 1017928116025

[5] Seredenin SB, Gudasheva TA, Boiko SS, Kovalev GI, Voronin MV, Yarkova MA. Endogenous dipeptide cycloprolylglycine shows selective anxiolytic activity in animals with manifest fear reaction. Bulletin of Experimental Biology and Medicine. 2002;**133**(4):360-362. DOI: 10.1023/a: 1016293904149

[6] Kolyasnikova KN, Gudasheva TA, Nazarova GA, Antipova TA, Voronina TA, Seredenin SB. Similarity of cycloprolylglycine to piracetam in antihypoxic and neuroprotective effects. Eksperimental'naia i Klinicheskaia Farmakologiia. 2012; **75**(9):3-6. (in Russ)

[7] Povarnina PY, Kolyasnikova KN, Nikolaev SV, Antipova TA, Gudasheva TA. Neuropeptide cycloprolylglycine exhibits neuroprotective activity after systemic administration to rats with modeled incomplete global ischemia and in vitro modeled glutamate neurotoxicity. Bulletin of Experimental Biology and Medicine. 2016;**160**(5):653-655. DOI: 10.1007/s10517-016-3241-5

[8] Ferro JN, de Aquino FL, de Brito RG, Dos Santos PL, Quintans Jde S, de Souza LC, et al. Cyclo-Gly-Pro, a cyclic dipeptide, attenuates nociceptive behavior and inflammatory response in mice. Clinical and Experimental Pharmacology and Physiology. 2015;**42**(12):1287-1295. DOI: 10.1111/1440-1681.12480

[9] Kovalev GI, Abdullina AA, Vasil'eva EV, Gudasheva TA, Seredenin SB. Antidepressant-like properties of cycloprolylglycine. Eksperimental'naia i Klinicheskaia Farmakologiia. 2018;**81**(11):3-6. (in Russ). DOI: 10.30906/0869-2092-2018-81-11-3-6

[10] Garibova TL, Gudasheva TA, Seredenin SB. A new component in the mechanism of regulation of endogenous depressive-like states. Doklady Biochemistry and Biophysics. 2019;**488**(1):324-326. DOI: 10.1134/ S1607672919050107

[11] Gudasheva TA, Grigoriev VV, Koliasnikova KN, Zamoyski VL, Seredenin SB. Neuropeptide cycloprolylglycine is an endogenous positive modulator of AMPA receptors. Doklady Biochemistry and Biophysics. 2016;**471**(1):387-389. DOI: 10.1134/S160767291606003X

[12] Gudasheva TA, Koliasnikova KN, Antipova TA, Seredenin SB.

Neuropeptide cycloprolylglycine increases the levels of brain-derived neurotrophic factor in neuronal cells. Doklady Biochemistry and Biophysics. 2016;**469**(1):273-276. DOI: 10.7868/S0869565216220254

[13] Ovchinnikov YA, Ivanov VT. Conformational states and biological activity of cyclic peptides. Tetrahedron. 1975;**31**:2177-2209. DOI: 10.1016/0040-4020(75)80216-X

[14] Baldoni HA, Zamarbide GN, Enriz RD, Jauregui EA, Farkas Ö, Perczel A, et al. Peptide models XXIX. Cis–trans isomerism of peptide bonds: Ab initio study on small peptide model compound; the 3D-Ramachandran map of formylglycinamide. Journal of Molecular Structure: THEOCHEM. 2000;**500**:97-111. DOI: 10.1016/S0166-1280(00)00372-9

[15] Rydon HN, Smith PWG. Polypeptides. Part IV. The self-condensation of the esters of some peptides of glycine and proline. Journal of the Chemical Society. 1956; **1956**:3642-3650. DOI: 10.1039/JR9560003642

[16] Manabe S, Machida H, Aihara Y, Yasunaga M, Ito Y, Matsumura Y. Development of a diketopiperazine-forming dipeptidyl Gly-pro spacer for preparation of an antibody–drug conjugate. MedChemComm. 2013;**4**(5): 792-796. DOI: 10.1039/C3MD00075C

[17] Young DW, Morecombe DJ, Sen PK. The stereochemistry of beta-lactam formation in penicillin biosynthesis. European Journal of Biochemistry. 1977; **75**(1):133-147. DOI: 10.1111/j.1432-1033.1977.tb11511.x

[18] Nazarova LS, Rozonov YB, Likhosherstov AM, Morozova TV, Skoldinov AP, Kaverina NV, et al. Azacycloalkanes. XXVII. Synthesis and antianginal activity of nonachlazine stereoisomers. Pharmaceutical Chemistry Journal. 1984;**18**(12):811-815. DOI: 10.1007/BF00768332

[19] Riveles K, Huang LZ, Quik M. Cigarette smoke, nicotine and cotinine protect against 6-hydroxydopamine-induced toxicity in SH-SY5Y cells. Neurotoxicology. 2008;**29**(3):421-427

[20] Longa EZ, Weinstein PR, Carlson S, Cummins R. Reversible middle cerebral artery occlusion without craniectomy in rats. Stroke. 1989;**20**(1):84-91. DOI: 10.1161/01.str.20.1.84

[21] Jolkkonen J, Puurunen K, Rantakömi S, Harkonen A, Haapalinna A, Sivenius J. Behavioral effects of the alpha(2)-adrenoreceptor antagonist, atipamezole, after focal cerebral ischemia in rats. European Journal of Pharmacology. 2000;**400**(2–3):211-219. DOI: 10.1016/s0014-2999(00)00409-x

[22] Bederson JB, Pitts LH, Germano SM, Nishimura MC, Davis RL, Bartkowski HM. Evaluation of 2,3,5-triphenyltetrazolium chloride as a stain for detection and quantification of experimental cerebral infarction in rats. Stroke. 1986;**17**(6):1304-1308. DOI: 10.1161/01.str.17.6.1304

[23] De Ryck M, Van Reempts J, Borgers M, Wauquier A, Janssen PA. Photochemical stroke model: Flunarizine prevents sensorimotor deficits after neocortical infarcts in rats. Stroke. 1989;**20**(10):1383-1390. DOI: 10.1161/01.str.20.10.1383

[24] Ader R, Weinen JAWM, Moleman P. Retention of a passive avoidance response as a function of the intensity and duration of electric shock. Psychonomic Science. 1972;**26**(3): 125-128. DOI: 10.3758/BF03335453

[25] Roshchina LF, Ostrovskaia RU. Effect of piracetam on the body's resistance to hypoxia. Farmakologiia i Toksikologiia. 1981;**44**(2):210-213

[26] Pellow S, Chopin P, File SE, Briley M. Validation of open:closed arm entries in an elevated plus-maze as a measure of anxiety in the rat. Journal of Neuroscience Methods. 1985;**14**(3):149-167

[27] Porsolt RD, Anton G, Blavet N, Jalfre M. Behavioural despair in rats: A new model sensitive to antidepressant treatments. European Journal of Pharmacology. 1978;**47**:379-391. DOI: 10.1016/0014-2999(78)90118-8

[28] Anderson GW, Zimmerman JE, Callahan FM. Reinvestigation of the mixed carbonic anhydride method of peptide synthesis. Journal of the American Chemical Society. 1967;**89**: 5012-5017

[29] Baumann E. Ueber eine einfache Methode der Darstellung von Benzoësäureäthern. Berichte der Deutschen Chemischen Gesellschaft. 1886;**19**:3218-3222. DOI: 10.1002/cber.188601902348

[30] Brenner M, Huber W. Herstellung von α-Aminosäureestern durch Alkoholyse der Methylester. Helvetica Chimica Acta. 1953;**36**:1109-1115. DOI: 10.1002/hlca.19530360522

[31] Xicoy H, Wieringa B, Martens GJ. The SH-SY5Y cell line in Parkinson's disease research: A systematic review. Molecular Neurodegeneration. 2017;**12**(1):10. DOI: 10.1186/s13024-017-0149-0

[32] Welch WJ, Suhan JP. Cellular and biochemical events in mammalian cells during and after recovery from physiological stress. Journal of Cell Biology. 1986;**103**(5):2035-2052. DOI: 10.1083/jcb.103.5.2035

[33] Gusev EI, Skvortsova VI. Ishemiya Golovnogo Mozga [Cerebral Ischemia] [in Russian]. Moscow: Meditsina; 2001. p. 248

[34] Lorenz J, Glatt HR, Fleischmann R, Ferlinz R, Oesch F. Drug metabolism in man and its relationship to that in three rodent species: Monooxygenase, epoxide hydrolase, and glutathione S-transferase activities in subcellular fractions of lung and liver. Biochemical Medicine. 1984;**32**(1):43-56

[35] Huang H, Chen Y-M, Zhu F, Tang S-T, Xiao J-D, Li L-L, et al. Down-regulated Na^+/K^+-ATPase activity in ischemic penumbra after focal cerebral ischemia/reperfusion in rats. International Journal of Clinical and Experimental Pathology. 2015;**8**(10): 12708-12717

[36] Kolyasnikova KN, Vichuzhanin MV, Konstantinopol'skii MA, Trofimov SS, Gudasheva TA. Synthesis and pharmacological activity of analogs of the endogenous neuropeptide cycloprolylglycine. Pharmaceutical Chemistry Journal. 2012;**46**(2):96-102

[37] Kolyasnikova KN, Nazarova GA, Gudasheva TA, Voronina TA, Seredenin SB. Antihypoxic activity of cycloprolylglycine analogs. Bulletin of Experimental Biology and Medicine. 2015;**158**:458-460. DOI: 10.1007/s10517-015-2784-1

[38] Can A, Dao DT, Arad M, Terrillion CE, Piantadosi SC, Gould TD. The mouse forced swim test. Journal of Visualized Experiments. 2012;**59**:e3638. DOI: 10.3791/3638

[39] Le Bars D, Gozariu M, Cadden SW. Animal models of nociception. Pharmacological Reviews. 2001;**53**(4): 597-652

[40] Konstantinopolsky MA, Gudasheva TA, Kolik LG. Experimental study of endogenous dipeptide cyclo-L-prolylglycine in aspects of opioid addiction and analgesia in rodents. European Neuropsychopharmacology. 2019;**29**:S180-S181. DOI: 10.1016/j.euroneuro.2018.11.305

Chapter 13

Aptamers and Possible Effects on Neurodegeneration

Fatma Söylemez and Çağatay Han Türkseven

Abstract

Aptamers are a new class of recognizing agents which are defined as short biomolecules like oligonucleotides and peptides that are used in diagnostics and therapeutics. They can bind to specific targets with extremely high affinity based on their structural conformations. It is believed that in the near future, aptamers could replace monoclonal antibody. The biggest advantage of using aptamers is that the process is in vitro in nature and does not require the use of animals and they also have unique properties, such as thermal stability, low cost, and unlimited applications. Aptamers have been studied as a biomaterial in numerous investigations concerning their use as a diagnostic and therapeutic tool and biosensing probe. DNA aptamers were also used for the diagnosis and treatment of neurodegeneration and neurodegenerative diseases. For example, functional nucleic acid aptamers have been developed to detect Aβ fragments in Alzheimer's brain hippocampus tissue samples. Aptamers are promising materials for diverse areas, not just as alternatives to antibodies but as the core components of medical equipment. Although they are in the preliminary stages of development, results are quite encouraging, and it seems that aptamer research has a very bright future in neuroscience.

Keywords: aptamers, neurodegeneration, diagnosis, biosensors, SELEX

1. Introduction

Aptamers, first introduced by Tuerk and Gold and Ellington and Szostak, are short chains of DNA or RNA oligonucleotides that bind to small molecules, peptides, and macromolecules, such as proteins of various sizes and conformations [1]. Aptamers are oligonucleotides that are possible of targeting specific molecules. The name aptamer is derived from the Latin word *aptus* which means to fit. A very interesting property of aptamers for therapeutic use is the ability of aptamers to bind with high selectivity. They are small double- or single-stranded DNA or RNA molecules. Aptamers have been extensively used in basic research, to ensure food safety and to monitor the environment. Furthermore, aptamers have a promising role in clinical diagnostics and as therapeutic agents [2].

1.1 Properties of aptamers

Aptamers are short single-chained oligonucleotides that fold into a defined 3D structure with which they bind specifically and with high affinity to defined target molecules (**Figure 1**) [3]. Aptamers usually consist of 15–50 nucleotides and have a molecular weight ranging from 5 to 15 kDa [4]. Multiple aptamers have been generated so far, successfully binding to a wide variety of different objects such as small molecules, proteins, and cells. Similar to the antibody-antigen interaction, the recognition between aptamers and their target is very specific.

Recently aptamers are capable of binding different targets such as large protein complexes, simple inorganic molecules, and total cells [5]. Thus, aptamers can be regarded as nucleotide analogues of antibodies [6]. However, the production of aptamers is easier and less expensive than antibodies.

Their binding properties are similar to those found for antibodies, being in the nanomolar to the picomolar range [7], and aptamers have been identified to distinguish between members of a protein family, as they recognize target structures in an epitope-specific manner [8]. Compared with antibodies, nucleic acid aptamers have many advantages in their suitability for clinical application and industrialization, including almost no immunogenicity, efficient penetration, less batch variation, easy modification, cost-effectiveness, and short production times [9] (**Table 1**).

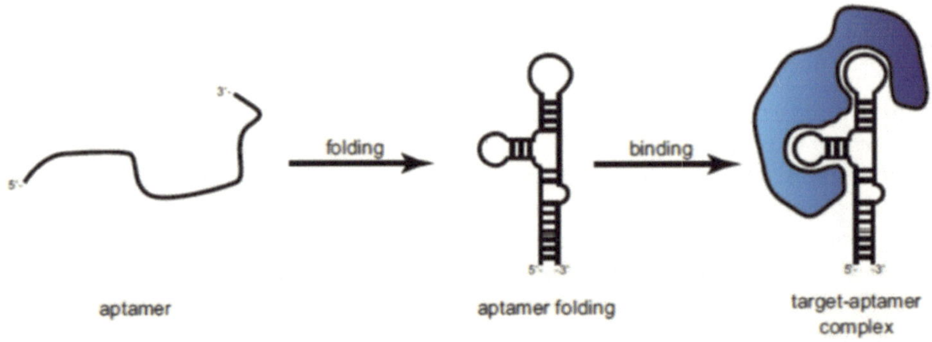

Figure 1.
Schematic representation of binding of an aptamer to a target protein. After binding, the aptamer interacts with a target molecule such as protein to fold into a 3D structure, which forms a stable target aptamer complex [3].

APTAMER	ANTIBODIES
Aptamers are oligonucleotide and protein.	Antibodies are protein in nature.
Uniform activity regardless of batch	Varies from batch to batch
Wide variety of chemical modifications to molecule for diverse functions.	Immune system determines target site of protein.
No evidence of immunogenicity	Significant immunogenicity
They are more stable at high temperature and they can be regenerated easily after denaturation	Temperature sensitive
Entire selection is a chemical process carried out in vitro and can therefore target any protein	Selection requires a biological system, therefore difficult to raise antibodies to toxins (not tolerated by animal) or non-immmunogenic target.
Aptamers are single stranted DNA or RNA oligonucleotide or peptides.	Antibodies are monoclonal or polyclonal.

Table 1.
Comparison between aptamer and antibody.

1.2 Types of aptamers

Nucleic acid aptamers are short single-stranded DNA or RNA molecules and can be selected from complex libraries by a technique called "systematic evolution of ligands by exponential enrichment" (SELEX). These aptamers are capable of binding to the target molecule with high affinity and specificity. Nucleic acid aptamers are functionally similar but have some differences in their stability and accessibility (**Table 2**). DNA aptamers are less reactive and relatively stable because of the C—H bonds at the 21st position of the deoxyribose sugar of DNA nucleotides. This chemical difference gives DNA aptamers an inherent advantage in stability over RNA aptamers [10].

RNA aptamers are defined as RNA oligonucleotides that bind to a specific target with high affinity and specificity, similar to how an antibody binds to an antigen [11]. RNA aptamers are less stable than DNA aptamers due to the presence of a reactive hydroxyl group (—OH) in the 21st position of the ribose sugar in the RNA nucleotides. This —OH group is especially deprotonated, particularly in alkali solutions. The resulting anionic 21-O can be nucleophilically attached to the phosphorus atom of the phosphodiester bond, leading to hydrolysis of RNA molecules. It was found that the nuclease resistance of RNA aptamers increased when the 21-hydroxyl group was removed from RNA sugars [10, 12]. Because of the C—H bonds of the DNA nucleotides at position 21 of the deoxyribose sugar, DNA aptamers are less reactive and relatively stable. Due to this chemical difference, DNA aptamers are more stable than RNA aptamers.

Another type of aptamer developed around 1996 was peptide aptamers. The concept, originally introduced by Roger Brent, proposed a short amino acid sequence embedded ("double constrained") within the context of a small and very stable protein backbone ("scaffold") [13, 14]. Peptide aptamers are conjugated protein molecules with specific binding affinity to target proteins formed under intracellular conditions. The typical structure of peptide aptamers is a short peptide region inserted within a scaffold protein. The short peptide region is responsible for binding with the target protein. The scaffold protein helps to increase binding affinity and specificity by a restriction on the conformation of the binding peptide [15]. Thus, peptide aptamer applications range from in vitro detection of various proteins in a complex mixture to in vivo modulation. In addition, peptide aptamers

RNA APTAMER	DNA APTAMER	PEPTİDE APTAMER
From complex secondary and tertiary structure	From complex secondary and tertiary structure	Structure constrains by scaffoled
From diverse 3D structure	Less diverse 3D structure than RNA aptamer	3D structure constraints by scaffold
Bind target with the entire sequence	Bind target with the entire sequence	Bind target variable region only
Biosenseor, diagnostic, therapeutics applications	Biosenseor, diagnostic, therapeutics applications	Biosenseor, diagnostic, therapeutics applications

Table 2.
Comparison of RNA, DNA, and peptide aptamers.

have been recognized as therapeutic molecules due to their anticancer and antivirus activities.

1.3 Aptamer production: selection and identification of aptamers

Aptamers are a new class of recognizing agents that came into light in 1990 [16]. Tuerk and Gold developed a method known as systematic evolution of ligands by exponential enrichment or popularly called as SELEX method for selection of aptamers against target [17]. The method is in vitro in nature and does not require the use of animals. Aptamers are chemically synthesized and selected for their high affinity and specificity for a certain target through the SELEX process (**Figure 2**).

The process starts with synthesizing a random DNA oligonucleotide library (**Figure 2**). This library consists of a diverse pool of ssDNA fragments (10^{15}). When selecting RNA aptamers, the library needs to be converted into an RNA library. Subsequently, the target is introduced in the pool, non-binding fragments are removed by several washing steps, and the remaining fragments are amplified by PCR or RT-PCR. A new pool of oligonucleotides is created using the selected fragments and another round is performed. Usually 8–15 rounds are performed in order to obtain a high-affinity aptamer.

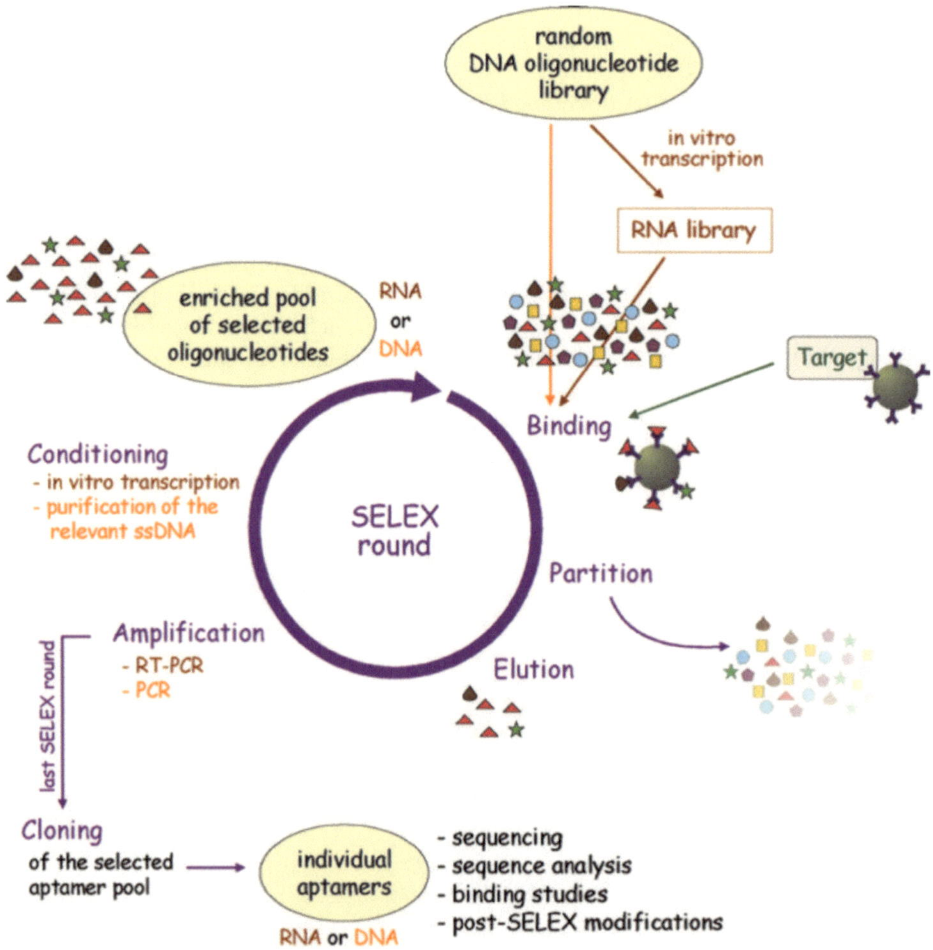

Figure 2.
Schematic illustration of an in vitro selection cycle.

Since the early 1990s, systematic evolution of ligands by exponential enrichment and similar methods have been reported to efficiently select RNA and DNA aptamers [10]. Thereafter, nucleic acid aptamers have been extensively researched and applied. The identification of aptamers is achieved by an in vitro selection process, also termed SELEX. In this method, a synthetic nucleic acid library that contains up to 1015 different sequences and structures is incubated with the desired target molecule, unbound sequences are removed, and target-linked sequences are recovered and amplified using PCR or RT-PCR [3, 18]. This cyclic process is repeated several times (5–16) until the nucleic acid population has been substantially enriched for target-specific sequences. Nucleic acid libraries offer the largest collection of compounds available so far for screening and selection purposes. The monoclonal aptamer sequences are accessible by cloning and sequencing these libraries. But the latest generation sequencing approaches allow in-depth evaluation of the selection process [19, 20]. A wide range of selection methods and strategies have been described since the first reports in 1990. The basis of these variations is based on the separation method used or chemical modifications added to the nucleic acid libraries.

2. The application of aptamers as molecular tools in neurosciences

Aptamers have a number of diagnostic and therapeutic applications, such as biosensors and target inhibitors. Due to simple preparation, easy modification, and stability, aptamers have been used in the diverse areas within molecular biology, biotechnology, and biomedicine [2]. In general, aptamers are used in diagnostics, pathogen recognition, cancer recognition, stem cell recognition, monitoring environmental contamination, biosensors, and therapeutics. Aptamers are being used in versatile applications. However, their use as a molecular research tool in neuroscience is limited. There are very few studies on the production of aptamers targeting neuroscience-related target proteins such as ion channels or application for neuronal cell behavior by inhibiting specific proteins.

Neurodegenerative diseases are defined as hereditary and sporadic conditions which are characterized by progressive nervous system dysfunction. These disorders are often associated with atrophy of the affected central or peripheral structures of the nervous system. Alzheimer's disease (AD) is the most common cause of dementia and is characterized by progressive loss of memory and other cognitive functions. It is considered a major epidemic worldwide, where currently more than 35 million people live with this disease. By 2050 it is estimated this figure will reach 115 million [21]. AD is characterized by two major abnormalities; abnormal extracellular amyloid β-protein (Aβ) disposition and intracellular neurofibrillary tangle (NFT) formation, both leading to neuronal degeneration. The generation of Aβ is triggered by B-site amyloid precursor protein cleaving enzyme 1 (BACE1). Thus, BACE1 is a prospective target for interfering with Aβ production and the treatment of AD [22]. A DNA aptamer selected by Liang et al. has been shown to bind to BACE1 with high affinity and good specificity, exhibiting a distinct inhibitory effect on BACE1 activity in an AD cell model [23].

Autoimmunity and autoantibodies play a role in the pathogenesis of many diseases. Recently, a research team in Germany demonstrated the presence of functional autoantibodies against G-protein bound receptors in the serum of Alzheimer's and vascular dementia patients [24]. And the aptamer BC007, which is selective for the GPCR-AAB FAB fragment as a "broad-spectrum neutralizer," has been developed based on binding and epitope mapping studies [24]. The fact that BC007 aptamer was successful in neutralization in an in vitro study revealed the possibility of being a potential therapeutic tool for dementia patients.

Parkinson's disease (PD), the second most common neurodegenerative disease after AD, affects over 7 million people worldwide. The pathology is characterized by loss of dopaminergic neurons, leading to decreased production of dopamine, a neurotransmitter that regulates movement and cognition. In the previous immunotherapy, targeting the α-syn in PD models with monoclonal antibodies has established α-syn protein as an effective target for neuronal cell death. The pathogenesis of Parkinson's disease involves the accumulation of α-synuclein protein in neurons. Anti-α-synuclein antibody treatment has achieved some success. However, this antibody-based immunotherapy is limited by the inherent immunogenicity of antibodies and the inability of antibodies to reach intracellular targets.

To date, there is no recognized cure for Parkinson's disease. Aptamer-based immunotherapy is an attractive alternative. Researchers in China have reported preliminary results for a selective aptamer to α-synuclein. The purified human α-syn was used as the target for in vitro selection of aptamers using systematic evolution by exponential enrichment in Zheng et al.'s study [25]. This resulted in the identification of two 58-base DNA aptamers with a high binding affinity and good specificity to the α-syn. Both aptamers could effectively reduce α-syn aggregation in vitro and in cells and target the α-syn to intracellular degradation through the lysosomal pathway. In vitro, the aptamer inhibited the accumulation of α-synuclein and its association with the mitochondria [26]. It also induced intracellular α-synuclein degradation, and the neuron maintained viability despite overexpression of α-synuclein. In vivo, the a-synuclein aptamer can potentially inhibit the accumulation of a-synuclein in the cell while at the same time promoting the destruction of existing aggregates and reducing the toxic effects of α-synuclein aggregates on neurons. These effects consequently rescued the mitochondrial dysfunction and cellular defects caused by α-syn overexpression [26].

Numerous examples in the literature have shown the efficacy of aptamers against several important targets. Aptamers have been developed to bind to α-synuclein monomers or its oligomer. These aptamers recognized β-sheet structure, the moiety though which they can bind not only to α-synuclein oligomer but also Aβ oligomer. This indicates that these aptamers could also potentially be deployed as drugs treat Parkinson's and Alzheimer's diseases (**Figure 3**).

Multiple sclerosis (MS) is a chronic inflammatory and demyelinating disorder of the nervous system. Currently, there is no cure for MS, and the available medications only shorten the duration of attacks to slow the progression of the disease. Remyelination is a naturally occurring process in the body to restore damaged myelin sheaths after an MS attack. Rozenblum et al. identified a 40-nucleotide DNA aptamer which exhibits affinity towards murine myelin and binds to multiple myelin components in vitro [27]. In mice, it has been shown that aptamer is introduced into CNS tissue by intraperitoneal (IP) injection and dispersed in the tissue [28]. In addition, the aptamer allowed remyelination of CNS lesions in mice infected with Theiler virus [29]. Therefore, this aptamer can be used for recovery following an episode of MS and may alleviate the symptoms of MS.

The toll-like receptor 4 (TLR4) plays a crucial role in the adaptive immune response. It plays a role in many pathologies including stroke, myocardial infarction, atherosclerosis, sepsis, multiple sclerosis, and chronic pain. A research group from Spain investigated TLR4 blocking DNA aptamers, especially for the treatment of stroke. In an in vivo study involving mice and rats exposed to permanent middle cerebral artery occlusion (pMCAO), the TLR4-blocking aptamer reduced ischemic brain injury 4–6 h after injury [30]. The presence of aptamer in the blood and brain has been demonstrated by imaging studies [30]. Although tissue plasminogen

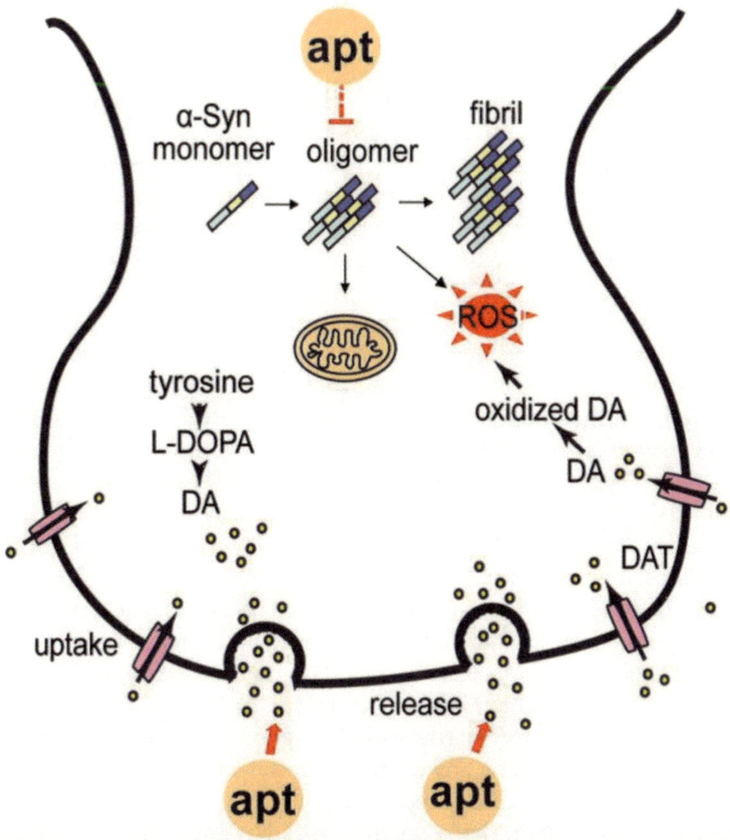

Figure 3.
Aptamers targeting α-Syn oligomers for diagnosing and preventing onset of PD and dopamine for diagnosing dopamine concentrations [26].

activator, tPA, is a viable option in only 5% of stroke treatment cases, TLR4 blocking aptamers have been shown to be a promising and nontoxic alternative.

Signal cascades play an important role in various aspects of cellular homeostasis and are also connected to several diseases [3, 31]. AMPA receptors are involved in excitatory synaptic transmission in the CNS and contribute to synaptic plasticity, as it is known in learning and memory processes [32]. They are hetero-oligomeric proteins, constituted of different combinations of four subunits GluR1-R4. The phosphorylation of GluR1 at the amino acid residues Ser831, Ser845, and Ser818 located at the receptor's intracellular domain has been found to have a strong impact on AMPA-mediated neurotransmission. Liu et al. identified an RNA aptamer, termed A2, which modulates the phosphorylation of the serine residue Ser845 of the GluR1, whereas the phosphorylation of the Ser831 and Ser818 has been found to be unaffected [33]. Another work identified an RNA aptamer, named C5, which specifically binds and inhibits the mitogen-activated protein kinase (MAPK) Erk1/2 [34].

Aptamers may be of therapeutic use in treating neurological diseases. One of its biggest advantages is that aptamers are better able to penetrate tissues, cells, and blood-brain barrier (BBB) because they are small. They are essentially non-immunogenic and chemically synthesized. Therefore, they eliminate concerns about biological contamination or long-term reagent formation that is often encountered in antibody treatments. Although new drug therapies are a risk to follow, there is a great potential in terms of increasing survival rates, decreasing healthcare costs, and high quality of life in aptamers.

3. Limitations and opportunities of aptamers

Around 50 million people worldwide have Alzheimer's disease, and more than 10 million people have Parkinson's disease. The most common type of cancer in children younger than 19 years is brain tumors and central nervous system tumors and is the leading cause of cancer-related deaths in children under 14 years of age in the United States. Although antibody drugs have taken major steps in cancer therapies, the passage of these drugs through the blood-brain barrier and proper cleansing of the brain limit the use of antibody drugs for the treatment of neurological diseases.

Aptamers have a number of advantages, such as their high specificity and affinity, their enzymatic or chemical production, and their high reliability and their renewability in simple ways. Furthermore, they have a higher inhibitory potential than monoclonal antibodies and have the possibility of wider chemical modification as they can be synthesized enzymatically or chemically. Aptamers can also remain stable in a wide variety of buffer environments without loss of activity and are more resistant to harsh processes such as physical or chemical denaturation. Since aptamers are developed completely in vitro without the need for cells or animal immune systems, aptamer production offers a wide variety of binding options. Aptamers can be produced against a large number of targets, such as molecules that are toxic to the cell, targets where an immune response does not occur, and compounds that are soluble only in solvents other than water [35]. Given the chemical and physical properties of aptamers, it is unlikely that they will enter the brain via paracellular aqueous pathways or transcellular lipophilic pathways. However, the aptamer may enter the brain by any of the pathways of adsorptive-mediated transcytosis and channels and/or receptors for absorption or liquid-phase pinocytosis. A recent study has shown that a quadruplex DNA aptamer binds to nucleotide by micropinocytosis [36]. Cheng et al. identified an aptamer that can enter brain endothelial cells under physiological conditions, and in vivo, into the brain parenchyma [36]. This development has shed light on the use of aptamers in the investigation of neurological diseases.

As all technologies and classes of substances, the use of aptamers has certain limitations as well as advantages. In vitro selection experiments are the major obstacle to success, which means whether a specific combination of the target protein and the nucleic acid library will produce an aptamer. Essentially, this limitation binds to a limited number of nucleotide groups and building blocks from which a nucleic acid library is made. The four canonical nucleotides, together with ribose (in the case of RNA) or deoxyribose (in the case of DNA) and phosphate backbone, are highly limited chemical diversity in comparison to 21 proteinogenic amino acids that are capable of forming a large number of molecular interactions and properties such as polar, charged, basic, acidic, aromatic, and aliphatic. Therefore, the success rate of in vitro selection experiments for protein targets was found to be 30% [37].

The inability of aptamers to cross cell membranes autonomously (e.g., passive diffusion represents a further limitation in their applicability and is mainly attributed to their macromolecules and polyanionic nature). Nevertheless, several options are available to overcome this restraint (e.g., transfection with liposomes, through plasmid or viral delivery or using nanoparticles). In experiments with isolated cells and cell culture, intracellular distribution of aptamers can be achieved, but this is more complicated in vivo, especially when the targeted tissue is CNS. The barrier (blood-brain barrier) cannot passively pass aptamers and other macromolecules. However, by performing in vivo experiments, aptamers that cross the blood-brain barrier in mice and penetrate into the brain parenchyma could be identified [36].

Aptamer technology has emerged into almost every field in the life sciences since its inauguration 25 years ago. To date, a wide variety of aptamers have been selected and characterized and also allowed to bind to a wide variety of target molecules. Aptamers are suitable for diagnostic and therapeutic applications because of their unique properties. In this chapter, we explained that because of the specific properties of aptamers, it can be a valuable tool for basic research in the field of neuroscience. In the future, neurobiology approaches will reveal a number of interesting target proteins in which specific and potent inhibitors are required. Analysis of target proteins in neurons and neuronal systems requires identification and availability of specific inhibitory compounds. Thus, the identification of new aptamers may be crucial for the timely acquisition of new inhibitors for the treatment of disorders in the neurological system. Together, we believe that aptamers will be a valuable research tool for neurological studies and that data from new studies in the field of aptamer and neuroscience will reveal the full potential of aptamers.

Author details

Fatma Söylemez[1*] and Çağatay Han Türkseven[2]

1 Department of Food Processing, Vocational School of Technical Sciences, Mersin University, Mersin, Turkey

2 Department of Biophysics, Faculty of Medicine, Mersin University, Mersin, Turkey

*Address all correspondence to: soylemez_fatma@yahoo.com

References

[1] Delac M, Motaln H, Ulrich H, Lah TT. Aptamer for imaging and therapeutic targeting of brain tumor glioblastoma. Cytometry Part A. 2015; **87A**:806-816

[2] Zhang Y, Lai BS, Juhas M. Recent advances in aptamer discovery and applications. Molecules. 2019;**24**:941

[3] Wolter O, Mayer G. Aptamers as valuable molecular tools in neurosciences. The Journal of Neuroscience. 2017;**37**(10):2517-2523

[4] Lakhin AV, Tarantul VZ, Gening LV. Aptamers: Problems, solutions and prospects. Acta Naturae. 2013;**4**(19):5

[5] Veedu RN. Aptamers: Tools for Nanotherapy and Molecular Imaging. Boca Raton, FL, USA: CRC Press; 2017

[6] Ali MH, Elsherbiny ME, Emara M. Updates on aptamer research. International Journal of Molecular Sciences. 2019;**20**:2511

[7] Meyer C, Hahn U, Rentmeister A. Cell-specific aptamers as emerging therapeutics. Journal of Nucleic Acids 2011:904750

[8] Michaud M, Jourdan E, Villet A, Ravel A, et al. ADNA aptamer as a new target-specific chiral selector for HPLC. Journal of the American Chemical Society. 2003;**125**:8672-8679

[9] Sun H, Zu YA. Highlight of recent advances in aptamer technology and its application. Molecules. 2015;**59**:1980

[10] Zhu Q, Liu G, Kai M. DNA aptamers in the diagnosis and treatment of human diseases. Molecules;**20**:20979-20997. DOI: 10.3390/molecules201219739

[11] Germer K, Leonard M, Zhang X. RNA aptamers and their therapeutic and diagnostic applications. International Journal of Biochemistry and Molecular Biology. 2013;**4**(1):27-40

[12] Adler A, Forster N, Homann M, Goringer HU. Post-SELEX chemical optimization of atrypanosome-specific RNA aptamer. Combinatorial Chemistry & High Throughput Screening. 2008;**11**: 16-23

[13] Reverdatto S, Burz DS, Shekhtman A. Peptide aptamers: Development and applications. Current Topics in Medicinal Chemistry. 2015; **15**(12):1082-1101

[14] Colas P, Cohen B, Jessen T, Grishina I, et al. Genetic selection of peptide aptamers that recognize and inhibit cyclin-dependent kinase 2. Nature. 1996;**380**:548-550

[15] Li J, Tan S, Chen X, Zhang CY, et al. Peptide aptamers with biological and therapeutic applications. Current Medicinal Chemistry. 2011;**18**(27): 4215-4222

[16] Tuerk C, Gold L. Systematic evolution of ligands by exponential enrichment: RNA ligands to bacteriophage T4 DNA polymerase. Science. 1990;**249**:505-510

[17] Parashar A. Aptamer and its role in diagnostics. International Journal of Bioassays. 2016;**5**(2):4799-4809

[18] Stoltenburg R, Reinemann C, Strehlitz B. SELEX: A (r)evolutionary method to generate high-affinity nucleic acid ligands. Biomolecular Engineering. 2007;**24**:381-403

[19] Schutze T, Wilhelm B, Greiner N, Braun H, et al. Probing the SELEX process with next-generation sequencing. PLoS One. 2011;**6**:e29604

[20] Tolle F, Mayer G. Preparation of SELEX samples for next-generation

sequencing. Methods in Molecular Biology. 2016;**1380**:77-84

[21] Robinson SW, Fernandes M, Husi H. Current advances in systems and integrative biology. Computational and Structural Biotechnology Journal. 2014;**11**(18):35-46

[22] Das U, Wang L, Ganguly A, Saikia JM, et al. Visualizing APP and BACE-1 approximation in neurons yields insight into the amyloidogenic pathway. Nature Neuroscience. 2016; **19**(1):55-64

[23] Liang H, Shi Y, Kou Z, Peng Y, et al. Inhibition of BACE1 activity by a DNA aptamer in an Alzheimer's disease cell model. PLoS One. 2015;**10**(10): e0140733

[24] Walukat G et al. Functional autoantibodies in patients with different forms of dementia. PLoS One. 2018; **13**(3):e0192778

[25] Zheng Y, Qu J, Xue F, Zheng Y, et al. Novel DNA aptamers for Parkinson's disease treatment inhibit α-synuclein aggregation and facilitate its degradation. Molecular Therapy. Nucleic Acids. 2018;**1**(11):228-242

[26] Qu J, Yu S, Zheng Y, Zheng Y, et al. Aptamer and its applications in neurodegenerative diseases. Cellular and Molecular Life Sciences. 2017; **74**(4):683-695

[27] Rozenblum GT, Kaufman T, Vitullo AD. Myelin basic protein and a multiple sclerosis-related MBP-peptide bind to oligonucleotides. Molecular Therapy. Nucleic Acids. 2014;**3**(9):e192

[28] Aaldering L, Krishnan S, Fletcher S, Wilton SD, et al. Aptamers as Therapeutic Tools in Neurological Diseases. Aptamers, Tools for Nanotherapy and Molecular Imaging. 1st ed, Chapter 6. 2016. ISBN: 9781315364780

[29] Nastasijevic B, Wright BR, Smestad J, Warrington AE, et al. Remyelination induced by a DNA aptamer in a mouse model of multiple sclerosis. PLoS One. 2012;7:e39595

[30] Fernandez G et al. TLR4-binding DNA aptamers show a protective effect against acute stroke in animal models. Molecular Therapy. 2018. DOI: 10.2016/ j.ymthe.2018.05.019

[31] Cohen P. The origins of protein phosphorylation. Nature Cell Biology. 2002;**4**:E127-E130

[32] Boudreau AC, Wolf ME. Behavioral sensitization to cocaine is associated with increased AMPA receptor surface expression in the nucleus accumbens. The Journal of Neuroscience. 2005;**25**: 9144-9151

[33] Liu Y, Sun QA, Chen Q, Lee TH, et al. Targeting inhibition of GluR1 Ser845 phosphorylation with an RNA aptamer that blocks AMPA receptor trafficking. Journal of Neurochemistry. 2009;**108**:147-157

[34] Lennarz S, Alich TC, Kelly T, Blind M, et al. Selective aptamer-based control of intraneuronal signaling. Angewandte Chemie (International Ed. in English). 2015;**54**:5369-5373

[35] Famulok M, Blind M, Mayer G. Intramers as promising new tools in functional proteomics. Chemistry & Biology. 2001;**8**(10):931-939

[36] Cheng C, Chen YH, Lennox KA, Behlke MA, et al. In vivo SELEX for identification of brain-penetrating aptamers. Molecular Therapy. Nucleic Acids. 2013;**8**(2):e67. DOI: 10.1038/ mtna.2012.59

[37] Gold L, Ayers D, Bertino J, Bock C, et al. Aptamer-based multiplexed proteomic technology for biomarker discovery. PLoS One. 2010;**5**(12):e15004

Chapter 14

Lifestyle Factors, Mitochondrial Dynamics, and Neuroprotection

Katheryn Broman, Abigail U. Davis, Jordan May and Han-A Park

Abstract

The brain requires vast amounts of energy to carry out neurotransmission; indeed, it is responsible for approximately one-fifth of the body's energy consumption. Therefore, in order to understand functions of brain cells under both normal and pathological conditions, it is critical to elucidate dynamics of intracellular energy. The mitochondrion is the key intercellular organelle that controls neuronal energy and survival. Numerous studies have reported a correlation between altered mitochondrial function and brain-associated diseases; thus mitochondria may serve as a promising target for treating these conditions. In this chapter, we will discuss the mechanisms of mitochondrial production, movement, and degradation in order to understand accessibility of energy during physiological and pathological conditions of the brain. While research targeting molecular dynamics is promising, translation into clinical relevance based on bench research is challenging. For these reasons, we will also summarize lifestyle factors, including interventions and chronic comorbidities that disrupt mitochondrial dynamics. By determining lifestyle factors that are readily accessible, we can propose a new viewpoint for a synergistic and translational approach for neuroprotection.

Keywords: mitochondria, neuroprotection, Bcl-2, exercise, diet

1. Introduction

Frequently referred to as the "the powerhouse of the cell," the mitochondrion is the key organelle that contributes to neuronal energy and viability through the production of adenosine triphosphate (ATP) via oxidative phosphorylation. During oxidative phosphorylation, electrons from $FADH_2$ or NADH travel across the electron transport chain (ETC) creating an electrical gradient along the inner mitochondrial membrane allowing protons to diffuse through the ATP synthase. This allows the ATP synthase to bind a phosphate group to adenosine diphosphate (ADP) creating ATP. Compared to other metabolic pathways such as fermentation and anaerobic respiration, oxidative phosphorylation is the most efficient process to generate ATP. Energy in the brain is used for overall maintenance of cellular processes, neuronal growth, and axonal branching [1]. However, a majority of the ATP produced is utilized to support one of the neuron's most essential functions, synaptic transmission [2]. For example, the Na^+, K^+ -ATPase or the Na^+, K^+-pump is responsible for approximately half of the energy consumed by the brain, through its use of active transport to pump out sodium ions while taking in potassium ions [3].

This pump is essential in neurotransmission through its regulation of membrane potential, cell volume, and intracellular Ca^{2+} homeostasis [4, 5]. Likewise, exocytosis requires sufficient energy to release neurotransmitters from presynaptic to postsynaptic vesicles [5].

Beyond the mitochondria's role in energy production, it is also a key regulator of apoptotic cell death [6]. Various proteins, such as cytochrome c, reside in the mitochondria and participate in apoptotic pathways. In normal physiological conditions, cytochrome c plays a role as an electron carrier in the ETC. However, during neurotoxic conditions, permeabilization of the mitochondrial membrane occurs, and cytochrome c is released into the cytoplasm. Upon release, cytochrome c binds to apoptotic protease activating factor 1 (Apaf-1) which, in turn, activates caspase-9, forming the apoptosome that then activates downstream caspases leading to cell death [7]. Second mitochondria-derived activator of caspase (Smac)/direct IAP-binding protein with low PI (DIABLO) is also a mitochondrial protein released during apoptosis. The N-terminus of Smac/DIABLO directly interacts with inhibitor of apoptosis proteins (IAPs), a family of proteins that inhibit caspase 3, 7, and 9 activities; thus Smac/ DIABLO exhibits pro-apoptotic roles [8].

It has been well studied that Bcl-2 family of proteins controls neuronal survival or death via regulating apoptotic pathways, i.e., pro-apoptotic proteins versus anti-apoptotic proteins [9]. The presence of at least one of the four Bcl-2 homology (BH) domains influences a Bcl-2 family member's role in apoptosis. Pro-apoptotic Bcl-2 family members include the multidomain homology proteins such as Bax and Bak as well as the BH3-only homology proteins such as Bid, Bim, Bad, PUMA, and NOXA. These pro-apoptotic Bcl-2 proteins enhance mitochondrial membrane permeabilization resulting in subsequent release of cytochrome c [10–14].

Anti-apoptotic proteins of the Bcl-2 family include Bcl-2, Bcl-xL, Bcl-w, Mcl-1, and Bfl-1. These proteins contain the BH4 homology, which is essential for anti-apoptotic functionality. Both Bcl-2 and Bcl-xL antagonize pro-apoptotic members to prevent apoptosis [15, 16]; for instance, Bcl-xL targets Bak, preventing its oligomerization and inhibiting it from damaging the mitochondrial outer membrane [17]. Similarly, the C-terminal of Bcl-xL binds to the BH3 domain of Bax, resulting in retro-translocation-activated Bax. [18]. Protein-protein binding is further demonstrated with additional members of Bcl-2 family. These observations suggest that the Bcl-2 family's role in mediating apoptosis and mitochondrial permeabilization is largely influenced by dynamic protein-protein interactions with each other [19–21].

The mitochondrion is also responsible for the production of reactive oxygen species (ROS), namely, superoxide and hydrogen peroxide, at Complex I and III of the ETC [22]. This occurs as a result of electron leakage from the complexes, which then allows oxygen to react [23]. Due to the high energy demands required by neuronal mitochondria, this results in increased ROS generation. Increased ROS activity contributes to lipid peroxidation, causing disruption of the hydrophobic interaction between cytochrome c and cardiolipin, thus releasing cytochrome c [24]. Furthermore, the brain is particularly susceptible to oxidative damage due to its composition of high lipid content. Indeed, ROS play a significant role in the regulation of cell death; however, ROS have recently been reported to induce DNA demethylation via 8-oxoguanine DNA glycosylase-1 (OGG1) [25]. As a result, DNA demethylation induces activation of the reelin gene [26], which has been implicated in enhancing synaptic plasticity by inducing long-term potentiation (LTP) [27], thus indicating that normal levels of ROS may play a role in supporting LTP. Additionally, elimination of ROS negatively impacted neural stem cell proliferation in hippocampal cells indicating that homeostatic levels of ROS may possibly be involved in cell proliferation during growth and development [28]; however additional information is needed in order to elucidate the mechanism behind this.

2. Mitochondrial dynamics

Mitochondria were previously thought of as static organelles. Due to advances in molecular biotechnologies, it has been revealed that mitochondria are indeed very dynamic; mitochondria undergo fission and fusion, can vary in morphology, and achieve intracellular movement. Precise execution of these processes is especially vital for proper ATP production, apoptosis, and ROS homeostasis in neurons to properly execute neurotransmission.

2.1 Fission and fusion

Fission and fusion are integral processes of cellular homeostasis that maintain proper mitochondrial morphology and turnover. Both are mediated by GTPases in the dynamin family, with rates of occurrence depending on changes in metabolic demands. Undoubtedly, fission is essential for dividing cells in order to maintain an adequate number of mitochondria; however, even in nonproliferating neurons, fission is necessary for cell survival [29]. Dynamin-related protein 1 (Drp1) is the primary GTPase that mediates fission, with its activity controlled by phosphorylation via kinases, primarily on two serine residues. Specifically, phosphorylation at Ser616 promotes fission, while phosphorylation at Ser637 inhibits fission, so balance of Drp1 phosphorylation is crucial for proper fission functionality [30]. Impairment in Drp1 leads to alterations in mitochondrial distribution, with mitochondria accumulation occurring at the soma and reduced density in the dendrites. Conversely, Drp1 overexpression yields an increase in dendritic mitochondria [31]. Hippocampal neurons lacking Drp1 display compromised function of axonal mitochondria due to the inability to maintain ATP levels, recycling at synapses [32]. Prominent regulators of fusion include mitofusion 1 and 2 (Mfn1 and Mfn2, respectively) and optic protein atrophy 1 (Opa1). Mitofusion proteins mediate the outer membrane, while Opa1 regulates the inner membrane; however, both work in coordination in a two-step process to carry out fusion [33, 34].

Both fission and fusion are enhanced by Bcl-xL, with fission being induced in a Drp1-dependent manner [35]. This is conclusive with a previous study demonstrating the direct interaction of Bcl-xL with Drp1, initiating Drp1-dependent synapse formation in hippocampal cells [36]. When investigated further, this Bcl-xL-Drp1 complex was found to be necessary for presynaptic plasticity by regulating endocytic vesicles [37].

2.2 Mitochondrial trafficking

Trafficking, mobility, and docking are intertwining processes that are vital to ensure neurons are equipped with the proper distribution and recycling of mitochondria at axons and synapses throughout the cell's life span. **Figure 1** demonstrates how mitochondria are motile and change morphology in primary hippocampal cells. Mitochondrial trafficking is mediated by intracellular signaling, physiological events, and alterations in metabolic demands. Approximately 70% of mitochondria are stationary, with the remaining 30% motile [38]. Furthermore, five distinct mitochondria motility patterns have been described by Sun's research group: stationary outside of synapses, docking at synapses, passing though synapses, pausing at synapses for a short amount of time, and pausing for a longer time [39].

Mechanisms of mitochondrial movement and transport are overall influenced by the polarity of axons, with the positive end directed toward the soma and the negative at the tips. Utilizing this consistent axonal polarity is how microtubule

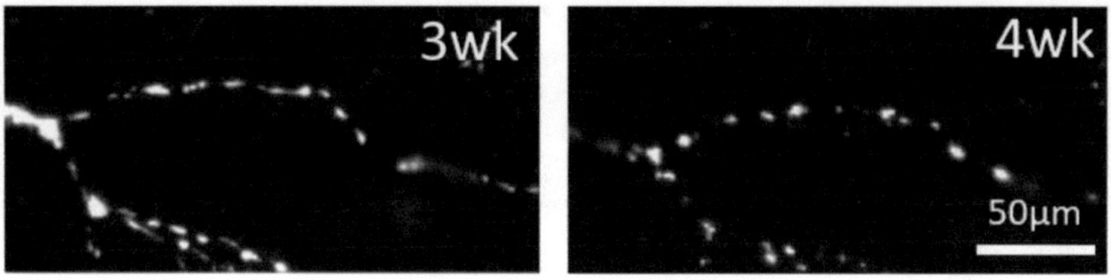

Figure 1.
Mitochondrial movement in primary hippocampal neurons. Primary hippocampal neurons were labeled with mitoRFP, a red fluorescent tag that labels mitochondria. Micrographs were taken at 3 and 4 weeks after seeding. Morphology and location of mitochondria change over time.

motors drive transport in two directions. Movement away from the soma or anterograde movement is conducted by the ATPase family of kinesins, with kinesin-1 being responsible for mitochondrial transport, specifically in neurons [38, 40]. Kinesin-1 consists of heavy chains (KHC) and light chains, with the heavy chains being the driving force that allows kinesin-1 to function as a motor protein [41]. Retrograde movement or movement toward the soma is driven by dynein. However, it is likely that these movements are coordinated rather than competitive toward each other, as it has been demonstrated that inhibiting kinesin-1 in *Drosophila* reduces retrograde movement [42].

Mitochondrial Rho-GTPase, or Miro, is an outer membrane receptor, Ca^{2+} sensor, and another pertinent regulator of mitochondrial motility due to its ability to anchor kinesin and dynein to the mitochondrial outer membrane [43]. Miro's anchoring role has been extensively studied in anterograde movement in the motor/adaptor complex formed between KHC and Miro, connected by the protein adaptor milton [44, 45].

Another important component of mitochondria trafficking is stationary docking. Mitochondrial docking is largely mediated by the axonal outer membrane protein syntaphilin (SNPH) and its interaction with microtubules in the cytoskeleton. This is demonstrated in rodent models in which deletion of the SNPH gene results in an increase in mitochondria motility and reduced density, while overexpression of endogenous or exogenous SNPH abolished mobility [46]. Along with decreasing the percentage of immobile mitochondria, loss of SNPH decreases axonal branching in cortical neurons [47]. This effect is comparable to neurons lacking LKB-1 and NUAK1, which is necessary for axonal specification [48]. The removal of either of these kinases leads to a decrease in the number of stationary mitochondria along with decreased branching. However, overexpression of SNPH in the LKB-1 and NUAK1-null neurons rescued these effects. Collectively, this implies that docking of mitochondria is required for axonal branching and growth [47]. Since Bcl-xL is required for neurite outgrowth [49], it is possible that Bcl-xL exerts this effect by interacting with docking proteins such as syntaphilin. However, the exact role of Bcl-xL in docking mechanisms must be further elucidated.

3. Alteration of mitochondrial function in brain-associated diseases

While various brain-associated diseases have different pathophysiologies, there is an underlying similarity that consistently occurs: mitochondrial dysfunction. Throughout these conditions, neurodegeneration is correlated with an energy deficit caused by inefficient operation of the ETC, activation of mitochondria-dependent apoptosis, and accumulation of ROS. In addition, excitotoxicity, which commonly occurs during cerebral ischemia and traumatic brain injury, impairs homeostasis of excitatory neurotransmitter glutamate [50–53]. Overstimulation of glutamate receptors further leads to Ca^{2+} release; because mitochondria are one of the key regulators of Ca^{2+}, excessive influx can consequently lead to mitochondrial dysfunction, altered membrane permeabilization, and subsequent cell death [50, 54–56]. Pathways such as these have been extensively explored in neurological conditions. However, research in the past decade has begun to determine the relationship between brain-associated conditions and mitochondrial dynamics.

3.1 Parkinson's disease

Parkinson's disease (PD) is a common neurodegenerative disease that has detrimental clinical effects including tremors, impaired gait, and stiffness of limbs [57]. These symptoms are often due to PD's hallmark characterization of degeneration of the dopaminergic neurons in the substantia nigra. Individuals with PD are vulnerable to increased ROS production due to reduced complex 1 activity, increased lipid oxidation, and altered antioxidant systems [58].

As several PD-specific proteins impact mitochondrial dynamics, it is possible that the neurodegeneration that occurs with PD is linked to alterations in fission and fusion [59, 60]. Dopaminergic neurons depleted of Drp1 demonstrated decreased mitochondrial mass, impaired motility, and overall neuron loss. Neurons depleted with Drp1 had less mitochondria in the soma and were almost completely depleted from the axons; by not having mitochondria at axons, this can lead to the neurodegeneration due to energy deficits, as synaptic transmission requires a high demand of ATP [61].

The PINK1/Parkin pathway has been traditionally studied with its roles in mitophagy. Under normal physiological conditions, PINK1 accumulates on the surface of dysfunctional mitochondria to signal Parkin translocation to initiate ubiquitination [62]. However, mutations in PINK1 and Parkin, which have been linked to early onset familial forms of PD, lead to loss of mitochondrial membrane potential, leading to impairment of Parkin's translocation and thus accumulation of dysfunctional mitochondria [63]. Research in recent years has begun to uncover the role of the PINK1/Parkin pathway in mitochondrial transport. Overexpression of PINK1 phosphorylates Miro, targeting it for ubiquitination and subsequent degradation. This results in the dismantling of the motor/adaptor complex, releasing kinesin and milton from the mitochondrial surface, and leads to halting of mitochondrial motility [64]. It is possible that this system may promote neuroprotection by preventing anterograde transport of mitochondria and allowing PINK1 to accumulate on damaged mitochondria to initiate mitophagy [65]. Furthermore, PINK1 may exert neuroprotection due to its interaction with Bcl-xL [66]. It has been shown that PINK1 phosphorylates Bcl-xL at its Ser62; as a result, this prevents N-terminal cleavage of Bcl-xL or formation of ΔN-Bcl-xL, which has been associated with neuronal death [67–69]. However, if altered PINK1 expression occurs as a result of genetic mutation, this may lead to dysregulated mitochondrial transport and promotion of apoptosis.

The presynaptic protein α-synuclein is a major constituent of Lewy bodies, with mutations in its encoding gene, SNCA, being linked to familial PD [70]. Some amount of α-synuclein can localize to the mitochondria, inducing mitochondrial fragmentation, dysfunction, and downregulation of complex 1 activity, potentially contributing to ROS production [71]. Overexpression of α-synuclein results in cytotoxicity due to decreased Bcl-xL expression and increased Bax expression [72]. Shaltouki's research group recently investigated the role of α-synuclein on mitochondrial dynamics by using multiple PD models. In the postmortem brains of humans with PD, it was observed that protein levels of α-synuclein and Miro were highly upregulated compared to the control brains, while KHC, VDAC, and Mfn2 remained unchanged. Additionally, the β-subunit of ATP synthase was upregulated in the PD brains. When this was further explored in human cell lines and in *Drosophila* bearing SNCA mutations, neurodegeneration and locomotion defects occurred as a result of the upregulated α-synuclein and subsequent upregulation of Miro. These effects were rescued with a partial reduction of Miro. Interestingly, upregulation of Miro led to delayed mitophagy implying that α-synuclein's impact on Miro is probably independent of the PINK1/Parkin pathways [73].

Recently, it was shown that the β-subunit of ATP synthase binds to DJ-1 suggesting that DJ-1 plays a role in increasing ATP efficiency [74]. Mutations in DJ-1 also demonstrate inefficient ATP production, alterations in mitochondrial morphology, and enhanced membrane permeability [74–76]. Although its functions are not completely understood, DJ-1 has been noted to prevent the aggregation of α-synuclein [77]. As Lewy bodies in PD are primarily a result of α-synuclein aggregation, inhibiting this aggregation may consequently delay Lewy body formation. Thus, therapies targeting DJ-1 may serve as a multi-faceted mechanism for PD treatment.

3.2 Alzheimer's disease

Alzheimer's disease (AD) is the most common neurodegenerative disease and the leading cause of dementia worldwide [78]. Two hallmark characteristics of AD are the presence of amyloid-beta peptide (Aβ) plaques and tau protein tangles. The formation of Aβ occurs as a consequence of cleavage of amyloid precursor protein (APP), where Aβ peptides can then aggregate into oligomers or fibrils [79]. In the brain, the typical role of tau proteins is to stabilize microtubules; however, in AD, it is suspected that hyperphosphorylation of tau leads to the formation of neurofibril tangles [80]. Both Aβ and tau tangles can cause impairments or interruptions in pathways essential for neuronal survival.

Reduced transport of axonal mitochondria has been documented in subjects with AD, but there may be multiple mechanisms to cause this disruption [81]. The presence of Aβ reduces bidirectional axonal mitochondrial motility but has a more significant impact on anterograde movement versus retrograde [82, 83]. This may be because Aβ activates GSK-3β, which is a negative regulator of kinesin-1. Phosphorylation of kinesin-1 by GSK-3β can lead to a reduction in mitochondria density [84]. Furthermore, mutations in presenilin-1 (PS1), which is linked to familial AD, promote GSK-3β-mediated kinesin-1 phosphorylation and reductions of anterograde mitochondria transport [84]. Overexpression of tau also has the ability to redirect mitochondrial transport; kinesin-1 encounters tau and is detracted from microtubule tracks, slowing down anterograde movement and increasing the favorability of dynein-mediated retrograde movement [85, 86]. Abnormal fission mechanics have also been observed in AD as a result of alteration in Drp1 function. Neurotoxicity via tau interrupts fission, causing elongated mitochondria and mislocalization of Drp1. This occurs because hyperphosphorylation of tau causes disruptions in actin, preventing actin-based translocation of Drp1 to the mitochondria [87].

3.3 Stroke

Cerebral ischemia, or more commonly stroke, is characterized by the decrease or cessation of blood flow to the brain. Consequently, the loss of oxygen and nutrients to neurons causes ATP deficits, apoptosis, and Ca^{2+} influx. It is not surprising then that mitochondrial dynamics are influenced after ischemic events. This is demonstrated by Zou's research group as they sought to elucidate how mechanisms of fission and mitophagy are impacted after ischemia [88]. Using a model of middle cerebral artery occlusion (MCAO), Drp1 initially increased but then decreased, implying that ischemia induced fission, but the process was disrupted due to abnormalities in translocation of Drp1 caused by MCAO. Mitophagy is also selectively induced by mild ischemia in a Drp1-dependent manner; this is evident by increased expressions of LC3B and Beclin-1 and decreased p62. Moreover, inhibition of Drp1 led to early onset of apoptotic pathways [88]. This may be supported by transient ischemia models, in which p-Drp1 is upregulated [89, 90]. Interestingly, evidence shows that p-Drp1 at Ser616 may be regulated by PINK1, establishing a link between fission and mitophagy [90]. Like fission, mechanisms of fusion are also impacted by ischemic insult. Mfn2 expression is decreased after MCAO and leads to apoptosis, but when overexpressed, Mfn2 shows an anti-apoptotic effect by modulating Bcl-2 and Bax [91]; these results are conclusive with a similar study, showing that Mfn2 expression is decreased after excitotoxic insult with a subsequent increase in Bax translocation to the mitochondria [92].

Excitotoxicity via overactivation of glutamate receptors, namely, N-methyl-D-aspartate (NMDA) receptors (NMDARs), is a key player of neuronal death after cerebral ischemia [93]. Thus, uncovering mechanisms effecting NMDARs is an attractive idea for therapeutic agents. While mechanisms of mitochondrial motility are less investigated in models of cerebral ischemia, a recent study has elucidated a novel role of kinesin-1 transport. The heavy chain of kinesin-1 has been shown to bind directly to NMDARs, mediating their transport. By either disassociating this bond or suppressing kinesin-1 expression, this can improve Ca^{2+} influx and NMDA excitotoxicity resulting from ischemia [94].

3.4 Traumatic brain injury (TBI)

Reducing excessive fission that occurs post-TBI is a potential target of neuroprotection to prevent neuronal impairments and death. In rodent models, TBI causes an increase in translocation of Drp1 to the mitochondria, increasing rates of fission. Consequently, this led to neuronal apoptosis, decreased neurogenesis, impaired cognition, and memory defects. When administered with Mdivi-1, a pharmacological inhibitor of Drp1, these negative effects were attenuated, confirming the role of increased Drp1 activity [95, 96]. Interestingly, Pietro's research group suggest that many molecular responses after severe TBI are opposite from that of mild TBI. Rodents with severe TBI presented with activation of fission as shown by overexpression of Drp1 and FIS1, a protein that binds to Drp1 for anchoring to the mitochondrial outer membrane. Furthermore, expressions of Mfn1 and Mfn2 were downregulated, and there were no changes in Opa1 gene and protein expressions, demonstrating an inhibition of fusion as a result of severe TBI. Additionally, the increase of dysfunctional mitochondria led to a subsequent overexpression of PINK1 and PARK2, triggering mitophagy. Conversely, mild TBI demonstrated activation of fusion with inhibition of fission; together, this did not change PINK1 or PARK2 gene expressions, thus showing no difference in mitophagy [97].

4. The effect of lifestyle factors on mitochondria function and dynamics

4.1 Exercise and mitochondria

Traditionally observed at a large, systemic level, research in recent years has begun to investigate the effect of exercise on mitochondrial function and dynamic processes. Furthermore, encouraging results have been observed by analyzing these effects in physiological processes in the brain and pathological conditions such as Alzheimer's disease and Parkinson's disease [98–101]. After old and young mice were subjected to 6 weeks of treadmill exercise, old mice were found to respond positively, showing attenuated activity of coupled complexes I–III of the ETC [99].

Exercise regulates mitochondrial fission and fusion proteins such as Opa1, Mfn2, and Drp1 and enhances mitochondrial biogenesis via upregulation of mitochondrial DNA. This suggests a role for exercise in maintaining a healthy population of mitochondria [98, 101]. In addition, rodents that undergo physical exercise demonstrate improved cognitive and exploratory behaviors along with improved mitochondrial redox homeostasis and mitochondria-mediated brain energy metabolism [102–104].

Exercise has been shown to regulate apoptosis through the regulation of the Bcl-2 family in various models and tissues. As previously discussed, age can have a significant role in mitochondrial dysfunction. A study conducted by Kim et al. investigated how hippocampal neurogenesis and apoptosis were affected by treadmill exercise in young and old-aged rats [105]. Expressions of caspase-3, Bax, Bid, and Bcl-2 were all increased in old mice. After being subjected to treadmill exercise for 30 minutes, once per day for 6 weeks, old rats exhibited further enhancement of Bcl-2 expression, along with decreased expressions of caspase-3, Bax, and Bid. Interestingly, exercise did not impact expressions of Bcl-2, Bax, or caspase-3 in young mice. These results implicate that aerobic exercise may be especially important during aging to exert neuroprotective properties. Aboutaleb et al. examined the effect exercise had on the ratio of Bax/Bcl-2 proteins in hippocampal CA3 cells after ischemia. Ischemic insult led to an increase in caspase-3 and decrease in Bcl-2, thus an increase in Bax/Bcl-2 ratio. However, rats pre-subjected to exercise showed reduced levels of caspase-3 and attenuation of Bax/Bcl-2 ratio [106]. Similar results have been seen in a rodent TBI model, in which treadmill exercise lowered the Bax/Bcl-2 ratio and decreased the levels of active caspase-3 [107]. Likewise, endurance exercise exerted neuroprotection in PD models by modulation of Mcl-1, Bcl-2, and apoptosis-inducing factor [108]. Although Bcl-2 has primarily been investigated in rodent exercise models, exercise results in a negative regulatory effect on caspase-3 [105–107] which may reduce post-translational cleavage of Bcl-xL supporting neuronal survival [67, 69].

Since the Bcl-2 family proteins are present in the mitochondria throughout all tissue types, it is plausible that protective effects observed in non-neuronal mitochondria are indeed simultaneously occurring in neuronal mitochondria. For example, due to the correlation between diabetes and cardiovascular disease, Cheng et al. examined the relationship between apoptosis, cardiomyocytes, and aerobic exercise in streptozotocin (STZ)-induced diabetic rats. The STZ rats had significantly lower amounts of Bcl-2, Bcl-xL, and p-Bad and higher levels of caspase-3 than controls. However, these levels were all rescued when subjected to aerobic exercise [109]. These results implicate the ability of aerobic exercise to regulate apoptosis and exert cellular protection, even during chronic conditions.

4.2 Non-neurological conditions and mitochondrial consequences

As chronic diseases such as diabetes and obesity become more prevalent worldwide, research is uncovering the relationship between traditional non-neurological and brain-associated diseases. However, many interventions in studies concerning chronic diseases observe outcomes on a macrolevel and may not consider molecular effects. For these reasons, it is important to uncover how these non-neurological chronic conditions are impacting the mitochondria. By elucidating these mechanisms, this can serve as an additional, albeit perhaps overlooked, means of prevention against brain pathology.

Besides disrupting the uptake of glucose, diabetes can also damage the function, population, and morphology of mitochondria in neurons, potentially contributing to impaired cognition later in life [110–113]. Metabolic pathways that can lead to energy failure in mitochondria as well as prevent antioxidant interception are affected by diabetes. In the diabetic brain, mitochondrial perturbation can result in a lack of neuronal energy that will alter synaptic function and eventually cause the neurons to degenerate [114]. The effect of energy impairments is demonstrated in a cross-sectional study in which adolescents with type 2 diabetes had slower conversion rates of ADP to ATP than obese and lean controls. The explanation for this effect was suspected to be due to decreased blood flow, thus causing alterations in oxygen delivery [115]. Studies have shown that diabetes can modify fission mechanisms in rodent models. Although amounts of Mfn1 and Opa1 remain unchanged during diabetes, Drp1 mRNA is increased. Furthermore, there is an increase of translocation of Drp1 to the mitochondria in diabetes [110, 113]. This increase in translocation is due to GSK3β-mediated phosphorylation at Ser616 of Drp1. The combination of unchanged Mfn1 and Opa1 with increased Drp1 proposes that the disproportion between fission and fusion proteins contributes to mitochondrial dysfunction in rats with diabetes. This was further evident by altered mitochondrial morphology and density. Elevated levels of Drp1 can lead to mitochondrial fragmentation that is conducive to damage in the synapses of neurons, contributing to impairments in learning and memory [116]. Beyond alterations in fission and fusion, decreased ATP production and activity of complex I were observed in the diabetic hippocampus. Moreover, glutathione and ascorbate levels were decreased, suggesting that diabetes impairs mitochondrial antioxidant systems [110]. These results are supported by a study that found decreased coenzyme Q9 and ATPase activity in the mitochondria of diabetic rats [117].

Obesity is known to increase the risk of developing diabetes, cardiovascular disease, and neurological conditions. Indeed, obese animal models are often utilized to study insulin resistance. A characteristic of obesity is chronic inflammation and oxidative stress, so it is not surprising that mitochondrial dysfunction occurs throughout the body, including the brain [114]. Specifically, brain mitochondria of obese rats induced via a high-fat diet have repeatedly demonstrated a shift to pro-apoptotic pathways, as shown by elevated Bax expressions, lowered Bcl-2, and a higher Bax/Bcl-2 ratio [118, 119]. The detrimental effects of obesity continue to be demonstrated in the brain by upregulating production of ROS and alteration of mitochondrial membrane potential [120–122].

4.3 Diet and mitochondria

Diet, including intake of specific nutrients and overall encompassing dietary patterns, is a driver of maintaining cellular processes throughout the body. Treatment of diseases via diet is appealing due to the ability of nutrients to cross the blood brain barriers and ease of accessibility. Specifically, it is important to consider how an individual's overall dietary pattern impacts cellular processes. Dietary patterns, including composition of macronutrients and caloric provision, have been studied regarding efficacy in neuroprotection [123–125].

Caloric restriction has been implicated in the protection against several pathological brain conditions in various animal models such as AD and PD and under conditions of excitotoxicity [126–130]. Caloric restriction has been shown to confer protection from neurodegeneration by improving mitochondrial redox status by reducing ROS production localized to complex I of the ETC [131]. Recent evidence suggests that caloric restriction may prevent formation of ROS via upregulation of antioxidants such as mitochondrial superoxide dismutase 2 (SOD2) and glutathione [132]. Caloric restriction has also been reported to upregulate antioxidants localized to the plasma membrane such as coenzyme Q10 and α-tocopherol via an increase in redox enzymes that are capable of reducing these molecules back to their antioxidant form [133]. Due to coenzyme Q10's pivotal role as an electron carrier in the ETC, we speculate that caloric restriction may be beneficial to maintain redox balance in the mitochondrial membrane. Additionally, mRNA expressions of Bcl-2 and Bcl-xL were also reported to be upregulated in the ipsilateral cortex region of mice placed on caloric restriction against TBI [134], indicating that caloric restriction may prevent TBI-induced neuronal loss. Furthermore, caloric restriction improves mitochondrial function by enhancing ATP levels in aging mice [135]. Mice placed on caloric restriction for 6 months had increased mitochondrial biogenesis and increased levels of cytochrome c oxidase and citrate synthase activity, enhancing mitochondrial respiration [136]. Caloric restriction may enhance mitochondrial metabolism by also upregulating the activity of complexes I, III, and IV [128]. Interestingly, recent evidence shows that caloric restriction enhances expression of brain-derived neurotrophic factor (BDNF) [137, 138], which has been reported to regulate mitochondrial mobility and enhance presynaptic docking [139]. However, the mechanisms of how caloric restriction mediates BDNF expression are still unclear. Clinical trials in which older adults are placed on caloric restriction consistently yield positive results, such as improved memory and enhanced gray matter [140, 141]. Additionally, caloric restriction attenuated behavioral dysfunction in a model of PD in adult rhesus monkeys [130]. Taken together, these studies point *toward* caloric restriction mediating biological markers of chronic disease such as oxidative stress and supporting mitochondrial function by enhancing ATP metabolism and possibly lessening clinical symptoms associated with neurodegeneration.

The ketogenic diet, popular for its high-fat and very low carbohydrate pattern, has recently been implicated in protection of the brain through apoptotic pathways. Various mammalian animals placed on the ketogenic diet show decreased rates of apoptotic stimuli in neuronal cells via downregulation of mitochondrial cytochrome c release and active caspase-3 both in seizures [142, 143] and TBI models [144], respectively. The decrease in translocation of cytochrome c from the mitochondria to the cytosol may be through the regulation of Bcl-2. One study found that both a high carbohydrate and a high ketogenic diet upregulate Bcl-2 in cortical neurons after focal cerebral ischemia; however, the ketogenic diet displayed higher upregulation [145], indicating that the ketogenic diet may be more efficient in regulating apoptosis than a high carbohydrate diet. The ketogenic diet may play an additional role in cell death and survival pathways, as it has been noted to protect hippocampal cells from death by preventing the interaction between Bad and Bcl-xL [146]. The ketogenic diet further supports neuronal energy metabolism by maintaining mitochondrial morphology, enhancing biogenesis of mitochondria, and improving mitochondrial respiration [147–151]. After neurotoxic insult, the ketogenic diet enhanced complex I-driven oxygen consumption and prevented loss of complex II–III function, implicating the ketogenic diet's ability to improve the activity of the ETC [147, 149]. Likewise, the ketogenic diet attenuates mitochondrial oxidative stress levels in both in vitro and in vivo model, which prevents energy deficit associated with brain cell damage [147, 149, 151]. Interestingly, the ketogenic diet has also been shown to upregulate Beclin-1 [142] and Drp1 [148], suggesting that the ketogenic diet may be able to control mitochondrial population by regulating autophagy and mitochondrial fission, respectively.

5. Conclusions

Mitochondria are well established in their role with ATP production, apoptosis, ROS homeostasis, and intracellular ion signaling. Research in recent years has recognized that proper execution of these processes is reliant on the mitochondria's dynamic capabilities. In this chapter we have discussed mechanisms of mitochondrial morphology, degradation, and trafficking, as well as the relationship between these processes and pathological brain conditions. Utilizing lifestyle factors, such as exercise and diet, can serve as a neuroprotective strategy by targeting neuronal mitochondrial dynamics. Implementing lifestyle changes serves as an accessible treatment that is easily translated from bench to bedside.

Acknowledgements

This research was funded by Summer Research Support by the College of Human Environmental Sciences, the University of Alabama.

Conflict of interest

The authors declare no conflict of interest.

Author details

Katheryn Broman, Abigail U. Davis, Jordan May and Han-A Park*
Department of Human Nutrition and Hospitality Management, College of Human Environmental Sciences, The University of Alabama, Tuscaloosa, AL, USA

*Address all correspondence to: hpark36@ches.ua.edu

References

[1] Smith GM, Gallo G. The role of mitochondria in axon development and regeneration. Developmental Neurobiology. 2018;**78**(3):221-237

[2] Harris JJ, Jolivet R, Attwell D. Synaptic energy use and supply. Neuron. 2012;**75**(5):762-777

[3] Skou JC. The identification of the sodium pump. Bioscience Reports. 2004;**24**(4-5):436-451

[4] Pivovarov AS, Calahorro F, Walker RJ. Na(+)/K(+)-pump and neurotransmitter membrane receptors. Invertebrate Neuroscience. 2018;**19**(1):1

[5] Pathak D, Shields LY, Mendelsohn BA, Haddad D, Lin W, et al. The role of mitochondrially derived ATP in synaptic vesicle recycling. The Journal of Biological Chemistry. 2015;**290**(37):22325-22336

[6] Kroemer G, Dallaporta B, Resche-Rigon M. The mitochondrial death/life regulator in apoptosis and necrosis. Annual Review of Physiology. 1998;**60**:619-642

[7] Zou H, Li Y, Liu X, Wang X. An APAF-1.cytochrome c multimeric complex is a functional apoptosome that activates procaspase-9. The Journal of Biological Chemistry. 1999;**274**(17):11549-11556

[8] Wu G, Chai J, Suber TL, Wu JW, Du C, et al. Structural basis of IAP recognition by Smac/DIABLO. Nature. 2000;**408**(6815):1008-1012

[9] Czabotar PE, Lessene G, Strasser A, Adams JM. Control of apoptosis by the BCL-2 protein family: Implications for physiology and therapy. Nature Reviews. Molecular Cell Biology. 2014;**15**(1):49-63

[10] Ren D, Tu HC, Kim H, Wang GX, Bean GR, et al. BID, BIM, and PUMA are essential for activation of the BAX- and BAK-dependent cell death program. Science. 2010;**330**(6009):1390-1393

[11] Desagher S, Osen-Sand A, Nichols A, Eskes R, Montessuit S, et al. Bid-induced conformational change of Bax is responsible for mitochondrial cytochrome c release during apoptosis. The Journal of Cell Biology. 1999;**144**(5):891-901

[12] Jurgensmeier JM, Xie Z, Deveraux Q, Ellerby L, Bredesen D, et al. Bax directly induces release of cytochrome c from isolated mitochondria. Proceedings of the National Academy of Sciences of the United States of America. 1998;**95**(9):4997-5002

[13] Kirkland RA, Franklin JL. Bax, reactive oxygen, and cytochrome c release in neuronal apoptosis. Antioxidants and Redox Signaling. 2003;**5**(5):589-596

[14] Wei MC, Lindsten T, Mootha VK, Weiler S, Gross A, et al. tBID, a membrane-targeted death ligand, oligomerizes BAK to release cytochrome c. Genes and Development. 2000;**14**(16):2060-2071

[15] Huang DC, Adams JM, Cory S. The conserved N-terminal BH4 domain of Bcl-2 homologues is essential for inhibition of apoptosis and interaction with CED-4. The EMBO Journal. 1998;**17**(4):1029-1039

[16] Cheng EH, Wei MC, Weiler S, Flavell RA, Mak TW, et al. BCL-2, BCL-X(L) sequester BH3 domain-only molecules preventing BAX- and BAK-mediated mitochondrial apoptosis. Molecular Cell. 2001;**8**(3):705-711

[17] Lee EF, Grabow S, Chappaz S, Dewson G, Hockings C, et al. Physiological restraint of Bak by Bcl-xL

is essential for cell survival. Genes and Development. 2016;**30**(10):1240-1250

[18] Todt F, Cakir Z, Reichenbach F, Youle RJ, Edlich F. The C-terminal helix of Bcl-x(L) mediates Bax retrotranslocation from the mitochondria. Cell Death and Differentiation. 2013;**20**(2):333-342

[19] Ku B, Liang C, Jung JU, Oh BH. Evidence that inhibition of BAX activation by BCL-2 involves its tight and preferential interaction with the BH3 domain of BAX. Cell Research. 2011;**21**(4):627-641

[20] Clohessy JG, Zhuang J, de Boer J, Gil-Gomez G, Brady HJ. Mcl-1 interacts with truncated bid and inhibits its induction of cytochrome c release and its role in receptor-mediated apoptosis. The Journal of Biological Chemistry. 2006;**281**(9):5750-5759

[21] Chen L, Willis SN, Wei A, Smith BJ, Fletcher JI, et al. Differential targeting of prosurvival Bcl-2 proteins by their BH3-only ligands allows complementary apoptotic function. Molecular Cell. 2005;**17**(3):393-403

[22] Murphy MP. How mitochondria produce reactive oxygen species. The Biochemical Journal. 2009;**417**(1):1-13

[23] Liu Y, Fiskum G, Schubert D. Generation of reactive oxygen species by the mitochondrial electron transport chain. Journal of Neurochemistry. 2002;**80**(5):780-787

[24] Ott M, Robertson JD, Gogvadze V, Zhivotovsky B, Orrenius S. Cytochrome c release from mitochondria proceeds by a two-step process. Proceedings of the National Academy of Sciences of the United States of America. 2002;**99**(3):1259-1263

[25] Zhou X, Zhuang Z, Wang W, He L, Wu H, et al. OGG1 is essential in oxidative stress induced DNA demethylation. Cellular Signalling. 2016;**28**(9):1163-1171

[26] Miller CA, Sweatt JD. Covalent modification of DNA regulates memory formation. Neuron. 2007;**53**(6):857-869

[27] Weeber EJ, Beffert U, Jones C, Christian JM, Forster E, et al. Reelin and ApoE receptors cooperate to enhance hippocampal synaptic plasticity and learning. The Journal of Biological Chemistry. 2002;**277**(42):39944-39952

[28] Yoneyama M, Kawada K, Gotoh Y, Shiba T, Ogita K. Endogenous reactive oxygen species are essential for proliferation of neural stem/progenitor cells. Neurochemistry International. 2010;**56**(6-7):740-746

[29] Youle RJ, van der Bliek AM. Mitochondrial fission, fusion, and stress. Science. 2012;**337**(6098):1062-1065

[30] Mishra P, Chan DC. Metabolic regulation of mitochondrial dynamics. The Journal of Cell Biology. 2016;**212**(4):379-387

[31] Li Z, Okamoto K, Hayashi Y, Sheng M. The importance of dendritic mitochondria in the morphogenesis and plasticity of spines and synapses. Cell. 2004;**119**(6):873-887

[32] Shields LY, Kim H, Zhu L, Haddad D, Berthet A, et al. Dynamin-related protein 1 is required for normal mitochondrial bioenergetic and synaptic function in CA1 hippocampal neurons. Cell Death and Disease. 2015;**6**:e1725

[33] Ranieri M, Brajkovic S, Riboldi G, Ronchi D, Rizzo F, et al. Mitochondrial fusion proteins and human diseases. Neurology Research International. 2013;**2013**:293893

[34] van der Bliek AM, Shen Q, Kawajiri S. Mechanisms of mitochondrial fission and fusion. Cold

Spring Harbor Perspectives in Biology. 2013;**5**(6):a011702

[35] Berman SB, Chen YB, Qi B, McCaffery JM, Rucker EB 3rd, et al. Bcl-x L increases mitochondrial fission, fusion, and biomass in neurons. The Journal of Cell Biology. 2009;**184**(5):707-719

[36] Li H, Chen Y, Jones AF, Sanger RH, Collis LP, et al. Bcl-xL induces Drp1-dependent synapse formation in cultured hippocampal neurons. Proceedings of the National Academy of Sciences of the United States of America. 2008;**105**(6):2169-2174

[37] Li H, Alavian KN, Lazrove E, Mehta N, Jones A, et al. A Bcl-xL-Drp1 complex regulates synaptic vesicle membrane dynamics during endocytosis. Nature Cell Biology. 2013;**15**(7):773-785

[38] Sheng ZH. Mitochondrial trafficking and anchoring in neurons: New insight and implications. The Journal of Cell Biology. 2014;**204**(7):1087-1098

[39] Sun T, Qiao H, Pan PY, Chen Y, Sheng ZH. Motile axonal mitochondria contribute to the variability of presynaptic strength. Cell Reports. 2013;**4**(3):413-419

[40] Saxton WM, Hollenbeck PJ. The axonal transport of mitochondria. Journal of Cell Science. 2012;**125** (Pt 9):2095-2104

[41] Jolly AL, Kim H, Srinivasan D, Lakonishok M, Larson AG, et al. Kinesin-1 heavy chain mediates microtubule sliding to drive changes in cell shape. Proceedings of the National Academy of Sciences of the United States of America. 2010;**107**(27):12151-12156

[42] Ligon LA, Tokito M, Finklestein JM, Grossman FE, Holzbaur EL. A direct interaction between cytoplasmic dynein and kinesin I may coordinate motor activity. The Journal of Biological Chemistry. 2004;**279**(18):19201-19208

[43] Tang BL. Miro-working beyond mitochondria and microtubules. Cell. 2018;**7**(3):18

[44] Schwarz TL. Mitochondrial trafficking in neurons. Cold Spring Harbor Perspectives in Biology. 2013;**5**(6):a011304

[45] Stowers RS, Megeath LJ, Gorska-Andrzejak J, Meinertzhagen IA, Schwarz TL. Axonal transport of mitochondria to synapses depends on Milton, a novel drosophila protein. Neuron. 2002;**36**(6):1063-1077

[46] Kang JS, Tian JH, Pan PY, Zald P, Li C, et al. Docking of axonal mitochondria by syntaphilin controls their mobility and affects short-term facilitation. Cell. 2008;**132**(1):137-148

[47] Courchet J, Lewis TL Jr, Lee S, Courchet V, Liou DY, et al. Terminal axon branching is regulated by the LKB1-NUAK1 kinase pathway via presynaptic mitochondrial capture. Cell. 2013;**153**(7):1510-1525

[48] Barnes AP, Lilley BN, Pan YA, Plummer LJ, Powell AW, et al. LKB1 and SAD kinases define a pathway required for the polarization of cortical neurons. Cell. 2007;**129**(3):549-563

[49] Park HA, Licznerski P, Alavian KN, Shanabrough M, Jonas EA. Bcl-xL is necessary for neurite outgrowth in hippocampal neurons. Antioxidants and Redox Signaling. 2015;**22**(2):93-108

[50] Wang R, Reddy PH. Role of glutamate and NMDA receptors in Alzheimer's disease. Journal of Alzheimer's Disease. 2017;**57**(4):1041-1048

[51] Johnson KA, Conn PJ, Niswender CM. Glutamate receptors

as therapeutic targets for Parkinson's disease. CNS and Neurological Disorders Drug Targets. 2009;**8**(6):475-491

[52] Lai TW, Zhang S, Wang YT. Excitotoxicity and stroke: Identifying novel targets for neuroprotection. Progress in Neurobiology. 2014;**115**:157-188

[53] Guerriero RM, Giza CC, Rotenberg A. Glutamate and GABA imbalance following traumatic brain injury. Current Neurology and Neuroscience Reports. 2015;**15**(5):27

[54] Onyango IG, Dennis J, Khan SM. Mitochondrial dysfunction in Alzheimer's disease and the rationale for bioenergetics based therapies. Aging and Disease. 2016;**7**(2):201-214

[55] Hiebert JB, Shen Q, Thimmesch AR, Pierce JD. Traumatic brain injury and mitochondrial dysfunction. The American Journal of the Medical Sciences. 2015;**350**(2):132-138

[56] Pivovarova NB, Andrews SB. Calcium-dependent mitochondrial function and dysfunction in neurons. The FEBS Journal. 2010;**277**(18):3622-3636

[57] DeMaagd G, Philip A. Parkinson's disease and its management: Part 1: Disease entity, risk factors, pathophysiology, clinical presentation, and diagnosis. Pharmacy and Therapeutics. 2015;**40**(8):504-532

[58] Hwang O. Role of oxidative stress in Parkinson's disease. Experimental Neurobiology. 2013;**22**(1):11-17

[59] Pozo Devoto VM, Falzone TL. Mitochondrial dynamics in Parkinson's disease: A role for alpha-synuclein? Disease Models and Mechanisms. 2017;**10**(9):1075-1087

[60] Santos D, Esteves AR, Silva DF, Januario C, Cardoso SM. The impact of mitochondrial fusion and fission modulation in sporadic Parkinson's disease. Molecular Neurobiology. 2015;**52**(1):573-586

[61] Berthet A, Margolis EB, Zhang J, Hsieh I, Zhang J, et al. Loss of mitochondrial fission depletes axonal mitochondria in midbrain dopamine neurons. The Journal of Neuroscience: The Official Journal of the Society for Neuroscience. 2014;**34**(43):14304-14317

[62] Pickrell AM, Youle RJ. The roles of PINK1, parkin, and mitochondrial fidelity in Parkinson's disease. Neuron. 2015;**85**(2):257-273

[63] Geisler S, Holmstrom KM, Treis A, Skujat D, Weber SS, et al. The PINK1/Parkin-mediated mitophagy is compromised by PD-associated mutations. Autophagy. 2010;**6**(7): 871-878

[64] Wang X, Winter D, Ashrafi G, Schlehe J, Wong YL, et al. PINK1 and Parkin target Miro for phosphorylation and degradation to arrest mitochondrial motility. Cell. 2011;**147**(4):893-906

[65] Liu S, Sawada T, Lee S, Yu W, Silverio G, et al. Parkinson's disease-associated kinase PINK1 regulates Miro protein level and axonal transport of mitochondria. PLoS Genetics. 2012;**8**(3):e1002537

[66] Arena G, Gelmetti V, Torosantucci L, Vignone D, Lamorte G, et al. PINK1 protects against cell death induced by mitochondrial depolarization, by phosphorylating Bcl-xL and impairing its pro-apoptotic cleavage. Cell Death and Differentiation. 2013;**20**(7):920-930

[67] Ofengeim D, Chen YB, Miyawaki T, Li H, Sacchetti S, et al. N-terminally cleaved Bcl-xL mediates ischemia-induced neuronal death. Nature Neuroscience. 2012;**15**(4):574-580

[68] Park HA, Jonas EA. DeltaN-Bcl-xL, a therapeutic target for neuroprotection. Neural Regeneration Research. 2017;**12**(11):1791-1794

[69] Park HA, Licznerski P, Mnatsakanyan N, Niu Y, Sacchetti S, et al. Inhibition of Bcl-xL prevents pro-death actions of DeltaN-Bcl-xL at the mitochondrial inner membrane during glutamate excitotoxicity. Cell Death and Differentiation. 2017;**24**(11):1963-1974

[70] Moon HE, Paek SH. Mitochondrial dysfunction in Parkinson's disease. Experimental Neurobiology. 2015;**24**(2):103-116

[71] Stefanis L. Alpha-synuclein in Parkinson's disease. Cold Spring Harbor Perspectives in Medicine. 2012;**2**(2):a009399

[72] Seo JH, Rah JC, Choi SH, Shin JK, Min K, et al. Alpha-synuclein regulates neuronal survival via Bcl-2 family expression and PI3/Akt kinase pathway. The FASEB Journal. 2002;**16**(13):1826-1828

[73] Shaltouki A, Hsieh CH, Kim MJ, Wang X. Alpha-synuclein delays mitophagy and targeting Miro rescues neuron loss in Parkinson's models. Acta Neuropathologica. 2018;**136**(4):607-620

[74] Chen R, Park HA, Mnatsakanyan N, Niu Y, Licznerski P, et al. Parkinson's disease protein DJ-1 regulates ATP synthase protein components to increase neuronal process outgrowth. Cell Death and Disease. 2019;**10**(6):469

[75] Hao LY, Giasson BI, Bonini NM. DJ-1 is critical for mitochondrial function and rescues PINK1 loss of function. Proceedings of the National Academy of Sciences of the United States of America. 2010;**107**(21):9747-9752

[76] Strobbe D, Robinson AA, Harvey K, Rossi L, Ferraina C, et al. Distinct mechanisms of pathogenic DJ-1 mutations in mitochondrial quality control. Frontiers in Molecular Neuroscience. 2018;**11**:68

[77] Shendelman S, Jonason A, Martinat C, Leete T, Abeliovich A. DJ-1 is a redox-dependent molecular chaperone that inhibits alpha-synuclein aggregate formation. PLoS Biology. 2004;**2**(11):e362

[78] Alzheimer's Association, editor. Alzheimer's Disease Facts and Figures. United States: Elsevier Science B.V. Amsterdam; 2018

[79] Hamley IW. The amyloid beta peptide: A chemist's perspective. Role in Alzheimer's and fibrillization. Chemical Reviews. 2012;**112**(10):5147-5192

[80] Kolarova M, Garcia-Sierra F, Bartos A, Ricny J, Ripova D. Structure and pathology of tau protein in Alzheimer disease. International Journal of Alzheimer's Disease. 2012;**2012**:731526

[81] Stokin GB, Goldstein LS. Axonal transport and Alzheimer's disease. Annual Review of Biochemistry. 2006;**75**:607-627

[82] Calkins MJ, Manczak M, Mao P, Shirendeb U, Reddy PH. Impaired mitochondrial biogenesis, defective axonal transport of mitochondria, abnormal mitochondrial dynamics and synaptic degeneration in a mouse model of Alzheimer's disease. Human Molecular Genetics. 2011;**20**(23):4515-4529

[83] Calkins MJ, Reddy PH. Amyloid beta impairs mitochondrial anterograde transport and degenerates synapses in Alzheimer's disease neurons. Biochimica et Biophysica Acta (BBA)—Molecular Basis of Disease. 2011;**1812**(4):507-513

[84] Rui Y, Tiwari P, Xie Z, Zheng JQ. Acute impairment of mitochondrial trafficking by beta-amyloid peptides in hippocampal neurons. The Journal of Neuroscience: The Official Journal of the Society for Neuroscience. 2006;**26**(41):10480-10487

[85] Chaudhary AR, Berger F, Berger CL, Hendricks AG. Tau directs intracellular trafficking by regulating the forces exerted by kinesin and dynein teams. Traffic. 2018;**19**(2):111-121

[86] Dixit R, Ross JL, Goldman YE, Holzbaur EL. Differential regulation of dynein and kinesin motor proteins by tau. Science. 2008;**319**(5866):1086-1089

[87] DuBoff B, Gotz J, Feany MB. Tau promotes neurodegeneration via DRP1 mislocalization in vivo. Neuron. 2012;**75**(4):618-632

[88] Zuo W, Zhang S, Xia CY, Guo XF, He WB, et al. Mitochondria autophagy is induced after hypoxic/ischemic stress in a Drp1 dependent manner: The role of inhibition of Drp1 in ischemic brain damage. Neuropharmacology. 2014;**86**:103-115

[89] Liu W, Tian F, Kurata T, Morimoto N, Abe K. Dynamic changes of mitochondrial fusion and fission proteins after transient cerebral ischemia in mice. Journal of Neuroscience Research. 2012;**90**(6):1183-1189

[90] Chen SD, Lin TK, Yang DI, Lee SY, Shaw FZ, et al. Roles of PTEN-induced putative kinase 1 and dynamin-related protein 1 in transient global ischemia-induced hippocampal neuronal injury. Biochemical and Biophysical Research Communications. 2015;**460**(2):397-403

[91] Peng C, Rao W, Zhang L, Wang K, Hui H, et al. Mitofusin 2 ameliorates hypoxia-induced apoptosis via mitochondrial function and signaling pathways. The International Journal of Biochemistry and Cell Biology. 2015;**69**:29-40

[92] Martorell-Riera A, Segarra-Mondejar M, Munoz JP, Ginet V, Olloquequi J, et al. Mfn2 downregulation in excitotoxicity causes mitochondrial dysfunction and delayed neuronal death. The EMBO Journal. 2014;**33**(20):2388-2407

[93] Wu QJ, Tymianski M. Targeting NMDA receptors in stroke: New hope in neuroprotection. Molecular Brain. 2018;**11**(1):15

[94] Lin R, Duan Z, Sun H, Fung ML, Chen H, et al. Kinesin-1 regulates extrasynaptic targeting of NMDARs and neuronal vulnerability toward excitotoxicity. iScience. 2019;**13**:82-97

[95] Song Y, Li T, Liu Z, Xu Z, Zhang Z, et al. Inhibition of Drp1 after traumatic brain injury provides brain protection and improves behavioral performance in rats. Chemico-Biological Interactions. 2019;**304**:173-185

[96] Fischer TD, Hylin MJ, Zhao J, Moore AN, Waxham MN, et al. Altered mitochondrial dynamics and TBI pathophysiology. Frontiers in Systems Neuroscience. 2016;**10**:29

[97] Di Pietro V, Lazzarino G, Amorini AM, Signoretti S, Hill LJ, et al. Fusion or fission: The destiny of mitochondria in traumatic brain injury of different severities. Scientific Reports. 2017;7(1):9189

[98] Chuang CS, Chang JC, Cheng FC, Liu KH, Su HL, et al. Modulation of mitochondrial dynamics by treadmill training to improve gait and mitochondrial deficiency in a rat model of Parkinson's disease. Life Sciences. 2017;**191**:236-244

[99] Gusdon AM, Callio J, Distefano G, O'Doherty RM, Goodpaster BH, et al.

Exercise increases mitochondrial complex I activity and DRP1 expression in the brains of aged mice. Experimental Gerontology. 2017;**90**:1-13

[100] E L BJM, Swerdlow RH. Effect of high-intensity exercise on aged mouse brain mitochondria, neurogenesis, and inflammation. Neurobiology of Aging. 2014;**35**(11):2574-2583

[101] SteinerJL, MurphyEA, McClellanJL, Carmichael MD, Davis JM. Exercise training increases mitochondrial biogenesis in the brain. Journal of Applied Physiology (Bethesda, MD: 1985). 2011;**111**(4):1066-1071

[102] Leem YH, Lim HJ, Shim SB, Cho JY, Kim BS, et al. Repression of tau hyperphosphorylation by chronic endurance exercise in aged transgenic mouse model of tauopathies. Journal of Neuroscience Research. 2009;**87**(11):2561-2570

[103] Garcia-Mesa Y, Gimenez-Llort L, Lopez LC, Venegas C, Cristofol R, et al. Melatonin plus physical exercise are highly neuroprotective in the 3xTg-AD mouse. Neurobiology of Aging. 2012;**33**(6):1124 e13-1124 e29

[104] Bo H, Kang W, Jiang N, Wang X, Zhang Y, et al. Exercise-induced neuroprotection of hippocampus in APP/PS1 transgenic mice via upregulation of mitochondrial 8-oxoguanine DNA glycosylase. Oxidative Medicine and Cellular Longevity. 2014;**2014**:834502

[105] Kim SE, Ko IG, Kim BK, Shin MS, Cho S, et al. Treadmill exercise prevents aging-induced failure of memory through an increase in neurogenesis and suppression of apoptosis in rat hippocampus. Experimental Gerontology. 2010;**45**(5):357-365

[106] Aboutaleb N, Shamsaei N, Khaksari M, Erfani S, Rajabi H, et al. Pre-ischemic exercise reduces apoptosis in hippocampal CA3 cells after cerebral ischemia by modulation of the Bax/Bcl-2 proteins ratio and prevention of caspase-3 activation. The Journal of Physiological Sciences. 2015;**65**(5):435-443

[107] Kim DH, Ko IG, Kim BK, Kim TW, Kim SE, et al. Treadmill exercise inhibits traumatic brain injury-induced hippocampal apoptosis. Physiology and Behavior. 2010;**101**(5):660-665

[108] Jang Y, Kwon I, Song W, Cosio-Lima LM, Taylor S, et al. Modulation of mitochondrial phenotypes by endurance exercise contributes to neuroprotection against a MPTP-induced animal model of PD. Life Sciences. 2018;**209**:455-465

[109] Cheng SM, Ho TJ, Yang AL, Chen IJ, Kao CL, et al. Exercise training enhances cardiac IGFI-R/PI3K/Akt and Bcl-2 family associated pro-survival pathways in streptozotocin-induced diabetic rats. International Journal of Cardiology. 2013;**167**(2):478-485

[110] Zhou Y, Lian S, Zhang J, Lin D, Huang C, et al. Mitochondrial perturbation contributing to cognitive decline in Streptozotocin-induced type 1 diabetic rats. Cellular Physiology and Biochemistry. 2018;**46**(4):1668-1682

[111] Moreira PI, Santos MS, Moreno AM, Seica R, Oliveira CR. Increased vulnerability of brain mitochondria in diabetic (Goto-Kakizaki) rats with aging and amyloid-beta exposure. Diabetes. 2003;**52**(6):1449-1456

[112] Moreira PI, Santos MS, Moreno AM, Proenca T, Seica R, et al. Effect of streptozotocin-induced diabetes on rat brain mitochondria. Journal of Neuroendocrinology. 2004;**16**(1):32-38

[113] Huang S, Wang Y, Gan X, Fang D, Zhong C, et al. Drp1-mediated

mitochondrial abnormalities link to synaptic injury in diabetes model. Diabetes. 2015;**64**(5):1728-1742

[114] Sripetchwandee J, Chattipakorn N, Chattipakorn SC. Links between obesity-induced brain insulin resistance, brain mitochondrial dysfunction, and dementia. Frontiers in Endocrinology (Lausanne). 2018;**9**:496

[115] Cree-Green M, Gupta A, Coe GV, Baumgartner AD, Pyle L, et al. Insulin resistance in type 2 diabetes youth relates to serum free fatty acids and muscle mitochondrial dysfunction. Journal of Diabetes and Its Complications. 2017;**31**(1):141-148

[116] Vantaggiato C, Castelli M, Giovarelli M, Orso G, Bassi MT, et al. The fine tuning of Drp1-dependent mitochondrial remodeling and autophagy controls neuronal differentiation. Frontiers in Cellular Neuroscience. 2019;**13**:120

[117] Moreira PI, Santos MS, Sena C, Seica R, Oliveira CR. Insulin protects against amyloid beta-peptide toxicity in brain mitochondria of diabetic rats. Neurobiology of Disease. 2005;**18**(3):628-637

[118] Sa-Nguanmoo P, Tanajak P, Kerdphoo S, Jaiwongkam T, Pratchayasakul W, et al. SGLT2-inhibitor and DPP-4 inhibitor improve brain function via attenuating mitochondrial dysfunction, insulin resistance, inflammation, and apoptosis in HFD-induced obese rats. Toxicology and Applied Pharmacology. 2017;**333**:43-50

[119] Sa-Nguanmoo P, Tanajak P, Kerdphoo S, Satjaritanun P, Wang X, et al. FGF21 improves cognition by restored synaptic plasticity, dendritic spine density, brain mitochondrial function and cell apoptosis in obese-insulin resistant male rats. Hormones and Behavior. 2016;**85**:86-95

[120] Pintana H, Sripetchwandee J, Supakul L, Apaijai N, Chattipakorn N, et al. Garlic extract attenuates brain mitochondrial dysfunction and cognitive deficit in obese-insulin resistant rats. Applied Physiology, Nutrition, and Metabolism. 2014;**39**(12):1373-1379

[121] Pratchayasakul W, Sa-Nguanmoo P, Sivasinprasasn S, Pintana H, Tawinvisan R, et al. Obesity accelerates cognitive decline by aggravating mitochondrial dysfunction, insulin resistance and synaptic dysfunction under estrogen-deprived conditions. Hormones and Behavior. 2015;**72**:68-77

[122] Wang D, Yan J, Chen J, Wu W, Zhu X, et al. Naringin improves neuronal insulin signaling, brain mitochondrial function, and cognitive function in high-fat diet-induced obese mice. Cellular and Molecular Neurobiology. 2015;**35**(7):1061-1071

[123] Wlodarek D. Role of ketogenic diets in neurodegenerative diseases (Alzheimer's disease and Parkinson's disease). Nutrients. 2019;**11**(1):169

[124] Agarwal P, Wang Y, Buchman AS, Holland TM, Bennett DA, et al. MIND diet associated with reduced incidence and delayed progression of Parkinsonism in old age. The Journal of Nutrition, Health and Aging. 2018;**22**(10):1211-1215

[125] Morris MC, Tangney CC, Wang Y, Sacks FM, Barnes LL, et al. MIND diet slows cognitive decline with aging. Alzheimer's and Dementia. 2015;**11**(9):1015-1022

[126] Duan W, Mattson MP. Dietary restriction and 2-deoxyglucose administration improve behavioral outcome and reduce degeneration of dopaminergic neurons in models of Parkinson's disease.

Journal of Neuroscience Research. 1999;**57**(2):195-206

[127] Anson RM, Guo Z, de Cabo R, Iyun T, Rios M, et al. Intermittent fasting dissociates beneficial effects of dietary restriction on glucose metabolism and neuronal resistance to injury from calorie intake. Proceedings of the National Academy of Sciences of the United States of America. 2003;**100**(10):6216-6220

[128] Amigo I, Menezes-Filho SL, Luevano-Martinez LA, Chausse B, Kowaltowski AJ. Caloric restriction increases brain mitochondrial calcium retention capacity and protects against excitotoxicity. Aging Cell. 2017;**16**(1):73-81

[129] Halagappa VK, Guo Z, Pearson M, Matsuoka Y, Cutler RG, et al. Intermittent fasting and caloric restriction ameliorate age-related behavioral deficits in the triple-transgenic mouse model of Alzheimer's disease. Neurobiology of Disease. 2007;**26**(1):212-220

[130] Maswood N, Young J, Tilmont E, Zhang Z, Gash DM, et al. Caloric restriction increases neurotrophic factor levels and attenuates neurochemical and behavioral deficits in a primate model of Parkinson's disease. Proceedings of the National Academy of Sciences of the United States of America. 2004;**101**(52):18171-18176

[131] Sanz A, Caro P, Ibanez J, Gomez J, Gredilla R, et al. Dietary restriction at old age lowers mitochondrial oxygen radical production and leak at complex I and oxidative DNA damage in rat brain. Journal of Bioenergetics and Biomembranes. 2005;**37**(2):83-90

[132] Hu Y, Zhang M, Chen Y, Yang Y, Zhang JJ. Postoperative intermittent fasting prevents hippocampal oxidative stress and memory deficits in a rat model of chronic cerebral hypoperfusion. European Journal of Nutrition. 2019;**58**(1):423-432

[133] Hyun DH, Emerson SS, Jo DG, Mattson MP, de Cabo R. Calorie restriction up-regulates the plasma membrane redox system in brain cells and suppresses oxidative stress during aging. Proceedings of the National Academy of Sciences of the United States of America. 2006;**103**(52):19908-19912

[134] Loncarevic-Vasiljkovic N, Milanovic D, Pesic V, Tesic V, Brkic M, et al. Dietary restriction suppresses apoptotic cell death, promotes Bcl-2 and Bcl-xl mRNA expression and increases the Bcl-2/Bax protein ratio in the rat cortex after cortical injury. Neurochemistry International. 2016;**96**:69-76

[135] Lin AL, Coman D, Jiang L, Rothman DL, Hyder F. Caloric restriction impedes age-related decline of mitochondrial function and neuronal activity. Journal of Cerebral Blood Flow and Metabolism. 2014;**34**(9):1440-1443

[136] Cerqueira FM, Cunha FM, Laurindo FR, Kowaltowski AJ. Calorie restriction increases cerebral mitochondrial respiratory capacity in a NO*-mediated mechanism: Impact on neuronal survival. Free Radical Biology and Medicine. 2012;**52**(7):1236-1241

[137] Duan W, Lee J, Guo Z, Mattson MP. Dietary restriction stimulates BDNF production in the brain and thereby protects neurons against excitotoxic injury. Journal of Molecular Neuroscience. 2001;**16**(1):1-12

[138] Stranahan AM, Lee K, Martin B, Maudsley S, Golden E, et al. Voluntary exercise and caloric restriction enhance hippocampal dendritic spine density and BDNF levels in diabetic mice. Hippocampus. 2009;**19**(10):951-961

[139] Su B, Ji YS, Sun XL, Liu XH, Chen ZY. Brain-derived neurotrophic factor (BDNF)-induced mitochondrial motility arrest and presynaptic docking contribute to BDNF-enhanced synaptic transmission. The Journal of Biological Chemistry. 2014;**289**(3):1213-1226

[140] Witte AV, Fobker M, Gellner R, Knecht S, Floel A. Caloric restriction improves memory in elderly humans. Proceedings of the National Academy of Sciences of the United States of America. 2009;**106**(4):1255-1260

[141] Prehn K, Jumpertz von Schwartzenberg R, Mai K, Zeitz U, Witte AV, et al. Caloric restriction in older adults-differential effects of weight loss and reduced weight on brain structure and function. Cerebral Cortex. 2017;**27**(3):1765-1778

[142] Wang BH, Hou Q, Lu YQ, Jia MM, Qiu T, et al. Ketogenic diet attenuates neuronal injury via autophagy and mitochondrial pathways in pentylenetetrazol-kindled seizures. Brain Research. 2018;**1678**:106-115

[143] Luan G, Zhao Y, Zhai F, Chen Y, Li T. Ketogenic diet reduces Smac/Diablo and cytochrome c release and attenuates neuronal death in a mouse model of limbic epilepsy. Brain Research Bulletin. 2012;**89**(3-4):79-85

[144] Hu ZG, Wang HD, Jin W, Yin HX. Ketogenic diet reduces cytochrome c release and cellular apoptosis following traumatic brain injury in juvenile rats. Annals of Clinical and Laboratory Science. 2009;**39**(1):76-83

[145] Puchowicz MA, Zechel JL, Valerio J, Emancipator DS, Xu K, et al. Neuroprotection in diet-induced ketotic rat brain after focal ischemia. Journal of Cerebral Blood Flow and Metabolism. 2008;**28**(12):1907-1916

[146] Noh HS, Kim YS, Kim YH, Han JY, Park CH, et al. Ketogenic diet protects the hippocampus from kainic acid toxicity by inhibiting the dissociation of bad from 14-3-3. Journal of Neuroscience Research. 2006;**84**(8):1829-1836

[147] Greco T, Glenn TC, Hovda DA, Prins ML. Ketogenic diet decreases oxidative stress and improves mitochondrial respiratory complex activity. Journal of Cerebral Blood Flow and Metabolism. 2016;**36**(9):1603-1613

[148] Hasan-Olive MM, Lauritzen KH, Ali M, Rasmussen LJ, Storm-Mathisen J, et al. A ketogenic diet improves mitochondrial biogenesis and bioenergetics via the PGC1alpha-SIRT3-UCP2 axis. Neurochemical Research. 2019;**44**(1):22-37

[149] Maalouf M, Sullivan PG, Davis L, Kim DY, Rho JM. Ketones inhibit mitochondrial production of reactive oxygen species production following glutamate excitotoxicity by increasing NADH oxidation. Neuroscience. 2007;**145**(1):256-264

[150] Nylen K, Velazquez JL, Sayed V, Gibson KM, Burnham WM, et al. The effects of a ketogenic diet on ATP concentrations and the number of hippocampal mitochondria in Aldh5a1(−/−) mice. Biochimica et Biophysica Acta. 2009;**1790**(3):208-212

[151] Yao J, Chen S, Mao Z, Cadenas E, Brinton RD. 2-Deoxy-D-glucose treatment induces ketogenesis, sustains mitochondrial function, and reduces pathology in female mouse model of Alzheimer's disease. PLoS One. 2011;**6**(7):e21788

Chapter 15

Hydrogen Sulfide as a Factor of Neuroprotection during the Constitutive and Reparative Neurogenesis in Fish Brain

Evgeniya V. Pushchina, Anatoly A. Varaksin and Dmitry K. Obukhov

Abstract

The H_2S-producing systems were studied in trout telencephalon, tectum, and cerebellum at 1 week after eye injury. The results of ELISA analysis have shown a 1.7-fold increase in the CBS expression at 1 week post-injury, as compared to the intact trout. In the ventricular and subventricular regions of trout telencephalon, CBS+ cells, as well as neuroepithelial and glial types, were detected. As a result of injury, the number of CBS+ neuroepithelial cells in the pallial and subpallial periventricular regions of the telencephalon increases. In the tectum, a traumatic damage leads to an increase in the CBS expression in radial glia with a simultaneous decrease in the number of CBS immunopositive neuroepithelial cells detected in intact animals. In the cerebellum, we revealed neuroglial interrelations, in which H_2S is probably released from the astrocyte-like cells with subsequent activation of the neuronal NMDA receptors. The organization of the H_2S-producing cell complexes suggests that the amount of glutamate produced in the trout cerebellum and its reuptake is controlled with the involvement of astrocyte-like cells, reducing its excitotoxicity. We believe that the increase in the number of H_2S-producing cells constitutes a response to oxidative stress, and the overproduction of H_2S neutralizes the reactive oxygen species.

Keywords: hydrogen sulfide, traumatic eye injury, oxidative stress, radial glia, excitotoxicity, reparative neurogenesis, adult neuronal stem cells, neuroepithelial cells, astrocyte-like cells, teleost fishes, CBS expression

1. Introduction

Hydrogen sulfide (H_2S) was initially considered as a gasotransmitter with antioxidant properties [1]. To date, the vasodilating, neuromodulating, and anti-inflammatory properties of H_2S have also been identified [2, 3]. In studies of the cardiovascular system, H_2S was assumed to act as a protective factor [4]; nevertheless, the effects of H_2S in the central nervous system (CNS) during stress or injury remain poorly understood. The involvement of H_2S, as well as other gaseous intermediaries such as NO, CO, and H_2, in the traumatic brain injury is now intensively investigated [5], but this question has not been completely clarified thus far. H_2S, like nitric oxide (NO), is known to mediate posttranslational modification of proteins by adding additional sulfur to reactive cysteine residues. This modification, referred to as S-sulfhydration, is required to activate or inactivate many classes of proteins, including the ion channels, such as the ATP-dependent potassium channels, TRPV3, TRPV6, TRPM [6], enzymes, and the transcription factors NF-kB and Nrf2 [7]. Modulation of ion channels, as well as the inflammatory and the antioxidant transcription factors, using H_2S after traumatic brain injury, can play a significant role in reducing edema and inflammation [8].

Recently, the involvement of H_2S in cerebral ischemia, traumatic brain injury (TBI), and decrease in reactive oxygen species in the H_2S-dependent mechanisms has been studied using different models [8–10]. The use of monoclonal antibodies against cystathionine β-synthase (CBS) in immunohistochemical (IHC) detection of the H_2S-producing complexes in the brain of juvenile trout showed an increase in hydrogen sulfide production in different parts of the brain and CBS induction in the radial glia cells after the damage of the optic nerve [11]. It was shown that the toxic and/or neuroprotective effects of hydrogen sulfide depended on concentration: lower concentrations play a physiological role, while very high concentrations cause cell death [12, 13]. Although hydrogen sulfide is considered a gasotransmitter, there is uncertainty about the total concentration of this volatile gas or highly active anionic particles (SH-) in both plasma and central nervous system tissues [14].

The progress in studies of the hydrogen sulfide biology has led to a conclusion that polysulfides are more significant sources of intermediate sulfhydration of proteins than H_2S [3]. The H_2S reactions with many signal mediators, transcription factors, and channel proteins in neurons and glial cells are known both in vivo and in vitro [7, 10]. However, still little is known about interaction of the H_2S intercellular communication and its consequences in the case of a traumatic cerebral injury. Such information is necessary to determine the cytoprotective or cytotoxic effects of H_2S in the brain injury and/or cerebral ischemia.

The study of biology of the neural stem cells, based on animal models, is becoming increasingly important, since the processes of constitutive neurogenesis occur in many areas of the animal brain [15], providing a high reparative potential of CNS. One of such models is fish, which is characterized by a high rate of reparative processes [16]. The results of preliminary studies showed an increase in proliferative activity of cells of the trout brain after damage to optic nerve [17]. To further characterize the cellular response in the trout brain after eye injury, the hydrogen sulfide-producing enzyme, cystathionine β-synthase (CBS), was analyzed using western immunoblotting, enzyme-linked immunosorbent assay (ELISA), and immunohistochemical labeling of CBS in various sections of the trout brain at 1 week after the traumatic eye injury.

2. Evaluation of CBS expression in the intact trout brain and after eye injury by the western blot analysis and ELISA immunosorbent assay

The cystathionine β-synthase enzyme has a tetramer binding with two substrates (homocysteine and serine) and three additional ligands (the coenzyme pyrodoxal 5′-phosphate, the allosteric activator S-adenosylmethionine, and heme). An assessment of CBS content by Western blot analysis showed the presence of protein with a molecular weight of 63 kDa in all the divisions of the trout brain. The quantitative CBS content in different divisions of the intact trout brain and after the mechanical eye injury is shown in **Figure 1A**. The maximum level of CBS

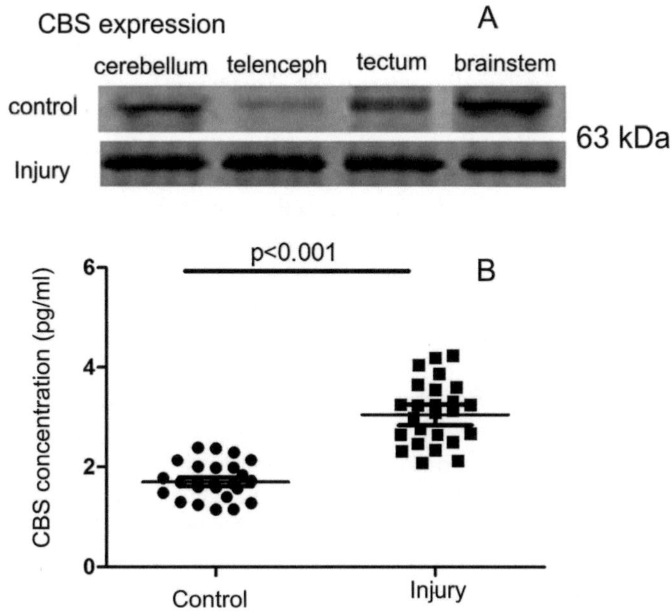

Figure 1.
Representation of western blots of cystathionine β-synthase content in the brain of the trout Oncorhynchus mykiss. *(A) the single protein band corresponding to a molecular weight of 63 kDa was present in the trout cerebellum, optic tectum, telencephalon, and brainstem in the control (intact) animals and at 1 week after the optic nerve damage. (B) ELISA assay of CBS in the rainbow trout brain at 1 week after UEI vs. control (intact) rainbow trout. Student's t-test was used to determine significant differences between the trout at 1 week after UEI vs. control (intact) fish (## P < 0.01); n = 20 in each group.*

expression in the intact animals was found in the brain stem, while the minimum was in the telencephalon. The cerebellum and tectum showed a medium level of CBS expression. A significant increase in the level of CBS expression was observed in all the brain divisions after the mechanical eye injury (**Figure 1A**). According to the enzyme immunosorbent assay, it was 1.86 ± 0.03 pg./mL and 3.12 ± 0.26 pg./mL after unilateral eye injury (UEI) ($P < 0.001$). Thus, within a week after the eye injury, the concentration of CBS increased 1.7 times compared with the control animals (**Figure 1B**).

3. Telencephalon

Results of the IHC CBS-labeling in the trout telencephalon showed the presence of intensely and moderately labeled cells in the pallial and subpallial regions. CBS-labeled cells were located in the superficial periventricular and subventricular pallial layers. In deep pallial areas, the number of intensively labeled cells was elevated. The presence of a H_2S-producing enzyme in the brain cells is associated with the process of neurochemical signaling and, in particular, with the activation of NMDA receptors. Activation of neurons in the brain of vertebrates leads to release of neurotransmitters, including glutamate, activating the NMDA receptors, which, in turn, leads to an increase in the astrocytic intracellular calcium and long-term potentiation [3, 18]. Thus, the presence of two levels of CBS activity in the trout telencephalon indicates the mediator/modulatory intercellular interactions, which agrees with the previously obtained data on fish [11].

In intact trout, when labeled with polyclonal antibodies against CBS, the CBS-labeled radial glia was detected particularly in the pallial and subpallial regions of the telencephalon, while labeling with monoclonal antibodies did not reveal similar structures [11]. The present data suggests that in the trout telencephalon CBS may label aNSCs with a glial phenotype (radial glia). Our assumption is consistent with the results of studies of the pallial neurogenic niche in adult zebrafish containing radial glia-like aNSCs with cellular bodies lining the walls of the ventricle [19]. Studies of the hydrogen sulfide biology in the mammalian brain have shown that astrocytes and glial cells constitute the main repositories of CBS in the brain [3]. In in vitro experiments, it was found that astrocytes produce 7.57 times more H_2S than the microglial cells [20]. However, in the fish brain, the detection of typical astrocytic glia gives controversial results [21, 22], and radial glia is detected frequently during attempts to identify the brain glial architectonics [23].

In the surface layer of different zones of the trout telencephalon, CBS+ cells and RG and cells of neuroepithelial type, representing a part of the constitutive matrix zones of the telencephalon, were also identified. Thus, CBS+ cells were detected in the zones of constitutive neurogenesis in the telencephalon of intact animals, which is consistent with the previously obtained data on the masu salmon and carp [24]. Studies on *D. rerio* have shown that aNSCs are associated with the ventricular system. In the fish telencephalon, aNSCs have a typical morphology of radial glial and/or neuroepithelium, which can be identified with several molecular markers of aNSCs [25, 26]. Thus, it is obvious that the CBS+ cells of the pallial and subpallial regions of the trout telencephalon are the aNSCs of the neuroepithelial and glial types. Earlier studies on trout have shown that after injury in the dorsal, medial, and lateral pallial zones, the number of the PCNA+ and HuCD+ cells significantly increases, indicating growth of proliferative and neurogenic activity in the telencephalon [17]. After the traumatic eye injury, the number of CBS+ cells increased in all areas of the telencephalon, with the exception of dorso-central zone (**Figure 2**). The number of H_2S-producing cells increases in the periventricular and subventricular regions of the telencephalon, which are characterized by intensification of proliferative processes that occur after the eye injury.

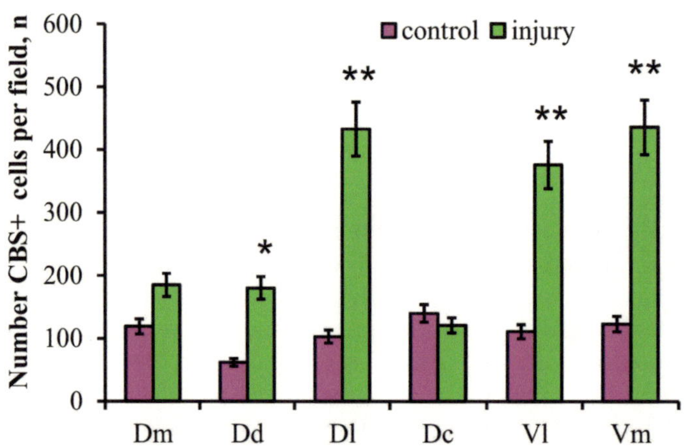

Figure 2.
Density of CBS+ cells in the telencephalon of the intact trout Oncorhynchus mykiss *and at 1 week post-injury. The one-way analysis of variance (ANOVA) followed by the student–Newman–Keuls post hoc test was used to determine significant differences between the control trout and fish after UEI (n = 5 in each group; * P < 0.01, ** P < 0.05 significant differences* vs. *the control group). Dm, Dd, Dl, and Dc are the medial, dorsal, lateral, and central parts of the dorsal telencephalic area; Vl and Vm are the lateral and medial parts of the ventral nucleus of telencephalon.*

4. CBS in the telencephalon parenchyma

An increase in another type of CBS+ cells, which are intensively labeled, having no processes, and adjacent to large moderately labeled neurons, in the telencephalon parenchyma suggests intercellular neuron/glial or neuron/microglial interactions associated with release of H_2S from intensively labeled astrocyte-like cells and/or microglia [18, 27]. In addition, after the injury, the patterns of distribution of the CBS+ radial glia cells in the telencephalon are retained, which indicates an additional production of H_2S in aNSCs of the glial phenotype. Studies showed that after ischemic brain damage, the additional production of H_2S is provided by sulfhydration [2]. In more recent studies, it has been shown that polysulfides are 300 times more active than H_2S in the TRPA1 receptor activation [3]. Polysulfides activate NMDA receptors, which is accompanied by the H_2S-dependent reduction of cysteine disulfide in extracellular domain of the receptor [3]. In this context, activation of the NMDA channels by H_2S is probably a detrimental condition arising from the excitotoxicity of glutamate causing calcium influx, which, in turn, leads to neuronal toxicity and cell death [1, 28].

The results of experimental in vitro studies have shown that the glutamate toxicity during a traumatic injury (ischemia) is attenuated by the effect of H_2S on ATP/K^+ and CFTR/Cl^- channels [29] and activation of the GLT1 transporters [30]. However, there is currently no consensus on the dual role of H_2S in the glutamate toxicity. Neurons that are formed in the matrix periventricular zones of the trout telencephalon represent the immature cell forms that migrate from the periventricular to subventricular layers of the brain. Such undifferentiated cells can express an incomplete set of glutamate NMDA receptors, and, therefore, those cascade processes that trigger apoptosis in mature neurons in immature cells cannot cause death. On the other hand, it is known that H_2S is metabolized by mitochondria through participation in the oxidation process of the H_2S-producing enzymes [13, 31]. The stress-induced H_2S production in mitochondria and a subsequent increase in the ATP production were demonstrated [32].

Changes in the mitochondrial membrane potential activate caspase-3 and then become attenuated with NaHS in the neuronal cell culture, which protects neurons from apoptosis [33]. Thus, the controversial role of H_2S in the mammalian brain neurons raises some questions about whether the excessive production of H_2S causes death of mature neurons in the trout brain as a result of eye injury. It is likely that H_2S has a protective effect on the immature telencephalic cells after the injury. What phenotype (glial or neuronal) does correspond to cells that produce H_2S after UEI in the trout brain? Considering our previous evidence that the cells of these zones in the trout telencephalon are HuCD+ [17], it is fair to assume that the H_2S-producing cells in the trout telencephalon can represent immature neurons. However, the detection of CBS expression in the radial glia cells indicates a glial phenotype. Thus, it can be concluded that as a result of UEI in the trout telencephalon, CBS expression is activated in both the neuronal and glial cell population.

5. Optic tectum

As a result of UEI in the trout tectum, the number of the CBS+ cells increases dramatically, the appearance of the dense CBS+ cell groups in different layers of the tectum is diagnosed, and the CBS expression is induced in the RG cells (**Figure 3A**). The present results of CBS labeling with polyclonal antibodies in the tectum of older trout confirm the IHC labeling data for a younger age group

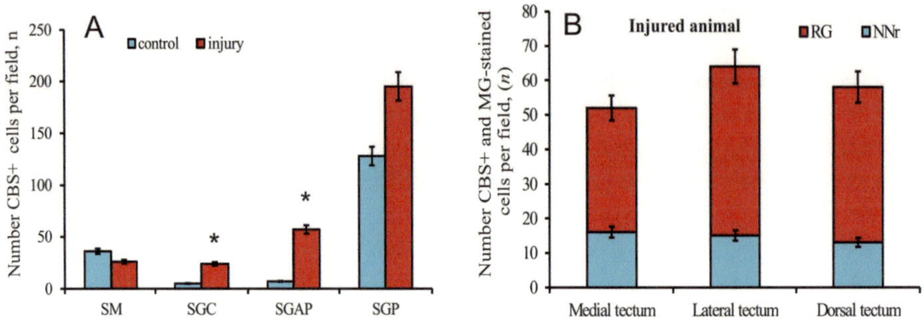

Figure 3.
Density of CBS+ cells in the optic tectum of the intact trout Oncorhynchus mykiss *and at 1 week post-injury. (A) Number of cells in the intact tectal layers and after UEI; the one-way analysis of variance followed by the student–Newman–Keuls post hoc test was used to determine significant differences between the control trout and fish after UEI (n = 5 in each group; (mean ± SD), * P < 0.05, vs. control group). SM, stratum marginale; SGC, stratum griseum centrale; SGAP, stratum griseum at album periventriculare; SGP, stratum griseum periventriculare. (B) Number of radial glia cells (RG) and reactive neurogenic niches (NNr) in different part of tectum after UEI (mean ± SD).*

of trout using monoclonal antibodies [11]. This indicates that at different periods of the trout constitutive ontogenesis, UEI leads to activation of expression in the aNSC radial glia cells against the background of a general decrease in the number of CBS immunopositive neuroepithelial cells, detected in the intact animals. Data of the quantitative analysis showed that in the lateral part of the tectum, the RG distribution density is greater than in the dorsal and medial parts, while the average number of reactive neurogenic niches in these areas remains approximately the same (**Figure 3B**). After UEI, an increase in the number of CBS+ cells is observed in all the tectum layers, reaching a maximum value in SGP (**Figure 3A**). In SGC and SGAP, a significant increase in the number of CBS+ cells ($P < 0.05$) was detected as compared with the control (**Figure 3A**).

Post-traumatic disorders of energy metabolism that occur in the trout tectum after UEI cause a number of changes resulting from the depletion of ATP. One of the main metabolic changes is glycolysis, which serves as the main factor of reduction in ATP-generating oxidative phosphorylation [4]. The loss of ATP leads to an imbalance in ionic homeostasis in the tectum cells due to the breakdown of ATPases or ATP-dependent ion transporters [9], which regulate the influx of calcium and sodium. These changes lead to an outflow of potassium due to the subsequent ATP depletion and calcium accumulation [28, 34]. The increase in intracellular calcium leads to growth of glutamate level, which increases calcium overload and activates calcium-dependent lipases and proteases [28]. Such shifts in ionic homeostasis lead to an increased production of reactive oxygen species (ROS), the opening of transitional pores of mitochondrial permeability, inflammation, and neuronal death [9, 35]. In intact animals, the astrocytes surrounding the neurons absorb extracellular glutamate and protect neurons from excitotoxicity [1, 4]. However, during the brain injury, the damaged astrocytes may exacerbate ischemic reperfusion injury due to the inhibition of the main glutamate transporter (GLT1) [1, 12].

Thus, as a result of UEI, a number of pathophysiological changes develop in the trout tectum, causing the oxidative stress. In vivo experiments indicate the important role of H_2S involved in many ways to control oxidative stress, including the glutathione cycle, activation of enzymes, and transcription factors related to the redox balance [3]. One of the pathophysiological effects in trout after UEI is assumed to be microglial polarization with appearance of clusters of activated microglia with a pro-inflammatory phenotype (**Figure 4**). Similar effects were also identified in a cell culture with exogenous administration of sodium hydrosulfide [36]. Thus, an

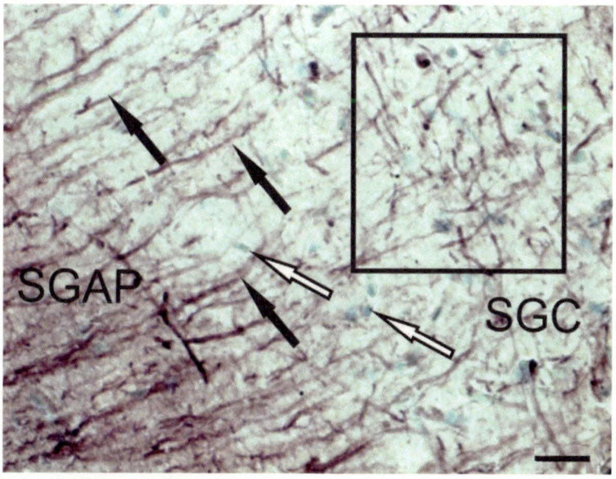

Figure 4.
CBS in the optical tectum of the trout Oncorhynchus mykiss *at 1 week after UEI. Clusters of tangentially located CBS+ reactive astrocytes (in black rectangle), radial glia (black arrows), and CBS- cells (white arrows). SGC, stratum griseum centrale; SGAP, stratum griseum at album periventriculare. Immunoperoxidase labeling of CBS in combination with methyl green staining. Scale bar: 20 μm.*

increase in the H_2S production in the trout brain after UEI should be considered in terms of maintaining cerebrovascular homeostasis, implying anti-apoptotic, anti-inflammatory, and antioxidant effects, and reducing the level of secondary neuronal damage that results from oxidative stress.

6. Cerebellum

The CBS localization was studied in the cerebellar body and granular eminences of trout. Earlier studies on juvenile trout using monoclonal antibodies against CBS showed the presence of H_2S-producing complexes in the granular layer and *valvula cerebelli* [11]. The data from this study allows a suggestion that the hydrogen sulfide production differs significantly between different neuroanatomical regions of *corpus cerebelli* (CCb), in particular, among granular cells. The highest number of CBS+ cells was found in the dorsolateral (DLP) and dorsomedial parts (DMP) of CCb, while in the basal part, the number of immunopositive cells was lower. In DLP, CBS+ Purkinje cells prevailed over negative cells; in the basolateral part (BLP), *vice versa* (**Figure 5**). In the medial zones of the trout CCb, dorsal and basal, typical CBS+ eurydendroid neurons (EDC) were revealed. The proportions of the CBS-positive and CBS-negative Purkinje cells (PC) in the basomedial part (BMP) and DMP were almost the same, and the number of CBS+ EDCs was higher in BMP (**Figure 5**). Thus, in the intact trout CCb, a heterogeneous population of PC was identified, some of which are CBS-positive and others are CBS-negative. The distribution of the CBS+ and CBS– Purkinje cells in CCb is characterized by a certain spatial specificity: most of the CBS+ PCs are localized in DLP. In the basal and dorsal parts of CCb, CBS+ eurydendroid neurons were found forming extracerebellar projections.

An essential feature of CBS-immunopositivity of projection cells in the trout ganglionic layer (GL) is their relationship with the CBS+ glial-like cells. Similar patterns of colocalization of the moderately labeled PCs and EDCs with small, intensely labeled cells were characteristic for all CCb areas and were also found in the adjacent areas of the granular layer (GrL) and molecular layer (ML). In most cases, we identified small, intensely labeled astrocyte-like cells and/or microglia

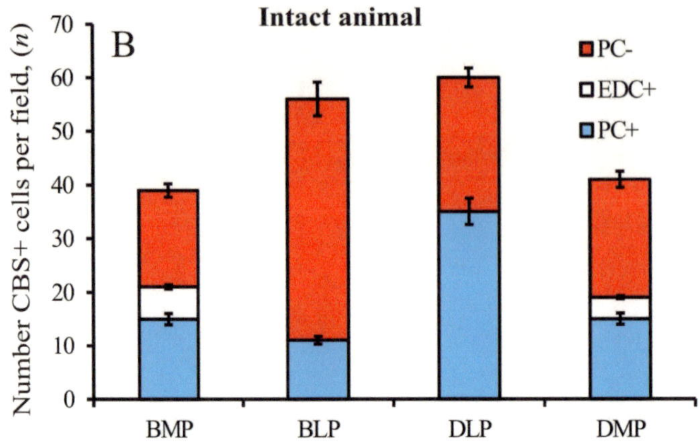

Figure 5.
Density of CBS+ cells in the cerebellum of the intact trout Oncorhynchus mykiss. *Ratio of Purkinje cells (PC) and eurydendroid cells (EDC) in different parts of the cerebellum (mean ± SD). BMP, basomedial part; BLP, basolateral part; DLP, dorsolateral part; DMP, dorsomedial part.*

attached to large EDCs or weakly or moderately labeled PC cells. Such a neuroglial/microglial construction corresponds to the established model of the intercellular relationships, in which glial cells are the main source of hydrogen sulfide for neurons [20, 27]. The relationship with neurons is a prerequisite for the release of H_2S from astrocytes and the increase in intracellular calcium in astrocytes [18]. H_2S activates the transition potential A1 channels (TRPA1) of the transition receptor, leading to an influx of calcium and activation of astrocytes by transmitting calcium waves after neuronal activation [37]. Further, D-serine is released from astrocytes, which subsequently activates the NMDA receptors [3]. Thus, the neuron-glial relationships were identified in CCb and granular eminences of the intact trout, in which H_2S is very likely to be released from the astrocyte-like cells with subsequent activation of the NMDA receptors in neurons. Such features of organization of the H_2S-producing cell complexes in trout correspond to physiological principles established in a mammalian model, according to which the astrocyte-like cells in the fish cerebellum regulate the amount of glutamate produced and its reuptake, preventing the excitotoxicity effects and providing the effective conditions for neurotransmission [2, 3].

After UEI in the trout cerebellum, the number of the CBS+ cells in ML increases dramatically, indicating a sharp activation of the ATP-dependent processes in this area. Along with the increase in the number of immunopositive cells, the number of the cellular CBS+ clusters also increases, both in the surface and deeper parts of ML. There is a reactivation of numerous neurogenic niches, with patterns of the neuron/glial/microglial colocation detected not only in GrL but also in ML. In ML, we found CBS+ fibers, which are absent in intact animals. In the neuron-glial complexes, glial cells are very intensely labeled, which indicates an increase in the CBS activity. We believe that this increase in the number of the CBS+ cells is due to the oxidative stress and the accumulation of ROS, which are neutralized by hydrogen sulfide. The sources of ROS generation in cell include mitochondria, superoxide-producing enzymes, such as xanthine oxide, NADPH oxidase, and hydrogen peroxide-producing enzymes, such as superoxide dismutase [12, 13]. ROS acceptors include antioxidants, such as glutathione, as well as enzymes superoxide dismutase and catalase. The modulation of ion channels and inflammatory and antioxidant transcription factors using H_2S after UEI may play a protective role in reducing edema and inflammation [20, 29, 30]. Similar effects have been reported in the culture of endothelial cells and hippocampal neurons with the addition of donors of hydrogen sulfide, Na_2S (50 μM) or NaHS (50 and 250 μM), which increase the activity of antioxidant enzymes such as superoxide dismutase, catalase, and glutathione peroxidase [27]. In vivo experiments indicate that the role of H_2S to control oxidative stress is expressed in many ways, including the glutathione cycle, enzyme activation, and transcription factors related to the redox balance [38]. Astrocytes provide cysteine as an important source of production in the GSH neurons [39]. In experiments on mammalian brain, the incorporation of the hydrogen sulfide donors, NaSH (100 μM), attenuated excitotoxicity and increased intracellular GSH levels in a dose-dependent manner in a primary culture of neurons [40]. Experiments with the inclusion of a metabolic radiolabel have confirmed the incorporation of L-cysteine generated by transulfuration of CBS and CSE into glutathione in astrocytes and neurons [41]. These studies suggest that H_2S may be useful to enhance the mechanism of cellular antioxidant protection in the brain.

Author details

Evgeniya V. Pushchina[1,2]*, Anatoly A. Varaksin[1] and Dmitry K. Obukhov[3]

1 Zhirmunsky National Scientific Center of Marine Biology, Far Eastern Branch, Russian Academy of Sciences, Vladivostok, Russia

2 Bogomolets Institute of Physiology, National Academy of Sciences of Ukraine, Kyiv, Ukraine

3 St. Petersburg State University, St. Petersburg, Russia

*Address all correspondence to: puschina@mail.ru

References

[1] Wang JF, Li Y, Song JN, Pang HG. Role of hydrogen sulfide in secondary neuronal injury. Neurochemistry International. 2014;**64**:37-47

[2] Kimura H, Shibuya N, Kimura Y. Hydrogen sulfide is a signaling molecule and a cytoprotectant. Antioxidants & Redox Signaling. 2012;**17**(1):45-57

[3] Kimura H. Physiological role of hydrogen sulfide and polysulfide in the central nervous system. Neurochemistry International. 2013;**63**(5):492-497

[4] Mergenthaler P, Dirnagl U, Meisel A. Pathophysiology of stroke: Lessons from animal models. Metabolic Brain Disease. 2004;**19**(3-4):151-167

[5] Deng J, Lei C, Chen Y, Fang Z, Yang Q, Zhang H. Neuroprotective gases–Fantasy or reality for clinical use? Progress in Neurobiology. 2014;**115**:210-245. DOI: 10.1016/j.pneurobio.2014.01.001

[6] Liu Y, Yang R, Liu X, Zhou Y, Qu C, Kikuiri T, et al. Hydrogen sulfide maintains mesenchymal stem cell function and bone homeostasis via regulation of Ca^{2+} channel sulfhydration. Cell Stem Cell. 2014;**15**(1):66-78

[7] Paul BD, Snyder SH. H_2S signalling through protein sulfhydration and beyond. Nature Reviews. Molecular Cell Biology. 2012;**13**(8):499-507

[8] Gopalakrishnan P, Shrestha B, Kaskas AM, Green J, Alexander JS, Pattillo CB. Hydrogen sulfide: Therapeutic or injurious in ischemic stroke? Pathophysiology. 2019;**26**:1-10

[9] Kalogeris T, Baines CP, Krenz M, Korthuis RJ. Cell biology of ischemia/reperfusion injury. International Review of Cell and Molecular Biology. 2012;**298**:229-317

[10] Che X, Fang Y, Si X, Wang J, Hu X, Reis C, et al. The role of gaseous molecules in traumatic brain injury: An updated review. Frontiers in Neuroscience. 2018;**12**:392. DOI: 10.3389/fnins.2018.00392

[11] Pushchina EV, Varaksin AA, Obukhov DK. Cystathionine β-synthase in the brain of the trout *Oncorhynchus mykiss* after unilateral eye damage and in conditions of *in vitro* cultivation. Russian Journal of Developmental Biology. 2019;**50**(2):39-58

[12] Li L, Rose P, Moore PK. Hydrogen sulfide and cell signaling. Annual Review of Pharmacology and Toxicology. 2011;**51**:169-187

[13] Jiang X, Huang Y, Lin W, Gao D, Fei Z. Protective effects of hydrogen sulfide in a rat model of traumatic brain injury via activation of mitochondrial adenosine triphosphate-sensitive potassium channels and reduction of oxidative stress. The Journal of Surgical Research. 2013;**184**:e27-e35. DOI: 10.1016/j.jss.2013.03.067

[14] Whitfield NL, Kreimier EL, Verdial FC, Skovgaard N, Olson KR. Reappraisal of H_2S/sulfide concentration in vertebrate blood and its potential significance in ischemic preconditioning and vascular signaling. American Journal of Physiology. Regulatory, Integrative and Comparative Physiology. 2008;**294**(6):R1930-R1937

[15] Than-Trong E, Bally-Cuif L. Radial glia and neural progenitors in the adult zebrafish central nervous system. Glia. 2015;**63**:1406-1428

[16] Zupanc GK, Sîrbulescu RF. Adult neurogenesis and neuronal regeneration in the central nervous system of teleost fish. The European Journal of Neuroscience. 2011;**3**:917-929

[17] Pushchina EV, Varaksin AA, Obukhov DK. Reparative neurogenesis in the brain and changes in the optic nerve of adult trout *Oncorhynchus mykiss* after mechanical damage of the eye. Russian Journal of Developmental Biology. 2016;**47**(1):11-32

[18] Nagai Y, Tsugane M, Oka J, Kimura H. Hydrogen sulfide induces calcium waves in astrocytes. The FASEB Journal. 2004;**18**(3):557-559

[19] Cuoghi B, Mola L. Macroglial cells of the teleost central nervous system: A survey of the main types. Cell and Tissue Research. 2009;**338**:319-332

[20] Lee M et al. Astrocytes produce the anti-inflammatory and neuroprotective agent hydrogen sulfide. Neurobiology of Aging. 2009;**30**(10):1523-1534

[21] Arochena M, Anadon R, Diaz Regueira SM. Development of vimentin and glial fibrillary acidic protein immunoreactivities in the brain of gray mullet (*Chelon labrosus*), an advanced teleost. The Journal of Comparative Neurology. 2004;**46**:413-436

[22] Alunni A, Vaccari S, Torcia S, Meomartini ME, Nicotra A, Alfei L. Characterization of glial fibrillary acidic protein and astroglial architecture in the brain of a continuously growing fish, the rainbow trout. European Journal of Histochemistry. 2005;**49**(2):51-60

[23] Kalman M. Astroglial architecture of the carp (*Cyprinus carpio*) brain as revealed by immunohistochemical staining against glial fibrillary acidic protein (GFAP). Anatomy and Embryology. 1998;**198**:409-433

[24] Pushchina EV, Varaksin AA, Obukhov DK. Cystathionine β-synthase in the CNS of masu salmon *Oncorhynchus masou* (Salmonidae) and carp *Cyprinus carpio* (Cyprinidae). Neurochemical Journal. 2011;5(1):24-34

[25] Ganz J, Kaslin S, Hochmann D, Freudenreich M, Brand M. Heterogeneity and independence of adult neural progenitors in the zebrafish telencephalon. Glia. 2010;**58**:1345-1363

[26] März M, Chapouton N, Diotel C, Vaillant B, Hesl M, Takamiya CS, et al. Heterogeneity in progenitor cell subtypes in the ventricular zone of the zebrafish adult telencephalon. Glia. 2010;**58**:870-888

[27] Hu R, Cai WQ, Wu XG, Yang Z. Astrocyte-derived estrogen enhances synapse formation and synaptic transmission between cultured neonatal rat cortical neurons. Neuroscience. 2007;**144**(4):1229-1240

[28] Mark LP, Prost RW, Ulmer JL, Smith MM, Daniels DL, Strottmann JM, et al. Pictorial review of glutamate excitotoxicity: Fundamental concepts for neuroimaging. AJNR. American Journal of Neuroradiology. 2001;**22**(10):1813-1824

[29] Kimura Y, Dargusch R, Schubert D, Kimura H. Hydrogen sulfide protects HT22 neuronal cells from oxidative stress. Antioxidants & Redox Signaling. 2006;**8**(3-4):661-670

[30] Xiao L, Lan A, Mo L, Xu W, Jiang N, Hu F, et al. Hydrogen sulfide protects PC12 cells against reactive oxygen species and extracellular signal-regulated kinase 1/2-mediated down regulation of glutamate transporter-1 expression induced by chemical hypoxia. International Journal of Molecular Medicine. 2012;**30**(5):1126-1132

[31] Hildebrandt TM, Grieshaber MK. Three enzymatic activities catalyze the oxidation of sulfide to thiosulfate in mammalian and invertebrate mitochondria. The FEBS Journal. 2008;**275**:3352-3361

[32] Fu M, Zhang W, Wu L, Yang G, Li H, Wang R. Hydrogen sulfide (H_2S)

metabolism in mitochondria and its regulatory role in energy production. Proceedings of the National Academy of Sciences of the United States of America. 2012;**109**(8):2943-2948

[33] Luo Y, Yang X, Zhao S, Wei C, Yin Y, Liu T, et al. Hydrogen sulfide prevents OGD/R-induced apoptosis via improving mitochondrial dysfunction and suppressing an ROS-mediated caspase-3 pathway in cortical neurons. Neurochemistry International. 2013;**63**(8):826-831

[34] Katsura K, Kristián T, Siesjö BK. Energy metabolism, ion homeostasis, and cell damage in the brain. Biochemical Society Transactions. 1994;**22**(4):991-996

[35] White BC, Sullivan JM, DeGracia DJ, O'Neil BJ, Neumar RW, Grossman LI, et al. Brain ischemia and reperfusion: Molecular mechanisms of neuronal injury. Journal of the Neurological Sciences. 2000;**179** (S 1-2):1-33

[36] Zhang M, Wu X, Xu Y, He M, Yang J, Li J, et al. The cystathionine β-synthase/hydrogen sulfide pathway contributes to microglia-mediated neuroinflammation following cerebral ischemia. Brain, Behavior, and Immunity. 2017;**66**:332-346

[37] Nagy P, Winterbourn C. Rapid reaction of hydrogen sulfide with theneutrophil oxidant hypochlorous acid to generate polysulfides. Chemical Research in Toxicology. 2010;**23**(10):1541-1543

[38] Islam KN, Polhemus DJ, Donnarumma E, Brewster LP, Lefer DJ. Hydrogen sulfide levels and nuclear factor-erythroid 2-related factor 2 (NRF2) activity are attenuated in the setting of critical limb ischemia (CLI). Journal of the American Heart Association. 2015;**4**(5):e001986. DOI: 10.1161/JAHA.115.001986

[39] Bridges RJ, Natale NR, Patel SA. System xc−cystine/glutamate antiporter: An update on molecular pharmacology and roles within the CNS. British Journal of Pharmacology. 2012;**165**(1):20-34

[40] Kimura Y, Kimura H. Hydrogen sulfide protects neurons from oxidative stress. The FASEB Journal. 2004;**18**(10):1165-1167

[41] Vitvitsky V, Thomas M, Ghorpade A, Gendelman HE, Banerjee R. A functional transsulfuration pathway in the brain links toglutathione homeostasis. The Journal of Biological Chemistry. 2006;**281**(47):35785-35793

Chapter 16

Neuroprotection: The Way of Anti-Inflammatory Agents

Patrice Mendel Nzogang and Martial Boris Donkeng

Abstract

Neurons are basic structural and functional units of the nervous system with major function being that of integration and interpretation of neuronal input or information. The lifespan of a nerve cell generally last throughout the individual lifetime. However, some physiologic or pathologic processes may affect the neuron causing premature death of this cell or tissue. This premature neurological death caused by pathologic circumstances is what we call neurotoxicity. The biochemical mechanisms put forward to explain neurotoxicity are not fully known. Nonetheless, whatever the mechanism involved, the outcome usually results in apoptosis, pyroptosis, or necrosis. Examples of these mechanisms include excitotoxicity, oxidative stress, glial cell destruction, vascular interruptions, and inflammation. The idea about possibly protecting neurons against insults using pharmacologic means leads to the birth of the neuroprotection concept. This new concept has emerged based on ongoing research, suggesting it is possible through physical and pharmacological means to prevent or avoid neurotoxicity by the abovementioned mechanisms but with the exception of vascular interruption mechanisms. We will present in this chapter a synoptic view of the inflammatory mechanisms implicated in neurotoxicity and bring out the possible implications in neuroprotection.

Keywords: neuroprotection, neurotoxicity, inflammation, inflammasome, NLRP3, metabolic syndrome

1. Introduction

Neurons represent the main component of the nervous system, and they are indispensable for integration and transcription of nerve impulses [1]. The central nervous system (CNS) is made up of about 100 billion neurons and approximately 10–50 times more glial cells [1]. Unlike glial cells, which maintain the ability to undergo cell division even after adult age, neurons are no more capable of mitosis at the adult age. Nevertheless, they are supposed to live all the life of an individual [1]. Unluckily, there are some pathologic and physiologic circumstances during which we observe a premature neuronal death [2]. These include stroke, head trauma, neurodegenerative disease, psychiatric disease, multiple sclerosis, aging, etc. This premature neurological death caused by pathologic circumstances is what we call neurotoxicity. The biochemical mechanisms of neurotoxicity are not all described yet. Nevertheless, no matter the mechanism, the result will be either apoptosis, pyroptosis, or necrosis [3]. Reviewing the literature, we found several biochemical pathways described as being implicated in the process of neurotoxicity. These include excitotoxicity, oxidative stress, glial cell destruction, vascularization interruption, and inflammation [3]. Being confronted with neurotoxicity, an idea emerged about possibly protecting neurons against insults using pharmacologic means. This was the birth of the neuroprotection concept.

The neuroprotection concept regroups all pharmacologic and/or physical resources capable of preventing or avoiding neurotoxicity by affecting one or more biochemical mechanisms of neurotoxicity [4, 5]. This definition excludes all therapeutics that lead to an improvement of the vascularization of the brain [4, 5]. The neuroprotection targets could therefore be avoidance of excitotoxicity, glial cell protection, oxidative stress reduction, and/or inhibition of inflammation. On the theoretical, logic and experimental fields, neuroprotection is evident; however, it remains a concept difficult to prove on the clinical field. Indeed, although many animal experimental researches on neuroprotection have been conclusive, this could not be confirmed in clinical trials. This could be explained by the difficulty to establish clinical criteria for the evaluation of neuroprotection in clinical researches. Despite this methodologic difficulty which tends to discredit the neuroprotection concept in clinical field, we propose to make an analysis of neuroprotection on the prism of inflammation. We will present a synoptic view of the inflammatory mechanisms implicated in neurotoxicity and bring out the possible implications in neuroprotection.

2. Inflammatory reaction and particularities in the central nervous system

Inflammation is the first step in the defense mechanism of the organism by which the actions of different components of the nonspecific immunity are put together in order to fight against an exogenous or endogenous aggression [6]. By definition, inflammation is a local process which takes place in the connective tissue of the organ affected. Nevertheless, according to the amplitude and duration of the local inflammation, it can be secondarily generalized through production of a systemic response such as the synthesis of acute-phase reactants or the endocrine effect of cytokines [6, 7].

2.1 Inflammation response mechanism

The first step of an inflammation reaction is the adhesion of leukocytes on the endothelial membrane. This step takes place essentially in the postcapillary venule. Activated endothelial cells are required for this step as they need to express adhesion molecules on their surfaces. These molecules serve as receptor for their complementary adhesive molecules present on the surface membrane of circulating leukocytes. Leukocyte adhesion to the vascular endothelium occurs in two phases which implicate both adhesion molecules. The first phase is the leukocytes rolling on the vascular endothelium. It involves the E-selectin (CD62E) and the P-selectin (CD62P) expressed on the vascular endothelium transiently interacting the P-selectin glycoprotein ligand-1 (PSGL-1), E-selectin ligand-1 (ESL-1), and L-selectin (CD62L) which are ligands expressed on leukocytes' surface. The second phase is the leukocyte-endothelium firm adhesion. It is realized by the interaction between the vascular endothelium adhesion molecules named vascular cell adhesion molecule-1 (VCAM-1) and intercellular adhesion molecule-1 (ICAM-1) and leukocyte integrins known as VLA-4 and LFA-1 (**Figure 1**). The leukocyte adhesion is preceded by a certain number of steps which aid the adhesion phase. These steps are endothelial activation, induced by interleukin-1β (IL-1β) and tumor necrotic factor α (TNFα); the activated endothelium secretes some agents such as

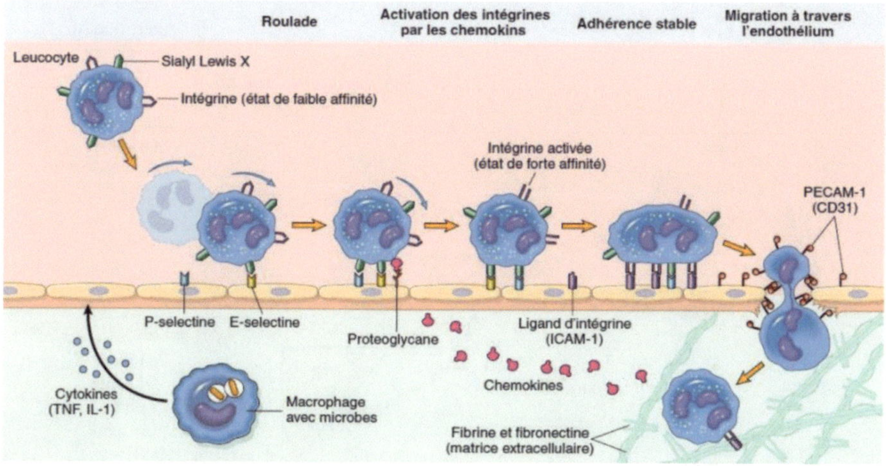

Figure 1.
Mechanism of inflammation reaction.

platelet-activating factor (PAF), prostaglandin E2 (PGE2), and azote monoxide (NO) which lead to a vasodilatation with reduction of blood flow aiding leukocyte rolling. Interleukin-1β and TNFα are also responsible for the adhesion molecules expressed on the endothelial surface and the liberation of chemotactic agents.

The second step of inflammation is diapedesis; it follows the leukocyte adhesion and refers to the passage of leukocytes from blood circulation to the connective tissue where the inflammation process has begun. This leukocyte migration is done across the intercellular endothelial junctions and is affected by chemotactic peptide concentration gradient at the inflammatory focal point. At the inflammatory focal point, leukocytes become activated and start to secrete oxygen-reactive substances, pro-inflammatory cytokines, and lipid inflammatory mediators. They also excrete the contents of their granules. All these actions lead to a systemic inflammatory response by endocrine effects of pro-inflammatory cytokines and also cessation of the cause of the inflammation. However, in certain cases the amplification of the inflammation by pro-inflammatory cytokines is responsible of destruction of the tissue where it takes place [7]. The endocrine effects of pro-inflammatory cytokines are multiple; the principal effects are observed on the liver and the brain [8]. In the liver, they induce the synthesis of acute-phase proteins; on the brain, they result in fever, asthenia, anorexia, and somnolence (**Figure 2**).

2.2 Inflammatory cytokines

The term cytokine regroups the low-molecular-weight glycoproteins implicated in cellular communication. They are active in the control of proliferation, maturation, and differentiation of hematopoietic cells and also in the regulation of inflammatory and immunologic responses. They exercise their regulatory activity through an autocrine, paracrine, juxtacrine, and endocrine mechanism via the membrane receptors present on focus cells. In the field of immunology, there exist two groups of cytokines: pro-inflammatory cytokines such as interleukins 1, 6, 8, and 18 (IL-1, IL-6, IL-8, IL-18), TNFα and anti-inflammatory cytokines such as interleukins 10, 4, and 13 (IL-10, IL-4, IL-13) transforming growth factor β (TGFβ). The balance between pro-inflammatory and anti-inflammatory cytokines regulates the local intensity of an inflammatory reaction and its duration. Among pro-inflammatory cytokines, IL-1β and TNFα have the central role in the initiation and chronicity

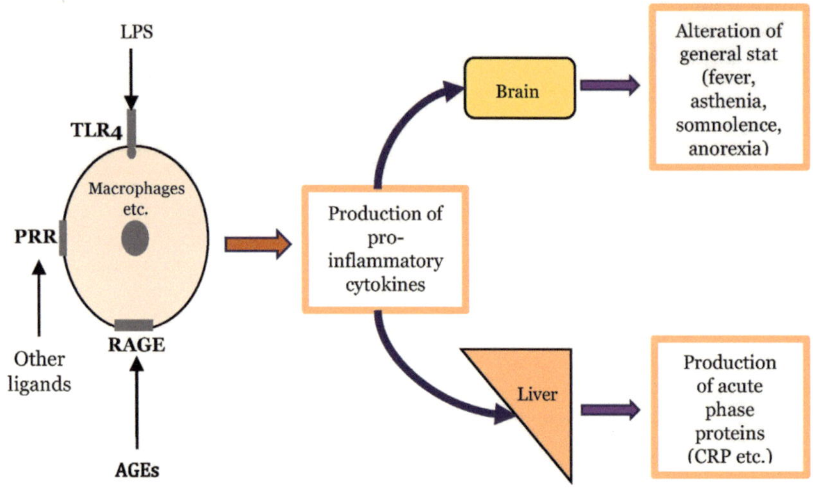

Figure 2.
Role of sentinel cells in the inflammatory response (modified from [8]). Sentinel cells (macrophage in this case) detects in its environment a potential danger by the pattern recognition receptors (PRR). This recognition active the inflammation signalization ways with the liberation of pro-inflammatory cytokines. PRRs considered in this example are toll like receptor 4 (TLR4) which recognize the lipo-poly-saccharide (LPS) of Gram negative bacteria and RAGE which recognize the ends products of glycation (AGEs).

of inflammation. These cytokines are synthetized in an inactive precursor form: pro-IL-1β and pro-TNFα. Activation of pro-IL-1β is done by a cysteine/aspartate-type membrane protease named caspase-1 or IL-1β converting enzyme (ICE). Concerning TNFα, its liberation and activation require an adamalysine family enzyme called TNFα- converting enzyme (TACE). Interleukin-1β and TNFα have a synergetic action at the inflammation focal point; they are implicated in the expression of cyclooxygenase 2 (COX2); production of PGE2, NO, and PAF; expression of adhesion molecules at the endothelium level membrane; production of other pro-inflammatory cytokines; liberation of chemotactic peptides and metalloproteases; etc. The activities of these major pro-inflammatory cytokines are under the control of many natural inhibitors. These inhibitors can be classified regarding their mode of action into three categories:

- The pro-inflammatory cytokine receptor antagonists: they compete with pro-inflammatory cytokines on their receptors.

- The pro-inflammatory cytokine soluble receptors: they inhibit pro-inflammatory cytokine activities binding them; this family is represented by truncated receptors of IL-1β (IL-1 R1 and R2) and TNFα (TNF R55 and R75).

- The anti-inflammatory cytokines: they act by inhibition of pro-inflammatory cytokine biosynthesis; this family is represented by IL-4, IL-10, IL-11, IL-13, and TGFβ.

Chemokines constitute another group of pro-inflammatory cytokines; they have chemotactic properties for the leukocytes. They are produced by all leukocytes, platelet, and connective tissue cells following stimulation by bacterial or viral products, IL-1β, TNFα, fragment C5a of complement, and leukotriene. Chemokine release leads to the degranulation and activation of leukocytes which provoke a massive release in the inflammatory focal point of lysosomal enzymes, oxidant, and lipid mediators [7].

2.3 Particularities of inflammation in the central nervous system

In the central nervous system (CNS), the same inflammatory mechanism previously described remains valid. However, because of the blood–brain barrier, the actors and kinetic of inflammation in the CNS are particular [9]. Furthermore, in the CNS, the immune reactions are molded by the presence of cellular and molecular factors slowing the immune response [9]. In the physiologic conditions, the blood–brain barrier is not permeable to blood constitutes including immune cells. This immune isolation of the CNS brings up the question about the actors implicated in an inflammatory reaction in this particular organ. Many studies prove that the microglial cells located in the periventricular spaces express the class II molecules of the major histocompatibility complex (class II MHC) and can play the role of macrophages in the initiation and amplification of inflammation [9, 10]. Hence, microglial cells can be activated in CNS by three ways: pathogen-associated molecular patterns (PAMPs), missing self, or danger-associated molecular patterns (DAMPs) [11, 12]. This microglial cell activation leads to phagocytosis, antigen presentation, and production of pro-inflammatory cytokines [13]. Furthermore, the active microglial cells express the co-stimulant molecules including CD45, B7–1, B7–2, LFA-1, CD40, ICAM-1, and VCAM-1 which increase the permeability of the blood–brain barrier resulting in the penetration of immune cells in the CNS [9, 13]. It is possible for the active T lymphocytes to cross the blood–brain barrier and penetrate into the brain parenchyma [14]. If these infiltrated T lymphocytes recognize their specific antigen, they will produce pro-inflammatory cytokines that further increase the permeability of the blood–brain barrier [9]. However, this inflammatory activity caused by activated microglial cells or activated T lymphocyte in the CNS remains strongly modulated and inhibited by many cells and molecular immunosuppressing factors present in the CNS.

In the CNS, they are unappropriated conditions for the development and amplification of an inflammatory reaction. Indeed, we observe in the CNS a reduction of the expression of class I and class II molecules of the major histocompatibility complex on the cells, a local production of anti-inflammatory cytokines and a continuous elimination, by apoptosis, of the active T lymphocytes that have crossed the blood–brain barrier [9]. This apoptotic elimination of infiltrated T lymphocyte is the result of an interaction between receptors Fas/Apo-1 (CD95) on the active T lymphocytes and ligands FasL (CD95L) on the CNS cells [15, 16]. This "inflammo-resistance" state of the CNS is not necessarily an advantage. Indeed, low expression of class I molecules of the major histocompatibility complex on the CNS cells leads to two potential consequences. Firstly, it may be possible for the active immune cells if they cross the blood–brain barrier to attack the self CNS cells following the "missing self" principle [11]. Secondly, it may be difficult for active cytotoxic T lymphocyte when they cross the blood–brain barrier to destroy infected CNS cells in the case of CNS viral infection [17]. These consequences make the CNS particularly susceptible to persistent inflammatory states once the pathogen or other cause of inflammation has circumvented all the anti-inflammatory processes present in CNS [17]. Furthermore, even if apoptotic elimination of infiltrated active T lymphocytes leads to a modulation of inflammation in the CNS, it also delays the elimination of the cause of inflammation and therefore prolongs the inflammatory state in the CNS. Apoptosis of infiltrated active T lymphocytes also leads to the release, in the CNS parenchyma, of anti-inflammatory cytokines notably IL-10 and TGFβ which inhibit the cytotoxic activity of active T lymphocytes and thus might perpetuate an eventual CNS viral infection [18, 19]. It appears that it is difficult for an inflammatory process to begin in the CNS, but if for one reason or the other an inflammatory process does begin in the CNS, it becomes very difficult to avert it completely and rapidly.

3. Inflammasome molecular platform

3.1 Description of an inflammasome

Inflammation is amplified and maintained by the activities of pro-inflammatory cytokines principally IL-1β and IL-18. However, the previously described inflammatory mechanism leads to the formation of these cytokines in an inactive form. In this part, we focus on the analysis of the molecular platform implicated in the activation of these cytokines called inflammasome. An inflammasome is an innate immune complex that recognizes pathogen-associated molecular patterns (PAMPs) and danger-associated molecular patterns (DAMPs) and leads to the activation of an inflammatory caspase: caspase-1 [20]. It is a macromolecule complex formed by oligomerization of a specific type pattern recognition receptor, an adaptor protein and caspase-1. This association results from the interaction between homotypic domains [20]. Pattern recognition receptors (PRRs) implicated in the inflammasome's structure are particular. Their activation leads specifically to the activation of caspase-1 rather than the activation of transcription factors such as nuclear factor kappa-B (NF-κB) or IFN regulatory factor 3/7 (IRF3/7) as well as protein synthesis [20]. Three receptors' families are actually descripted as principal activators of the inflammasome: nucleotide-binding domain and leucine-rich repeats containing receptors (NLR), AIM2 {absent in melanoma 2}-like receptors (ALR), and RIG {retinoic acid inducible gene}-I-like receptor (RLR) [20]. The implication of the RLR in the activation of inflammasome is still debated.

Twenty-two NLR types have been identified in humans. They have a structural organization with a leucine-rich repeat (LRR) domain, which interacts with the ligand; a nucleotide-binding domain (NBD), which permits the ATP depending oligomerization of NLR into an hexameric form that activates the inflammasome; and an effector domain, which permits the transduction of signals (**Figure 3**) [21]. The effector domain is different for each NLR receptors and aids in their distinction. The NLRP have as effector domain the pyrin domain (PYD); the NLRC have as

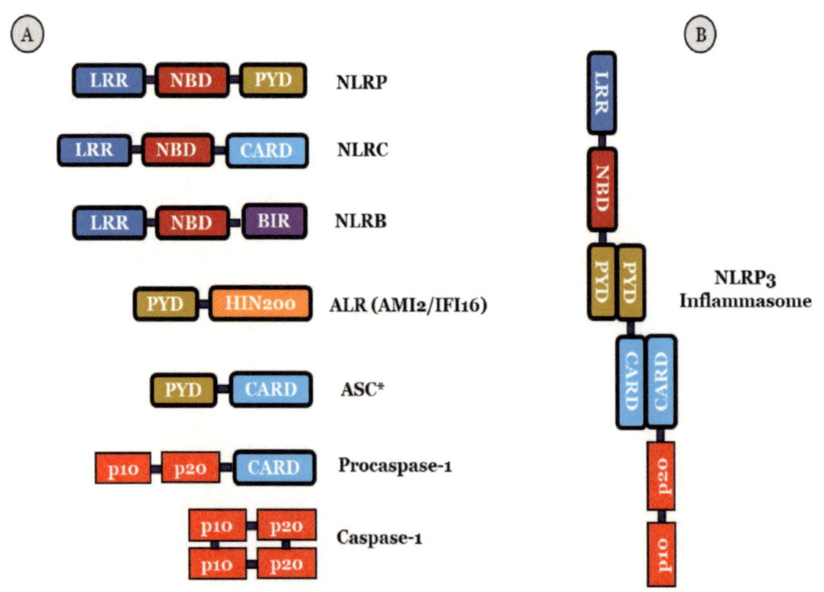

Figure 3.
*Inflammasome structure (modified from [20]) (A) structure of Inflammasome domains (B) NLRP3 Inflammasome. *Apoptosis-associated speck-like protein containing a CARD plays the role of adaptor protein.*

effector domain the caspase activation and recruitment domain (CARD); and the NLRB or NAIP (NLR family apoptosis inhibitory protein) have as effector domain the baculoviral inhibitor of apoptosis protein repeat (BIR) [21]. AIM2-like receptors (ALR) are formed by four receptors: the AIM2, interferon-γ- inducible antigen 16 (IFI16), myeloid cell nuclear differentiation antigen (MNDA), and interferon-inducible protein X (IFIX). The end carboxyl extremity of these receptors is formed by an HIN200 domain which reacts with double-stranded DNA, and the end amino extremity is formed by a pyrin domain [20].

3.2 Activation of the inflammasome

Activation of inflammasome requires the interaction between its receptors and the specific ligands grouped in the name of pathogen-associated molecular patterns (PAMPs) and danger-associated molecular patterns (DAMPs) [11, 12]. A large number of inflammasome ligands have been identified; the major ones are presented in **Table 1**. Receptors implicated in the inflammasome structure are located on the intracellular site of cell membrane. This localization means that the inflammasome's receptors are activated by ligands present on the inner aspect of the cell [20]. In other words, an inflammasome is activated in a cell only if the considered cell is infected, mutated, or damaged. The most studied inflammasome platform is the NLRP3 or cryopirine; its activation can be mediated by a double stimulus. The first is the stimulation of a toll-like receptor (TLR) which leads to the activation of the transcription pathway of pro-IL-1β that raises the transcription of the genes of NLRP3 and its deubiquitination [22]. The second stimulus is

Receptors	Stimuli	DAMPs/PAMPs
NLRP1	Anthrax toxin	PAMP
	Myramyl dipeptide of peptidoglycan bacterial wall	PAMP
NLRP3	Extracellular ATP	DAMP
	Reactive oxygen species	DAMP
	Asbestos fiber	DAMP
	Potassium ions efflux	DAMP
	Urate crystal	DAMP
	Silica crystal	DAMP
	Aluminum salt	DAMP
	Cholesterol crystal	DAMP
	β-amyloid protein	DAMP
	Pore forming bacteria toxin	PAMP
NLRP6	Unknown	Unknown
NLRP7	Bacteria lipopeptide	PAMP
NLRP12	*Yersinia pestis* unknown pattern	PAMP
NLRC4	Flagellin	PAMP
	Type 3 and 4 secretion system	PAMP
AIM2	Bacterial and viral DNA	PAMP
IFI16	Viral nuclear DNA	PAMP

Table 1.
Major Inflammasome activators (modified from [20]).

done directly on the NLRP3 through its receptors by a DAMP expressed by the cell secondary to the first stimulus and linked to a cell membrane damage, trouble of cell ionic or metabolic homeostasis, etc. Another activation mechanism of NLRP3 is described in Alzheimer's disease and implicates the β-amyloid protein [23]. Beta-amyloid proteins activate the inflammasome pathway in the microglial cells and thus provoke the liberation of IL-1β and its pyropoptosis which lead to neural cell death. Inflammasomes are also activated by reactive oxygen species resulting from mitochondrial malfunctioning or destruction [20].

Regardless of the inflammasome receptor activating stimulus, it causes a conformational modification of the receptor with liberation of the NBD domain. This liberation of the NBD domain permits the oligomerization of the inflammasome receptor into a hexamer or heptamer and recruitment of an adaptor protein by homotypic PYD-PYD interaction in the case of NLRP3. The recruited adaptor protein also recruits the procaspase-1 by homotypic CARD-CARD interaction. The obtained conformational two-by-two rapprochement of procaspase-1 leads to their autoproteolytic cleavage and their autoactivation [20]. On active form, caspase-1 is a tetramer formed by two pairs P10 and P20 subunits. Active caspase-1 produces activation of IL-1β and IL-18 and the outbreak of pyropoptosis by induction of cell membrane pore formation, which leads to water influx into the cell, swelling, and then osmotic lysis. Interleukin-1β and IL-18 amplify inflammation reaction and activities of all types of lymphocyte. Pyropoptosis, defined as inflammatory programmed cell death, has been found in macrophages, dendritic cells, and neurons [24]. So, in the CNS, inflammation through inflammasome and caspase-1 activation leads to pyroptosis of neurons and microglial cells that play the role of macrophages. This cellular death occurs indirectly in the case of microglial cell death or directly in the case of neuronal death resulting in significant neurotoxicity observed in many diseases.

4. Inflammation in neurotoxicity and neuroprotection

4.1 Inflammation in neurotoxicity

At the level of the central nervous system (CNS) as we have shown previously, the inflammasome effects are much more detrimental than beneficial for its homeostasis. This detrimental effect has been observed in many neurological disorders where inflammasomes seem to provoke neurotoxicity, both directly or indirectly [2]. Among these disorders we have Alzheimer's disease, bacterial meningitis, mouse's equivalent multiple sclerosis, depression, etc. [2, 23, 25]. This evidence, built from clinical and experimental researches, is more often based on the observation of a rise in the expression of inflammasome NLRP3 in the CNS or in the peripheral blood or on the discovery of an anti-inflammasome activity of the drugs used in the treatment of these disorders. **Table 2** summarizes for each neurological disorder the role played by inflammasome and inflammation in its pathogenesis. Another fact is that a unique neuron culture treatment with IL-1β does not produce deleterious effect; however, when the administration is prolonged for several days, it leads to neurotoxicity [34]. The negative impact of pro-inflammatory cytokines on the CNS is also seen on glial cells. Indeed, glial cells are the targets of pro-inflammatory cytokines and are activated by an inflammatory stimulus (PAMPs or DAMPs). This glial cell activation leads to the production of cytokines responsible of a local inflammatory response. Astrocytes activated by inflammation produce neurotrophins and growth factors like nerve growth factor (NGF), brain-derived neurotrophic factor (BDNF), and glial cell

Neurological pathologies	Inflammasome actors	Experimental justifications	References
Alzheimer's disease	NLRP3, IL-1β	Activation of inflammasome NLRP3 by β-amyloid protein and production IL-1β by microglial cell leading to neuro-inflammation and neurons death.	[23, 25]
Multiple sclerosis	NLRP3, ASC, IL-1β	Presence of SEP-like lesions in Muckle-Wells syndrome. Rise of gene's expression and concentrations of caspase-1, IL-18 in peripheral mononuclear cells. Gene's polymorphisms of caspase-1 is associated with SEP.	[26–28]
Amyotrophic lateral sclerosis	Caspase-1, IL-1β	Activation of caspase-1 and IL-1β by a mutant of superoxide dismutase in microglial mouse cell provokes neuro-inflammation.	[29]
Parkinson's disease	NLRP3, IL-1	Activation of inflammasome NLRP3 by α-synuclein protein. Neuro-degenerescence is accelerated by excess IL-1.	[30, 31]
Pneumococci meningitis	NLRP1, NLRP3, CARD8, ASC, IL-1β, IL-18	Gene's polymorphisms of NLRP1 and CARD8 and spinal fluid concentration of IL-1β and IL-18 are associated to clinical prognostic of meningitis. Low severity of meningitis in mouse's models deficient to NLRP3and ASC or after inhibition of IL-1 or IL-18.	[32, 33]

Table 2.
Implication of inflammasome in neurological pathologies (modified from [2]).

line-derived neurotrophic factor (GDNF) [34]. These trophic factors have a neuroprotective effect. In contrast, microglial cell activation leads to the release of neurotoxic factors such as pro-inflammatory cytokines, chemokines, free radicals, nitric oxide, and metalloproteases [34]. For example, in the case of stroke, vascular interruption provokes an ischemia with neural lysis. This neural lysis is associated with a massive release of intracellular contents into the extracellular compartment, among which is glutamate. At this stage two neurotoxicity pathways are triggered: the excitotoxicity pathway by massive glutamate release and the inflammation pathway by activation of microglial cells. Microglial cells are activated by the ischemic danger signal or through N-Methyl-D-aspartate (NMDA) receptors on their surface membrane that are sensible to glutamate [34]. This microglial cell activation leads to the production and release of pro-inflammatory cytokines and other molecules as specified previously. The consequences are neurotoxicity and in stroke an increase of the core ischemia at the expense of ischemic penumbra.

4.2 Metabolic syndrome as a cause of inflammation in neurotoxicity

Neurotoxicity as we aforementioned results from multiple biochemical processes including inflammation. Whether it is initiated and amplified at the level of the CNS or at the periphery, inflammation remains harmful to the CNS. As a matter of fact, when it comes to inflammation, there is a communication between the periphery and the CNS [34]. Before addressing, at the end of this section, this connection between CNS and periphery, we would first of all want to present the metabolic syndrome as a cause of peripheral inflammation that could have an impact on the CNS. The metabolic syndrome is in fact a metabolic disorder characterized by a group of conditions that increase the risk of developing cardiovascular diseases and type 2 diabetes mellitus. Two mechanisms are suggested in an attempt to explain the genesis of inflammation in metabolic syndrome. The first is a dysfunction of the organelles of adipocytes, observed in obesity; the second is adipose tissue hypoxia also observed in obesity [35]. The first mechanism suggests that hypertrophic adipose tissue found in obesity undergoes excessive lipolysis resulting in hyperlipidemia and an increase in circulating fatty acid levels. This increase in circulating levels of fatty acids, coupled with an abundance of carbohydrates, results in an increase in the oxidative activity of mitochondria that produce excess energy. As time goes by, this state results in a dysfunction of the mitochondria freeing a large quantity of electrons responsible for an increased production of reactive oxygenated compounds. This oxidative stress can subsequently activate the innate immune system and thus cause inflammation. Furthermore, the excess of nutrients overruns the endoplasmic reticulum, resulting in a faulty plication of proteins which activates the response to faulty plication of proteins. This response stimulates the activation of three membranous proteins: PKR-like eukaryotic initiation factor 2-alpha kinase (PERK), inositol requiring enzyme-1 (IRE-1), and activating transcription factor-6 (AFT-6). PERK, IRE-1, and AFT-6 significantly enhance inflammation by activating the signaling pathway NF-kB [35].

Concerning the second mechanism, it is suggested that a localized hypoxia could initiate a dysregulation of adipokines in obesity. As a matter of fact, adipose tissue is mainly made up of adipocytes, but also preadipocytes, resident macrophages, fibroblasts, and endothelial cells. With the increase in adipose tissue observed in obesity, there is a need for a significant angiogenesis. The hypoxic signal present during this expansion results in the activation of transcription factors like the hypoxia-inducible factors which are required in the activation of genes associated with angiogenesis, glucose metabolism, stress, and inflammation. Moreover, in vitro data reveal that human preadipocytes, when exposed to hypoxia, increase their expression of leptin and reduce their expression of the peroxisome proliferator-activated receptor gamma (PPARγ). Yet, agonists of the PPARγ stimulate insulinosensitivity and reduce inflammation. Furthermore, exposed to hypoxia, resident macrophages produce pro-inflammatory cytokines [35]. In type 2 diabetes, coupled with the mechanisms mentioned above, chronic hyperglycemia maintains a vicious circle. In fact, chronic hyperglycemia is responsible for an increase in glycation end products (AGEs) whose receptors belong to the family of PRRs. So, glycated plasma proteins, glycated lipids, or nucleic acids bind to AGE receptors present at the surface of macrophages and provoke a pro-inflammatory and pro-oxidative response [35].

Therefore, the metabolic syndrome induces a state of peripheral inflammation that becomes chronic because it is maintained by its causative process. This peripheral inflammation can directly affect the CNS through produced and circulating inflammatory mediators. These mediators penetrate the CNS via areas without a blood–brain barrier like the periventricular choroid plexuses following which they cause the aforementioned neurotoxic effects [34]. Furthermore, the blood–brain barrier is capable of transmitting an inflammatory message from the vascular endothelium to the CNS via active mechanisms involving cyclooxygenases [34]. Through these mechanisms, an inflammation at the periphery, if it lasts long enough, can extend to the CNS and result in neurotoxicity and subsequent neurologic disorders.

4.3 Inflammation and neuroprotection

Actually, even if some anti-inflammatory strategies have proven their efficacy in animal models, none have demonstrated efficacy in humans in the prevention or treatment of neurological diseases associated with neurotoxicity. However, with conclusive experimental results on the use of anti-inflammatory drugs in neuroprotection, this therapeutic approach presents encouraging prospects for clinical research. In doing so, after bringing out the negative impact of inflammation on the central nervous system (CNS), it seems appropriate to present some strategies explored or still to be explored in an attempt to inhibit neuro-inflammation and prevent or treat neurotoxicity associated with many neurological disorders. Glucocorticoid and general anesthesia products have stimulated a strong interest in neuroprotection in the cases of stroke on experimental animal models; this has not been demonstrated yet in humans [34]. Indeed, glucocorticoids have been found to be ineffective in stroke, head trauma, and meningeal hemorrhage [34]. And classic hypnotic agents like thiopental, midazolam, or propofol have peripheral immune-modulatory effects and are capable of inhibiting inflammatory response. They inhibit chemotaxis, adherence of neutrophils, phagocytosis, and liberation of free radicals and pro-inflammatory cytokines like IL-1β and TNFα in experimental mouse model; however, these activities have not been demonstrated in humans yet [34]. In general, having in mind previously described inflammation and inflammatory neurotoxicity mechanisms, we can conclude that neuroprotection strategies based on modulation of inflammation have to maintain the beneficial roles of immunological defense and healing of inflammation while neutralizing its neurotoxic consequences. Thus, three anti-inflammatory strategies for neuroprotection axis can be developed: the modulation of the communication between peripheral inflammation and CNS, the modulation of interaction between pro-inflammatory cytokines and their intracerebral targets, and the modulation of inflammasome expression in CNS cells.

In relation to the first axis, namely, the modulation of the communication between peripheral inflammation and CNS and the COX inhibitors (nimesulide and indomethacin) has shown a neuroprotective activity in baby mice with brain lesions. This neuroprotective activity is made possible by inhibition of the communication through the blood–brain barrier between activated peripheral inflammatory cells and the CNS [34]. With the same idea, the COX inhibitors have been presented as potentially beneficial in the treatment of major depression and other psychiatric disorders. Indeed, celecoxib has presented a beneficial effect in the treatment of major depression and schizophrenia especially in early stages [36]. Acetyl salicylic acid in particular seems to have both a preventive and therapeutic effect on schizophrenia [36]. Communication between peripheral inflammation and the CNS does not occur solely via the blood–brain barrier as it can also be done through the parasympathetic and sympathetic systems. Indeed, immune cells present at their surfaces nicotinic receptors for acetylcholine and β-adrenergic receptors for catecholamine [34]. These receptors link immune cells to parasympathetic and sympathetic systems respectively. Thus, a pharmacologic vagal or noradrenergic stimulation could represent a potential target for neuroprotection. For this purpose, vagal stimulation potentially passing through the modulation of lipocalin prostaglandin D2 synthase (L-PGDS) has shown in rat models with ischemic stroke a neuroprotective effect against ischemia reperfusion [37]. Also, a noradrenergic stimulation has shown, in Parkinson's disease, a neuroprotective effect by inhibition of inflammation [38].

Concerning the modulation of interaction between pro-inflammatory cytokines and their intracerebral target strategy, specific receptor antagonist of IL-1 appears to be the most conclusive therapeutic approach. This antagonist is produced endogenously following brain injury, and its administration by systemic or intracerebral route leads to a reduction in the size of lesions in mouse models [34]. Furthermore, Veltkamp et al. report the use, via general route of anakinra, of an antagonist of IL-1 receptors in a clinical trial on a patient having stroke [39]. This clinical trial has shown a great reduction of national institute of health stroke scale (NIHSS), and it also shows more patient with modified Rankin score (mRS) of 0–1 in 3 months [39].

Also based on this axis, sitagliptin, a molecule used in the treatment of type 2 diabetes since the discovery of incretin effect, has shown a great anti-inflammatory capacity. This anti-inflammatory activity of sitagliptin is linked to the inhibition of synthesis of pro-inflammatory cytokine and a raise in anti-inflammatory cytokine synthesis [40]. This property has been exploited in the treatment of Alzheimer's disease in mouse models, and the results were conclusive [40]. In humans, the administration of sitagliptin was associated with an amelioration of the mini-mental state examination (MMSE) score used to evaluate dementia [40]. All these axes remain focused on more or less advanced stages of inflammation. For this reason, they carry the risk of possibly altering the beneficial effects of inflammation. Thus, to reduce this intrinsic risk, it seems necessary to develop more specific methods to modulate the inflammation. One method could be the inhibition of inflammasomes. However, because of the lack or incomplete knowledge on inflammasome structure and activation, this approach remains difficult. Nevertheless, the inhibition of NLRP3, the most studied inflammasome, has been subjected to several studies in psychiatric disorders [41]. A specific inhibitor of NLRP3 has been developed which lays the foundation for further exploration of this axis [42].

5. Conclusion

Neuroprotection is both a topical problem and a realistic dream for the researchers and clinicians. By this analysis, the immune system no more seems to only be a tool useful in the protection against endogenous and exogenous offenders. As a matter of fact, its role could be understood as defense against all sorts of disorders, including infectious, metabolic, degenerative, etc. and even aging. Indeed, the role of the immune system and inflammation in disease-associated neurotoxicity is more and more highlighted in present literature. This evidence justifies the outbreak of an inflammatory approach to develop a neuroprotection strategy in the fight against neurotoxicity. All this evidence does not only provide hope for the future development of neuroprotective strategies, but also invite us to reflect on the possibility that failure of the immune system may be implicated as primary cause of any human pathology. In experimental research, this is in the process of being demonstrated for neurologic and psychiatric disorders. Even though clinically the results of the researches are not yet irrevocable, the inflammatory pathway in neuroprotection remains a good approach in the fight against these main neurological ailments.

Acknowledgements

We wish to give thanks to Tchinda Fomekong Gérald, a resident of internal medicine, e-mail: fomekonggt@gmail.com, for all his support in the redaction of this chapter; Nana Rudy Arnaud, a resident of internal medicine, faculty of medicine and biomedical sciences University of Yaoundé 1, e-mail: arnaud.nana@yahoo.com; and Fombong T. Fombong, a resident of gynecology and obstetrics, faculty of medicine and biomedical sciences University of Yaoundé 1, e-mail: tfombongjnr@gmail.com.

Conflict of interest

The authors declare that they have no competing interests.

Author details

Patrice Mendel Nzogang* and Martial Boris Donkeng
Circle for Research, Development and Innovation (CIRDI), Yaoundé, Cameroon

*Address all correspondence to: nzogangmendel@gmail.com

References

[1] Ganong WF, Barret KE, Barman SM, Boitano S, Brooks HL. Physiologie médicale. 3rd ed. Bruxelles: De Boerks; 2012

[2] Jamilloux Y, Sève P, Henry T. Les inflammasomes et les maladies humaines. Revista Médica. 2014;**35**(11):730-741

[3] Brouns R, De Deyn PP. The complexity of neurobiological processes in acute ischemic stroke. Clinical Neurology and Neurosurgery. 2009;**111**(6):483-495

[4] Ginsberg MD. Neuroprotection for ischemic stroke: Past, present and future. Neuropharmacology. 2008;**55**(3):363-389

[5] Onteniente B, Onteniente P, Bordet R. Médicaments neuroprotecteurs, neurogenèse, définitions, évaluations pré-cliniques, cliniques, guidelines... Communication à la: XXIèmes Rencontres de Pharmacologie Clinique; 5-18 octobre 2005; Giens

[6] Burmester G, Pezzutto A. Atlas de poche d'immunologie: Bases, analyses biologiques, pathologies. Paris: Flammarion Médecine-Sciences; 2000

[7] Henrotin Y, Deby-Dupont G, ReginsterJY.Lesmédiateursbiochimiques de l'inflammation. Revue Médicale de Liège. 2001;**56**(6):433-442

[8] Pickup J. Inflammation and activated innate immunity in the pathogenesis of type 2 diabetes. Diabetes Care. 2004;**27**(3):813-823

[9] Lau P, Joly E. Le contexte immunologique très particulier du système nerveux central. Médecine/sciences. 2001;**17**:395-401

[10] Perry VH, Andersson PB, Gordon S. Macrophages and inflammation in the central nervous system. Trends in Neurosciences. 1993;**16**:268-273

[11] Medzhitov R, Janeway CA Jr. Decoding the patterns of self and nonself by the innate immune system. Science. 2002;**296**(5566):298-300

[12] Matzinger P. The danger model: A renewed sense of self. Science. 2002;**296**(5566):301-305

[13] Audinat E, Arnoux I. La microglie: des cellules immunitaires qui sculptent et contrôlent les synapses neuronales. Medical Science. 2014;**30**(2):153-159

[14] Hickey WF, Hsu BL, Kimura H. T-lymphocyte entry into the central nervous system. Journal of Neuroscience Research. 1991;**28**(2):254-260

[15] Flügel A, Schwaiger FW, Neumann H, Medana I, Willem M, Wekerle H, et al. Neuronal FasL induces cell death of encephalitogenic T lymphocytes. Brain Pathology. 2000;**10**(3):353-364

[16] Griffith TS, Brunner T, Fletcher SM, Green DR, Ferguson TA. Fas ligand-induced apoptosis as a mechanism of immune privilege. Science. 1995;**270**(5239):1189-1192

[17] Joly E, Mucke L, Oldstone MB. Viral persistence in neurons explained by lack of major histocompatibility class I expression. Science. 1991;**253**(5025):1283-1285

[18] Chen JJ, Sun Y, Nabel GJ. Regulation of the proinflammatory effects of Fas ligand (CD95L). Science. 1998;**282**(5394):1714-1717

[19] Li XC, Wells AD, Strom TB, Turka LA. The role of T cell apoptosis in transplantation tolerance. Current Opinion in Immunology. 2000;**12**(5):522-527

[20] Jamilloux Y, Henry T. Les inflammasomes Plates-formes de

l'immunité innée. Médecine/sciences. 2013;**29**(11):975-984

[21] Ting JP, Lovering RC, Alnemri ES, Bertin J, Boss JM, Davis BK, et al. The NLR gene family: A standard nomenclature. Immunity. 2008;**28**(3):285-287

[22] Poeck H, Bscheider M, Gross O, Finger K, Roth S, Rebsamen M, et al. Recognition of RNA virus by RIG-I results in activation of CARD9 and inflammasome signaling for interleukin 1 beta production. Nature Immunology. 2010;**11**(1):63-69

[23] Halle A, Hornung V, Petzold GC, Stewart CR, Monks BG, Reinheckel T, et al. The NALP3 inflammasome is involved in the innate immune response to amyloid-beta. Nature Immunology. 2008;**9**(8):857-865

[24] Miao EA, Rajan JV, Aderem A. Caspase-1-induced pyroptotic cell death. Immunological Reviews. 2011;**243**(1):206-214

[25] Nakanishi A, Kaneko N, Takeda H, Sawasaki T, Morikawa S, Zhou W, et al. Amyloid β directly interacts with NLRP3 to initiate inflammasome activation: Identification of an intrinsic NLRP3 ligand in a cell-free system. Inflammation and Regeneration. 2018;**38**:27

[26] Compeyrot-Lacassagne S, Tran TA, Guillaume-Czitrom S, Marie I, Koné-Paut I. Brain multiple sclerosis-like lesions in a patient with Mückle–Wells syndrome. Rheumatology (Oxford, England). 2009;**48**(12):1618-1619

[27] Jha S, Srivastava SY, Brickey WJ, Iocca H, Toews A, Morrison JP, et al. The inflammasome sensor, NLRP3, regulates CNS inflammation and demyelination via caspase-1 and interleukin-18. The Journal of Neuroscience. 2010;**30**(47):15811-15820

[28] Ming X, Li W, Maeda Y, Blumberg B, Raval S, Cook SD, et al. Caspase-1 expression in multiple sclerosis plaques and cultured glial cells. Journal of the Neurological Sciences. 2002;**197**(1-2):9-18

[29] Meissner F, Molawi K, Zychlinsky A. Mutant superoxide dismutase 1-induced IL-1beta accelerates ALS pathogenesis. Proceedings of the National Academy of Sciences of the United States of America. 2010;**107**(29):13046-13050

[30] Codolo G, Plotegher N, Pozzobon T, Brucale M, Tessari I, Bubacco L, et al. Triggering of inflammasome by aggregated α-synuclein, an inflammatory response in synucleinopathies. PLoS One. 2013;**8**(1):e55375

[31] Pott Godoy MC, Tarelli R, Ferrari CC, Sarchi MI, Pitossi FJ. Central and systemic IL-1 exacerbates neurodegeneration and motor symptoms in a model of Parkinson's disease. Brain: A Journal of Neurology. 2008;**131**(7):1880-1894

[32] Geldhoff M, Mook-Kanamori BB, Brouwer MC, Valls Seron M, Baas F, van der Ende A, et al. Genetic variation in inflammasome genes is associated with outcome in bacterial meningitis. Immunogenetics. 2013;**65**(1):9-16

[33] Hoegen T, Tremel N, Klein M, Angele B, Wagner H, Kirschning C, et al. The NLRP3 inflammasome contributes to brain injury in pneumococcal meningitis and is activated through ATP-dependent lysosomal cathepsin B release. Journal of Immunology. 2011;**187**(10):5440-5451

[34] Degosa V, Chhora V, Gressensa P, Mantza J. Neuroprotectrive strategies and acute neuro-inflammation. Réanimation. 2009;**18**:556-565

[35] Calle M, Fernandez M. Inflammation and type 2 diabetes.

Diabetes and Metabolism. 2012; **38**(3):183-191

[36] Müller N. COX-2 inhibitors, aspirin, and other potential anti-inflammatory treatments for psychiatric disorders. Psychiatry. 2019;**10**:375

[37] Zhang L, Ma J, Jin X, Jia G, Jiang Y, Li C. L-PGDS mediates vagus nerve stimulation-induced neuroprotection in a rat model of ischemic stroke by suppressing the apoptotic response. Neurochemical Research. 2017;**42**(2):644-655

[38] O'Neill E, Harkin A. Targeting the noradrenergic system for anti-inflammatory and neuroprotective effects: Implications for Parkinson's disease. Neural Regeneration Research. 2018;**13**(8):1332-1337

[39] Veltkamp R, Gill D. Clinical trials of immunomodulation in ischemic stroke. Neurotherapeutics. 2016;**13**(4):791-800

[40] WiciNski M, Wódkiewicz E, Słupski M, Walczak M, Socha M, Malinowski B, et al. Neuroprotective activity of sitagliptin via reduction of neuroinflammation beyond the incretin effect: Focus on Alzheimer's disease. BioMed Research International. 2018;**2018**:9

[41] Herman FJ, Pasinetti GM. Principles of inflammasome priming and inhibition: Implications for psychiatric disorders. Brain, Behavior, and Immunity. 2018;**73**:66-84

[42] Ludwig-Portugall I, Bartok E, Dhana E, Evers BD, Primiano MJ, Hall JP, et al. An NLRP3-specific inflammasome inhibitor attenuates crystal-induced kidney fibrosis in mice. Kidney International. 2016;**90**(3):525-539